D1267300

Date Due

6·15·11			
9·15·11			

1302065

Live/Real Time 3D
Echocardiography

This book is dedicated to my late parents, Balwant Rai Nanda, MD, and Mrs. Maya Vati Nanda; my wife, Kanta Nanda, MD; our children, Nitin Nanda, Anita Nanda Wasan, MD, and Anil Nanda, MD; their spouses Sanjeev Wasan, MD, and Seema Tailor Nanda; and our very cute grandchildren Vinay and Rajesh Wasan and Nayna Nanda.

Navin C. Nanda, MD

I dedicate this book to my parents, the late Yuan Hsiung, MD, and Wei Lee; and to my wife, Wen Hsiung; and sons, Teddy, Richard, and Jerry.

Ming C. Hsiung, MD

I dedicate this book to my mother and father, Linda and Gordon Miller, who made all things possible.

Andrew P. Miller, MD

This book is dedicated to my parents, Gabriel and Aida Hage, who have made me who I am; my wife, Sulaf Mansur Hage, MD, for her never-ending support, encouragement, and inspiration over the years; my son, Alexander F. Hage, for making it all worthwhile; and to my colleagues and patients who I hope will benefit from this book.

Fadi G. Hage, MD

Live/Real Time 3D Echocardiography

Navin C. Nanda, MD, FACC, FAHA

Professor of Medicine, Division of Cardiovascular Diseases
Director, Heart Station/Echocardiography Laboratories
University of Alabama at Birmingham and
Director, Echocardiography Laboratory, The Kirklin Clinic
University of Alabama Health Services Foundation
Birmingham, AL, USA

Ming Chon Hsiung, MD

Physician, Division of Cardiology
Associate Researcher, Department of Medical Research and Education
Cheng Hsin General Hospital
Taipei, Taiwan, Republic of China

Andrew P. Miller, MD, FACC, FAHA

CardioVascular Associates, PC, Birmingham, AL, USA
and
formerly, Assistant Professor of Medicine
Division of Cardiovascular Diseases
University of Alabama at Birmingham
Birmingham, AL, USA

Fadi G. Hage, MD

Assistant Professor of Medicine
Division of Cardiovascular Disease
University of Alabama at Birmingham
Birmingham, AL, USA
and
Section of Cardiology
Birmingham Veteran's Administration Medical Center
Birmingham, AL, USA

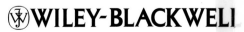

WILEY-BLACKWELL

A John Wiley & Sons, Ltd., Publication

Contents

Companion DVD

This book is accompanied by a DVD with:
- A database of 384 movie clips
- Movie clips are all referenced in the text where
  you see this symbol: 👁

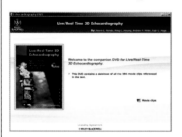
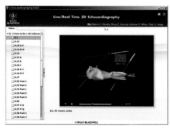
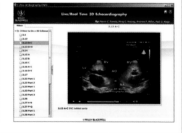

Preface

Echocardiography has progressed to become the most cost-effective noninvasive modality in the assessment of cardiovascular disease entities. It began in the 1950s and 60s as 1D A-mode and M-mode techniques, wherein a single pencil thin ultrasonic beam was used to image the heart. This limited modality was replaced in the early seventies by real time 2D echocardiography which revolutionized the field of noninvasive cardiac diagnosis. It did not take long before practically every large hospital in the United States, and soon after elsewhere in the world, offered this modality. The 2D technique essentially consisted of rapidly moving the single ultrasonic beam (mechanically in the beginning and later on electronically) so that larger segments of various cardiac structures could be visualized simultaneously. However, it provided visualization of only thin slices through the heart and it became apparent to many of us as soon as it was developed that even though it was a huge improvement over M-mode, it still did not give us full structural information. For example, the mitral leaflets appeared only as two thin "lines" moving in the cardiac cycle and the entire extent of leaflet surfaces could not be viewed. In essence, the images still bore no similarity whatsoever to the mitral valve visualized at surgery or anatomically, which was our pursuit. In developing 3D technology, early attempts were made to stitch the thin 2D planes together to reconstruct full-volume 3D images, but the enormous computer time taken to do this precluded its widespread clinical use. The advent of transesophageal echocardiography in the late 1980s provided further impetus to the development of 3D echocardiography because of superior quality images obtained by this technique and advances in computer technology. This resulted in several publications from investigators in many countries demonstrating the advantages of viewing various cardiac structures and chambers in three dimensions. A major advancement in 3D technology occurred a few years ago with the introduction of live/real time 3D transthoracic echocardiography. This innovative technique utilizes a transducer which broadcasts hundreds of ultrasound beams through the heart simultaneously resulting in a large 3D dataset that can then be cropped to provide a comprehensive view of different cardiac structures from any desired angle. The transducer was subsequently miniaturized leading to the development of live/real time transesophageal echocardiography in 2007. Both of these modalities supplement conventional 2D imaging by providing additional information in a variety of clinical scenarios.

The aim of this book is to provide a comprehensive, state-of-the-art review of both live/real time 3D transthoracic and transesophageal echocardiography illustrating both normal and pathologic cardiovascular findings. This book predominantly describes our experience with these two new modalities in the clinical setting in our Echocardiography Laboratories at the University of Alabama at Birmingham and the Kirklin Clinic and Cheng-Hsin Medical Center, Taipei, Taiwan, Republic of China. It also covers the contributions of other investigators in the field. A major highlight of the book is the large number of illustrations, over 800, which detail the technique of performing live/real time 3D echocardiograms and demonstrate the various cardiovascular pathologies encountered by us. These also serve to emphasize the superiority of 3D echocardiography over conventional 2D imaging in several clinical situations. Since the echo images we obtain and interpret in our day-to-day clinical practice are moving images and not static ones, we have also prepared a DVD to accompany this book. The DVD contains a large number of movie clips, over

350, which serve to supplement the static illustrations in the book.

The book is organized into 16 chapters. The first chapter provides a brief glimpse of the historical aspects of 3D echocardiography. The second chapter written by Dr. Ivan Salgo of Philips Medical Systems describes the basics and technical aspects of live/real time 3D transthoracic and transesophageal echocardiography. We are grateful to him for preparing this chapter for the book. Chapter 3 details normal anatomy, examination protocols, and the technique for performing live/real time 3D transthoracic echocardiography. This should prove especially useful to the beginners. Abnormalities affecting the mitral, aortic, tricuspid, and pulmonary valves and the aorta are described in Chapters 4 through 6. Prosthetic heart valves are discussed in Chapter 7. This is followed by Chapters 8–10, which cover 3D echocardiographic assessment of left and right ventricular function, ischemic heart disease, and cardiomyopathies. The largest chapter, Chapter 11, deals with congenital cardiac lesions. Another large chapter, Chapter 12, deals with tumors and other mass lesions. We are most grateful to Dr. Michael Faulkner, Internal Medicine Resident, for his help in writing the text portion of Chapter 12. Pericardial disorders are described in Chapter 13. One of the newest innovations, live/real time 3D transesophageal echocardiography is covered in detail in Chapter 14. Some of the most recent advances in 3D technology, real time full-volume imaging, and 3D wall tracking, including 3D assessment of strain, strain rate, twist, and torsion, are discussed in Chapters 15 and 16. These were written by Kutay Ustuner and Matthew Paul Esham of Siemens Healthcare and Tetsuya Kawagishi, William Kenny, Berkley Carpenter, and Willem Gorissen of Toshiba Medical Systems Corporation. We would like to express our heartfelt gratitude to all of them for doing this.

We must also thank several individuals in our universities who have contributed directly or indirectly to the growth and development of 3D echocardiography in our Echocardiography Laboratories. First and foremost, we are grateful to all present and past members of the Division of Cardiovascular Disease at the University of Alabama at Birmingham headed by Dr. Robert Bourge and at the Cheng Hsin General Hospital, Taipei, Taiwan

(Dr. Wei-Hsian Yin, head, Dr. Mason S. Young, and Dr. Shen Kou Tsai) for providing us full clinical support. Most of all, we are grateful to the Division of Cardiovascular Surgery, especially Dr. James K. Kirklin, Dr. Albert D. Pacifico, Dr. David McGiffin, Dr. James Holman, and Dr. Octavio E. Pajaro from the University of Alabama at Birmingham as well as Dr. Jeng Wei, Dr. Yi-Cheng Chuang, Dr. Chung-Yi Chang, and Dr. Sung-How Sue from the Division of Cardiovascular Surgery of Cheng Hsin General Hospital, Taipei, Taiwan, not only for facilitating the performance of 3D intraoperative transesophageal echocardiography but also for providing us surgical correlation in the patients operated upon by them. We also thank Dr. Pohoey Fan, Associate Professor of Medicine in the Division of Cardiovascular Disease at the University of Alabama at Birmingham, for his help and support.

We are most grateful to the Clinical and Research Fellows, Medical Residents, and Observers, both past and present, from the Echocardiography Laboratories at the University of Alabama at Birmingham who directly or indirectly helped in the performance of 3D echocardiography and in preparation of this book. They are: Elsayed Abo-Salem, Gopal Agrawal, Sujood Ahmed, Raed A. Aqel, Naveen Bandarupalli, Oben Baysan, Ravindra Bhardwaj, Monodeep Biswas, Kunal N. Bodiwala, Hari Bogabathina, Marcus L. Brown, Todd M. Brown, Manjula V. Burri, Preeti Chaurasia, Anand Chockalingam, Bryan Cogar, Onkar Deshumkh, Harvinder S. Dod, Christopher Douglas, Kurt Duncan, Rajarshi Dutta, Sibel Enar, Ligang Fang, William S. Fonbah, William A. A. Foster, Ebenezer Frans, Sujit R. Gandhari, Isha Gupta, Mohit Gupta, Sachin Hansalia, Thein Htay, T. Fikret Ilgenli, Vatsal Inamdar, Gultekin Karakus, Saritha K. Kesanolla, Deepak Khanna, Visali Kodali, William D. Luke, Jr, Pavan Madadi, Edward F. Mahan III, Ravi K. Mallavarapu, Jayaprakash Manda, Carlos Martinez-Hernandez, Farhat Mehmood, Anjlee Mehta, Deval Mehta, Vijay K. Misra, Virenjan Narayan, Sadik Raja Panwar, Vinod Patel, Koteswara R. Pothineni, Ganga Prabhakar, A. N. Ravi Prasad, Xin Qi, Sanjay Rajdev, Barugur S. Ravi, Venkataramana K. Reddy, Venu Sajja, Kumar Sanam, Upasana Sen, Maninder S. Sidhu, Anurag Singh, Harpreet Singh, Preeti Singh, Vikramjit Singh, Ashish Sinha, Thouantosaporn Suwanjutah, Sailendra K. Upendram, Dasan

E. Velayudhan, Srinivas Vengala, Bryan J. Wells, and Pridhvi Yelamanchili.

We deeply appreciate the help of Lindy Chapman, Administrative Associate at the University of Alabama at Birmingham, who provided excellent editorial and secretarial assistance, and Diane Blizzard, Office Associate, for her help. We would also like to thank our clinical sonographers for their help. These are: Beverly Black, Latonya Bledsoe, Rosalyn Boatwright, Audrey Brown, Lynn Devor, Cynthia Dudley, RN, Crystal Green, May Hullett, Emily Milhouse, Peggy Perry, Lucia Sanderson, Sharon Shirley, RN, Octavia Story, Gayle Williams, and Denise Usrey all from the University of Alabama Hospital and The Kirklin Clinic as well as Hsin-Hsien Tseng, Chi-Yeh Teng, and Li-Na Lee from Cheng Hsin General Hospital, Taiwan, Taipei.

Finally, we are grateful to our families for their support during the innumerable hours we spent on this project: Dr. Nanda's wife, Kanta K. Nanda, MD, sons, Nitin Nanda and Anil Nanda, MD, and daughter Anita Nanda Wasan, MD; Dr. Hsiung's wife Wen Hsiung and sons Teddy, Richard, and Jerry; Dr. Miller's wife, Jane Emmerth, and children Aaron and Sarah Miller; and Dr. Hage's wife, Sulaf Mansur Hage, MD, and son Alexander F. Hage.

Navin C. Nanda, MD
Ming C. Hsiung, MD
Andrew P. Miller, MD
Fadi G. Hage, MD

CHAPTER 1

Historical Perspective

The history of echocardiography is a series of successful advancements in the technology to image the heart. This started with A-mode images derived by a thin ultrasound beam and advanced to M-mode displays and then to 2D examination of the heart in motion. This was followed by the addition of Doppler and color Doppler, the recent introduction of tissue Doppler, speckle imaging, contrast echocardiography, and 3D reconstruction, and ultimately the development of real time 3D transthoracic echocardiography (3DTTE) [1–3]. It is, therefore, not surprising that on top of its predecessors, this new technique has proven useful, versatile, and revolutionary in the assessment of cardiovascular diseases. In this book, we will discuss in detail the benefits of this developing technology and its incremental value on top of 2DTTE and/or 2D transesophageal echocardiography (2DTEE).

Although 2DTTE revolutionized noninvasive imaging, its limitations in clinical practice soon became clear. 2DTTE provides real time tomographic images resembling thin slices of cardiac structures that require mental reconstruction of 3D cardiac structures. This has shown clinical value but has been imperfect due to the complex geometrical anatomy of most cardiac structures. Since this imaging modality is noninvasive, does not utilize harmful radiation, and is portable unlike many of its competitors, there has been a great interest in further development of this technology. This led to several attempts to develop 3D echocardiography [4–10]. Morris and Shreve [11] introduced the spark gap position-locating approach (an acoustic spatial locating system) to provide 3D coordinates,

but this method could not record or view 3D images. This method was further developed by other investigators to allow for the ability to model organs and calculate volumes [12]. Ghosh *et al.* [9] developed a simple approach that was able to image the left ventricle (LV) in 3D. This approach used a 2D transducer that was mounted on a mechanical arm that allowed it to rotate around its axis and measured the degrees of rotation. Placement of the transducer in this way ensured that any other form of motion or tilting was not allowed. This transducer could then be placed on the patient's chest wall at the cardiac apex and rotated every few degrees in a sequential manner to obtain multiple slices of the heart, at end systole and end diastole, which were then computer-reconstructed to obtain 3D images of the LV (Figure 1.1). The volumes obtained using this method were validated by angiography [9]. This work was further extended by Raqueno *et al.* [13] and Schott *et al.* [14] to successfully incorporate velocity information and color-coded reconstruction. This allowed 3D imaging of the magnitude of flow disturbance that accompanies valvular regurgitation. Similarly, data on flow patterns obtained by color Doppler could be easily merged with the 3D-reconstructed images of the LV since both datasets were obtained in the same coordinate system (Figure 1.2) [13].

The field of 3D echocardiography was further strengthened by the introduction of TEE with its superior 2D image quality (compared to 2DTTE) due to the close proximity of the probe in the esophagus to the heart, allowing the use of higher frequency and higher resolution transducers, which led to the development of 3DTEE. Investigators used a monoplane TEE probe mounted on a sliding carriage within a casing. Transverse sections

Live/Real Time 3D Echocardiography, 1st edition.
By Navin C. Nanda, Ming Chon Hsiung, Andrew P. Miller, and Fadi G. Hage. Published 2010 by Blackwell Publishing Ltd.

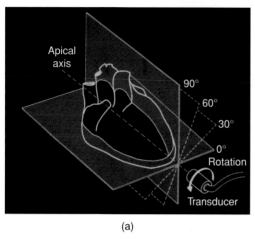

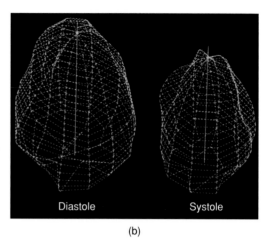

(a)

(b)

Figure 1.1 3D reconstruction of the left ventricle. (a) The apical axis rotation method is shown in which the transducer is rotated in few degree increments to obtain multiple 2D images of the heart. (b) These images were then reconstructed by the computer to form 3D end-diastolic (left) and end-systolic (right) views of the left ventricle. (Reproduced from Ghosh *et al.* [9], with permission.)

at various parallel cardiac levels were obtained by moving the probe up and down the esophagus in small increments by a computerized system, and the images were then reconstructed to provide 3D images (Figure 1.3) [15,16]. Electrocardiographic and respiratory gating was performed to allow for the spatial and temporal registration of images [15]. The large size of the probe, however, precluded routine clinical use. Attempts were then made to use a regular biplane TEE probe for 3D imaging [17]. A protractor mounted on the bite guard was used to accurately determine the probe rotation angle.

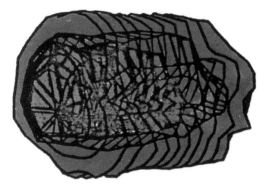

Figure 1.2 Overlay of the high- and the low-velocity isopleths obtained by color Doppler with the reconstructed image of the left ventricular endocardium is shown. Blue, low-velocity isopleth; Red, high-velocity isopleth. (Reproduced from Raqueno *et al.* [13], with permission.)

The probe was angulated at 90° and manually rotated in a clockwise direction in small increments to provide sequential longitudinal images, which were then reconstructed in 3D since their spatial orientation and relationship to each other was known. Offline, the endocardial surface and the intima of the great vessels were manually traced to allow the conversion of the images to a digital format which was reconstructed in 3D (Figure 1.4) [17]. Nanda *et al.* [18] then used a multiplane TEE transducer to reconstruct 3D images by ensuring that the probe remains stationary at a given level and rotating it at 18° intervals at a time (Figure 1.5). Offline, the images were digitized by using a frame grabber and the digitized frames were imported into a 3D modeling program which provided a 3D-reconstructed image of the LV (Figure 1.6) [18]. The superior image quality of TEE images allowed for a much better quality of reconstructed 3D images, and this reignited the interest in 3D echocardiography (Figure 1.7) [19]. Furthermore, the ability to slice the 3D dataset using dissecting planes in any direction allowed for the accurate measurement and the visualization of defects and masses from any direction (Figures 1.8 and 1.9) [20]. The 3D reconstruction of images from multiplane TEE was widely utilized by multiple investigators to provide clinically useful incremental information over 2D imaging and even resulted in the publication of a book with

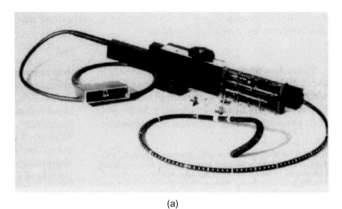
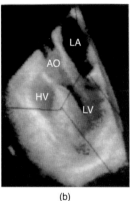

(a)

(b)

Figure 1.3 (a) Probe used for 3D transesophageal echocardiographic (3DTEE) reconstruction. It was mounted on a sliding carriage within a casing (TomTec, Munich, Germany) and interfaced with a computed tomography ultrasound system for data acquisition and 3D reconstruction. (b) A tangential section of a 3D image of the heart during diastole displays open mitral valve and the left ventricle (LV). Portions of the left atrium (LA), right ventricle (RV), and aorta (AO) are also seen. (Reproduced from Pandian et al. [15], with permission.)

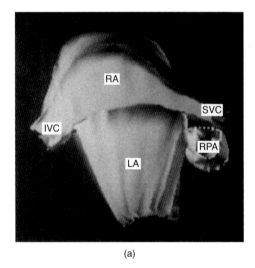
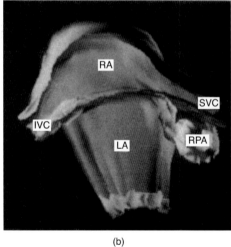

(a)

(b)

Figure 1.4 Regional display of 3D-reconstructed image. (a) 3D image of superior vena cava zone, showing 3D-reconstructed longitudinal structures of superior vena cava (SVC), inferior vena cava (IVC), right atrium (RA), left atrium (LA), and right pulmonary artery (RPA). (b) Stereo-sectional display of the structures shown in Figure 1.3a. (Continued on next page)

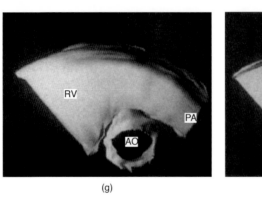

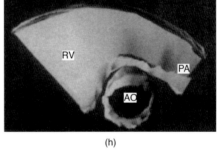

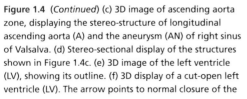

Figure 1.4 (*Continued*) (c) 3D image of ascending aorta zone, displaying the stereo-structure of longitudinal ascending aorta (A) and the aneurysm (AN) of right sinus of Valsalva. (d) Stereo-sectional display of the structures shown in Figure 1.4c. (e) 3D image of the left ventricle (LV), showing its outline. (f) 3D display of a cut-open left ventricle (LV). The arrow points to normal closure of the mitral valve in systole. (g) 3D image of right ventricular outflow tract (RV)–pulmonary artery (PA) zone, showing the longitudinal outline of these structures which are oriented perpendicular to the aortic root (AO). (h) Display of cut-open structures shown in Figure 1.4g (stereo-sectional display). (Reproduced from Li *et al.* [17], with permission.)

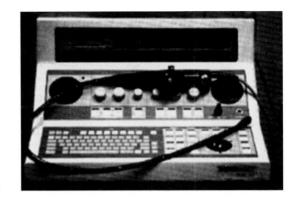

Figure 1.5 Multiplanar transesophageal probe. (Reproduced from Nanda *et al.* [18], with permission.)

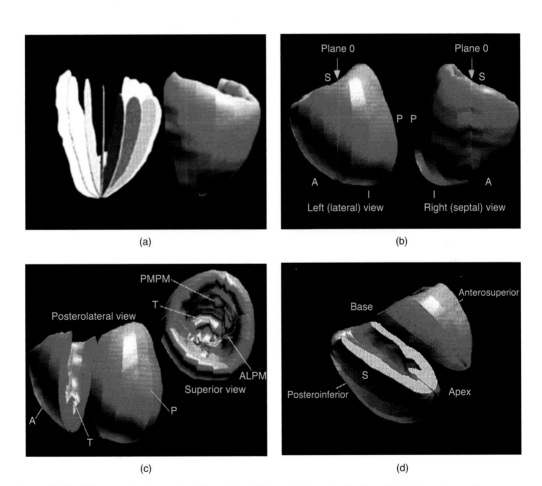

(a)

(b)

(c)

(d)

Figure 1.6 (a–f) 3D reconstruction of the left ventricle (LV) using sequential planes obtained from multiplane transesophageal examination in one of the patients. For 3D reconstruction, all frames were obtained in mid-diastole using the mitral valve motion as the reference. (a) Shows the "rib cage" on the left. (*Continued on next page*)

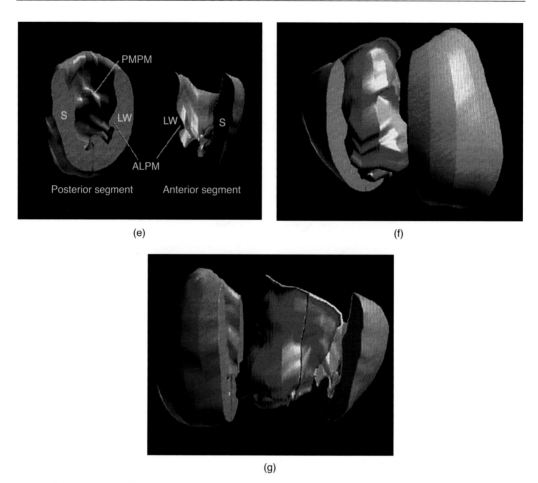

(e)

(f)

(g)

Figure 1.6 (*Continued*) (f, g) Show the "volume cast" of the left ventricular cavity. A, anterolateral wall; ALPM, anterolateral papillary muscle; I, inferior wall; LA, lateral wall; P, posterior wall; PMDM, posteromedial papillary muscle; S, ventricular septum; T, trabeculation. (Reproduced from Nanda *et al.* [18], with permission.)

contributions from many investigators around the world [21]. With further development of these techniques and applying them to color Doppler data, 3D imaging of dynamic abnormal intracardiac blood flow was possible (Figure 1.10) [22].

A limitation of this method was the introduction of artifact due to the time needed for the acquisition of images over several cardiac cycles with patient and/or probe motion during the procedure in addition to inevitable changes in heart rate. To obviate this problem, live/real time 3DTTE and subsequently 3DTEE imaging were developed, and remain the mainstay of 3D echocardiography as it is currently practiced in the clinical setting today. Initial attempts at the development of 3DTTE resulted in a standalone system which was able to provide B-mode images only [23]. The advantage of live/real time 3D imaging is that an entire volume of heart is obtained using one cardiac cycle which is a major advancement from the thin slice, sector imaging that 2D provided [24]. A matrix probe was then developed and incorporated into the regular ultrasound system to provide not only B-mode images but also color Doppler live/real time 3D images, therefore facilitating its use in day-to-day clinical practice [25]. Subsequently, the transducer was miniaturized and incorporated in the TEE probe, providing superior quality 3D images [26]. With these advancements, 3D echocardiography evolved from predominantly a research tool in its early development to a modality that is highly valuable and useful in everyday clinical practice.

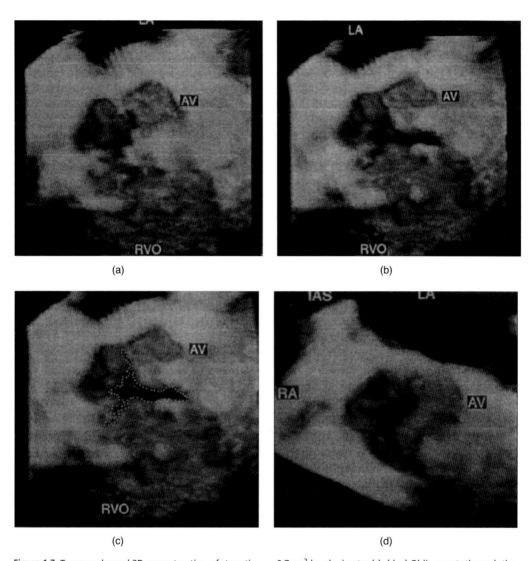

(a)

(b)

(c)

(d)

Figure 1.7 Transesophageal 3D reconstruction of stenotic aortic valve (AV). (a–c) The AV shows multiple echodense areas in both diastole (a) and systole (b, c) indicative of severe thickening and calcification. Although the AV is considerably distorted, three leaflets are easily identified in systole (b, c). The AV orifice is very small and measured 0.7 cm^2 by planimetry (c). (d, e) Oblique cuts through the data cube of the same patient resulting in incomplete visualization of the AV orifice (arrows in (e)). D, diastolic image; E, systolic image. Transverse cuts (as in (a–c)) are essential for complete and accurate delineation of the AV orifice. (*Continued on next page*)

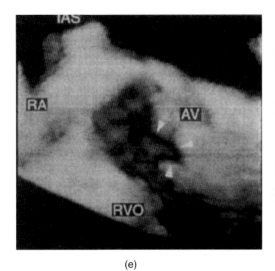

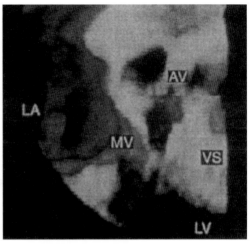

(e)   (f)

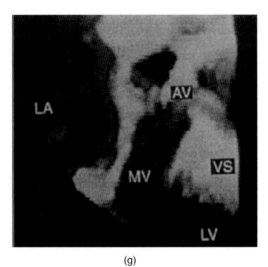

(g)

Figure 1.7 (*Continued*) (f, g) Visualize the AV and the left ventricle (LV) in long axis. Note the markedly restricted opening of the AV in systole (g) and the hypertrophied ventricular septum (VS) seen in both diastole (f) and systole (g). IAS, interatrial septum; LA, left atrium; MV, mitral valve; RA, right atrium; RVO, right ventricular outflow tract. (Reproduced from Nanda *et al.* [19], with permission.)

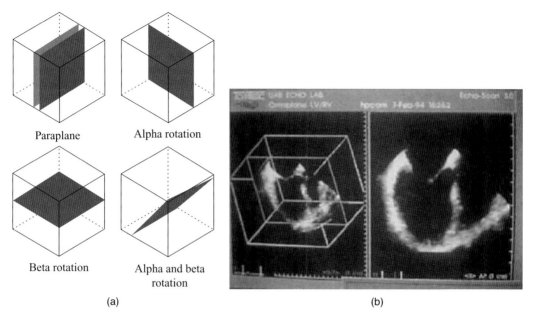

(a)

(b)

Figure 1.8 (a) Various techniques used to "slice" and obtain 2D sections from 3D-reconstructed images. (b) A 2D image using the paraplane technique. (Reproduced from Nanda *et al.* [20], with permission.)

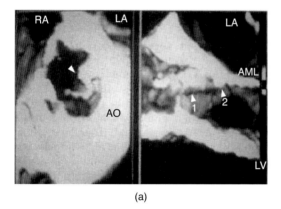

(a)

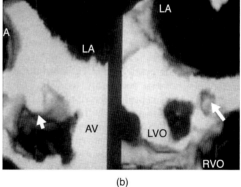

(b)

Figure 1.9 (a) Large vegetations (arrows) are seen involving the aortic valve (AV) reconstructed in short-axis (left) and long-axis (right) views. (b) A large vegetation (left, arrow) is noted on the AV together with an abscess cavity (right, arrow) involving the mitral-aortic intervalvular fibrosa. (*Continued on next page*)

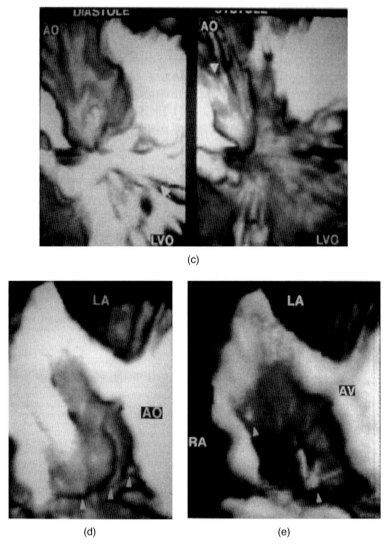

(c)

(d)   (e)

Figure 1.9 (*Continued*) (c–e) "Peeling off of layers" of the aortic root and valve to delineate more clearly AV vegetations (arrows). In (c), both diastolic (left) and systolic (right) frames are shown. AO, aorta; AML, anterior mitral leaflet; LA, left atrium; LVO, left ventricular outflow tract; RA, right atrium; RVO, right ventricular outflow tract. (Reproduced from Nanda *et al.* [20], with permission.)

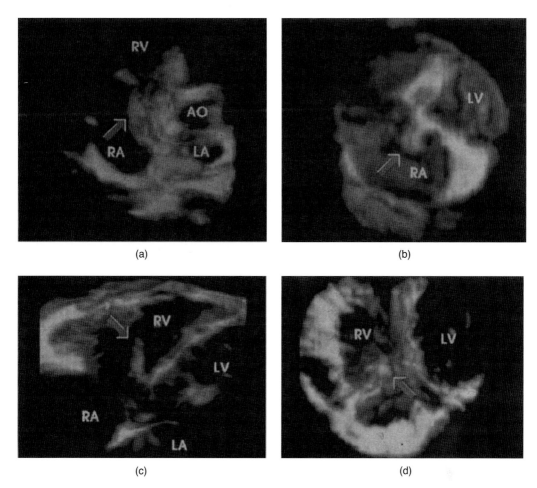

(a)

(b)

(c)

(d)

Figure 1.10 Dynamic 3D images of intracardiac shunt. (a) Shunt jet (arrow) from the left atrium (LA) to the right atrium (RA) and then through the tricuspid valve into the right ventricle (RV) in atrial septal defect. (b) Cross-sectional view of shunt jet (arrow) from the RA in the same patient, as shown in (a). (c) Shunt jet (arrow) from the left ventricle (LV) to RV in another patient with a ventricular septal defect. (d) Cross-sectional view of shunt jet (arrow) from the RV in the same patient shown in (c). AO, aorta. (Reproduced from Li *et al.* [22], with permission.)

References

1. Krishnamoorthy VK, Sengupta PP, Gentile F, Khandheria BK. History of echocardiography and its future applications in medicine. *Crit Care Med* 2007;35:S309–13.

2. Feigenbaum H. Evolution of echocardiography. *Circulation* 1996;93:1321–7.

3. Pandian NG, Roelandt J, Nanda NC, *et al.* Dynamic three-dimensional echocardiography: methods and clinical potential. *Echocardiography* 1994;11:237–59.

4. Dekker DL, Piziali RL, Dong E, Jr. A system for ultrasonically imaging the human heart in three dimensions. *Comput Biomed Res* 1974;7:544–53.

5. Geiser EA, Lupkiewicz SM, Christie LG, Ariet M, Conetta DA, Conti CR. A framework for three-dimensional time-varying reconstruction of the human left ventricle: sources of error and estimation of their magnitude. *Comput Biomed Res* 1980;13:225–41.

6. King D, Al-Bana S, Larach D. A new three-dimensional random scanner for ultrasonic/computer graphic imaging of the heart. In: White DN, Barnes R, eds. *Ultrasound in Medicine*. New York: Plenum Press; 1975:363–72.

7. Moritz WE, Pearlman AS, McCabe DH, Medema DK, Ainsworth ME, Boles MS. An ultrasonic technique for imaging the ventricle in three dimensions and calculating its volume. *IEEE Trans Biomed Eng* 1983;30:482–92.

8. Matsumoto M, Matsuo H, Kitabatake A, *et al.* Three-dimensional echocardiograms and two-dimensional echocardiographic images at desired planes by a computerized system. *Ultrasound Med Biol* 1977;3:163–78.

9. Ghosh A, Nanda NC, Maurer G. Three-dimensional reconstruction of echo-cardiographic images using the rotation method. *Ultrasound Med Biol* 1982;8:655–61.

10. Handschumacher MD, Lethor JP, Siu SC, *et al.* A new integrated system for three-dimensional echocardiographic reconstruction: development and validation for ventricular volume with application in human subjects. *J Am Coll Cardiol* 1993;21:743–53.

11. Moritz WE, Shreve PL. A microprocessor based spatial locating system for use with diagnostic ultrasound. *Proc IEEE* 1976;64:966–74.

12. King DL, King DL, Jr., Shao MY. Three-dimensional spatial registration and interactive display of position and orientation of real time ultrasound images. *J Ultrasound Med* 1990;9:525–32.

13. Raqueno R, Ghosh A, Nanda NC. Four-dimensional reconstruction of two-dimensional echocardiographic images. *Echocardiography* 1989;6:323–37.

14. Schott JR, Raqueno R, Ghosh A, *et al.* Four-dimensional cardiac blood flow analysis using color Doppler echocardiography. In: Nanda NC, ed. *Textbook of Color Doppler Echocardiography.* Philadelphia: Lea & Febiger; 1989:332–41.

15. Pandian NG, Nanda NC, Schwartz SL, *et al.* Three-dimensional and four-dimensional transesophageal echocardiographic imaging of the heart and aorta in humans using a computed tomographic imaging probe. *Echocardiography* 1992;9:677–87.

16. Wollschlager H, Zeiher AM, Klein H, *et al.* Transesophageal echo computer tomography: a new method for dynamic 3-D imaging of the heart (Echo-CT). *Computers in Cardiology* 1990:39.

17. Li ZA, Wang XF, Nanda NC, *et al.* Three dimensional reconstruction of transesophageal echocardiographic longitudinal images. *Echocardiography* 1995;12:367–75.

18. Nanda NC, Pinheiro L, Sanyal R, *et al.* Multiplane transesophageal echocardiographic imaging and three-dimensional reconstruction. *Echocardiography* 1992;9:667–76.

19. Nanda NC, Roychoudhury D, Chung SM, Kim KS, Ostlund V, Klas B. Quantitative assessment of normal and stenotic aortic valve using transesophageal three-dimensional echocardiography. *Echocardiography* 1994;11:617–25.

20. Nanda NC, Abd El-Rahman SM, Khatri GK, *et al.* Incremental value of three-dimensional echocardiography over transesophageal multiplane two-dimensional echocardiography in qualitative and quantitative assessment of cardiac masses and defects. *Echocardiography* 1995;12:619–28.

21. Nanda NC, Sorrell VL. *Atlas of Three-Dimensional Echocardiography.* Armonk: Futura Publishing Company; 2002.

22. Li Z, Wang X, Xie M, Nanda NC, Hsiung MC. Dynamic three-dimensional reconstruction of abnormal intracardiac blood flow. *Echocardiography* 1997;14:375–81.

23. Sheikh K, Smith SW, von Ramm O, Kisslo J. Real time, three-dimensional echocardiography: feasibility and initial use. *Echocardiography* 1991;8:119–25.

24. von Ramm OT, Smith SW, Pavy HR. High-speed ultrasound volumetric imaging system. II. Parallel processing and image display. *IEEE Trans Ultrason Ferroelectr Freq Control* 1991;38:109–15.

25. Salgo I, Bianchi M. Gong "live" with 3-D cardiac ultrasound. *Today Cardiol* 2002;5.

26. Pothineni KR, Inamdar V, Miller AP, *et al.* Initial experience with live/real time three-dimensional transesophageal echocardiography. *Echocardiography* 2007;24:1099–104.

CHAPTER 2

3D Echocardiographic Technology

Ivan S. Salgo, MD, MS
Philips Healthcare, Andover, MA, USA

Introduction

Echocardiography remains the most commonly requested imaging study of the heart. Furthermore, recent insights into our understanding of the sophistication of the structural and functional mechanisms of the heart have come from advances in this area. Combined with portability, safety, low cost, and widespread availability, it is a tribute to the evolution of ultrasound technology that echo's role in deciphering clinical problems in cardiac physiology has kept pace with the ever-increasing demands of a busy practice. This chapter addresses the current state-of-the-art technology in 3D echocardiography as it applies to transducer design, beamforming, display, and quantification. Since 3D echocardiography encompasses many technical and clinical areas, we will review the strengths and limitations of 3D echocardiography and conclude with an analysis of what to use when. In this survey, we will be precise about the terminology related to "3D" imaging and utilize dimension to refer to one, two, or three spatial dimensions.

Transducer design

The ultrasound transducer keeps echo unique amongst its siblings in imaging technology. It converts electrical energy into mechanical vibrations and vice versa. In order to understand what sets 3D systems apart from conventional scanning systems, we need to review some acoustic principles. Convention holds that we refer to one, two, or three

Live/Real Time 3D Echocardiography, 1st edition.
By Navin C. Nanda, Ming Chon Hsiung, Andrew P. Miller, and Fadi G. Hage. Published 2010 by Blackwell Publishing Ltd.

spatial scanning dimensions. Current 2D systems transmit and receive acoustic beams in a flat 2D scanning plane. As opposed to M-mode (one spatial and one temporal dimension), 2D scanning systems sweep a "scan line" to and fro within this 2D imaging plane; the angular position of the beam is said to vary in the "azimuthal" dimension. Even though traditional, flat 2D scanning comprises two spatial dimensions plus one temporal dimension, we do not call this "3D imaging." The transducer itself consists of elements working in unison to create a scan line. Typically, a conventional transducer consists of 64–128 elements spaced according to the ultimate frequency (and hence wavelength) of the acoustic vibrations; these propagate radially along the direction of the scan line. This array of elements steers the outward ultrasound beam or scan line by utilizing interference patterns generated by varying the spatiotemporal phase of each element's transmit event. These principles comprise the underpinnings of any phased array system.

Armed with this knowledge, let us survey the key differences pertinent to 3D ultrasound imaging. First, these 64–128 elements of a conventional cardiac transducer for 2D imaging are arranged along a single row. Technically this is referred to as a 1D array of elements intended for 2D scanning. (Remember that the two spatial dimensions in the image come from sweeping the beam by firing along this 1D row of piezoelectric elements at different times.) Nonetheless, we live in a world with three, not two, spatial dimensions. Note that this "flat" scanning plane of ultrasound energy is not perfectly flat, even though the image appears so on the scanning system. Conventional systems make no use of this elevational direction. To be true to our 3D world, we must sweep the beam efficiently in 3D

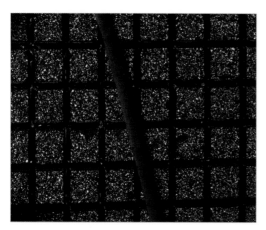

Figure 2.1 Scanning electron micrograph of a fully sampled 2D matrix array used for 3D beam steering. A human hair is shown within the view for comparison.

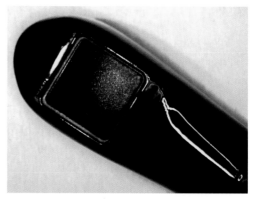

Figure 2.2 A matrix array transesophageal transducer distal tip. The active aperture is 10 mm   10 mm. Note that this supports 2D and 3D imaging, as well as spectral and color Doppler modes.

space. An innovation applied in the last decade was to take just five to seven rows of elements to keep the beam "flatter." These few stacks of rows now comprise, e.g., a 5   64 or 320 element or primitive matrix array transducer. However, these rows were not electrically independent from each other. These primitive matrix array transducers thinned the beam by growing the aperture in the elevation dimension. They did not, however, steer in the third dimension.

True 3D ultrasound steering has been the subject of much academic and industrial research that began in the 1980s. In order to steer an ultrasound beam, a 2D matrix array comprising as many elements in the elevational as azimuthal dimension needed to be fabricated. In order to do this, a block of transducer material is "diced" by a diamond-tipped saw to create each element (Figure 2.1). Today's transducers comprise more than 3000 elements and can have row and column sizes >60. Note that this is a "2D matrix array" that generates "3D images." This concept was known for decades. The significant innovation that actually allows steering is making the elements electrically independent from each other. This allows generating a scan line that varies both azimuthally and elevationally. Thus, a true 3D scan line is born. Early transducers, while having electrically independent rows, did not have every element electrically active as the technology to connect such a dense array was not known yet. Newer types of electrical circuitry connecting each element were first commercialized in 2002. Today, miniaturization has allowed fitting

thousands of fully sampled elements into the tip of a transesophageal transducer (Figure 2.2). It is important to realize that the physical aperture needs to be designed according to the application. The wider the aperture in each dimension, the better the scan line can be focused. However, transthoracic and transesophageal imaging techniques are physically limited by the width and length of the transducer surface, and frequency aperture trade-offs are taken into account when the transducer is designed for each application.

Modern 2D transducers, therefore, consist of thousands of electrically active elements that steer a scan line "left and right" as well as "up and down." New materials that allow more bandwidth (simultaneous high and low frequencies) allow these matrix array transducers to obtain both penetration and high-resolution imaging.

Miniaturization of 3D transducers entails designing smaller integrated circuits with less dissipation of thermal energy. Since signal-to-noise ratio is paramount to the formation of any image, newer designs that allow a full suite of modes while working within acoustic and thermal power constraints continue to push the envelope of innovation.

Beamforming in three spatial dimensions

Beamforming constitutes the steering and focusing of transmitted and received scan lines. Since each element must have independent electrical control by the ultrasound system, a conventional cable that would be used to connect each element would make the transducer cable unwieldy. In order to reduce the size of the cable and reduce power consumption, a significant portion of the beam steering is done within the transducer in highly specialized integrated circuits. The main system steers at coarse angles but the transducer circuits steer in fine increments in a process termed *microbeamforming*. Summing is the act of combining raw acoustic information from each element to generate a scan line, and by summing these in a sequence (first in the transducer and then subsequently in the system), both the transducer connectors and cables are reduced in size dramatically. The 3D beamformer steers both in azimuth and elevation. This creates a 3D spherical wedge of acoustic information that is subsequently processed.

The radio frequency (RF) data are summed and processed using various signal techniques and finally put into rectangular (Cartesian) space by a 3D scan converter. Note that this is an extension of the traditional phased array approach. Older 3D techniques used in the 1990s did not steer electronically but rather involved combining 45–100 cardiac loops and recombining them to create a 3D dataset [1,2]. While this works for static structures, irregular rhythms spell the downfall of gated reconstruction of many beats. Any transducer movement during acquisition of these many gates created artifacts and required a significant amount of smoothing of the data. While this helped reduce attention to "slippage" or misalignment, it reduced the overall image quality if significant stitching needed to be done.

There are two major black and white modes that run in an electronically steered 3D system. The first is a "live" mode where the system scans in real time 3D. The test of this mode is as follows: if the transducer comes off the chest, the image disappears. As with sector scanning, the volume pyramid may be reduced to "zoom" in 3D. This is again a "live" mode. Today, computer and beamforming processing power are not the limiting items for 3D ultrasound image generation; *it is the speed of sound*. Gating, this time only four to eight beats, allows a technique to generate wider volumes while maintaining frame rate. It is done by stitching four (or more) gates together in "full-volume" mode. This can generate >90° scanning volumes at frame rates > 30 Hz. In patients with arrhythmias, RR intervals that fall out of a set range cause the discard of the

errant subvolume and the system scans again until all subvolumes are generated from suitable beat intervals. Thus, in patients with irregular intervals, as long as the average RR rate falls within a reasonable range, a full volume can be reconstructed. Since Doppler methods require many transmit events to be fired along a single path, color Doppler methods use gating. These multiple events are compared or cross-correlated to find the velocity of moving structures. The true 3D spatial modes may be summarized as follows (Figures 2.3–2.5):

1 Live 3D—instantaneous
2 3D zoom—instantaneous
3 Full volume—gated
4 3D color Doppler—gated

A variant of pyramidal 3D beamforming is to scan simultaneous planes in a process known as bi- and triplane imaging. Since this process requires firing fewer scan lines, frame rate is increased at the cost of spatial resolution. This brings us to a point worth emphasizing: *all 3D echocardiography is subject to the laws of physics*. Artifacts such as ringing, reverberations, shadowing, and attenuation occur in 3D as well as 2D imaging. The system must play within these constraints. The numbers and densities of scan lines can be traded off to increase temporal resolution.

Receive parallelism is a beamforming technique in which "virtual" receive lines are constructed in the imaging system as part of the imaging process. For every transmit line, extra receive lines are created around this to boost resolution. Since this is a part of the beamforming process, there are no losses to frame rate because no extra lines are acoustically transmitted. Systems can generate synthetic receive lines (4 , 16 , 32 , or 64) for each transmit line by increasing beamforming parallelism. Note that as the "synthetic" receive line is pointed farther and farther away from the transmitted scan line, the signal-to-noise ratio drops. Increasing the parallelism of a system must account for this effect. Thus, there is a practical limit to receive parallelism. The benefit is that it can increase the density of received lines, thereby improving resolution.

Ultimately, the laws of physics must be obeyed in the design of any system. This can be thought of as living within a triangular "acoustic" playing field bounded by (1) image resolution, (2) frame or volume scanning rate, and (3) sector or volume

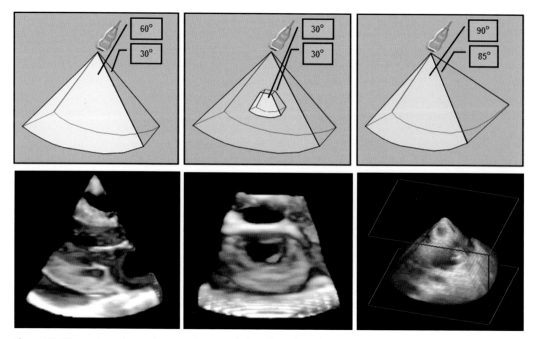

Figure 2.3 3D scanning volumes show as volume rendering. These show the extent of the 3D scan line steering limits in each case. Ultimately, these will constitute a voxel dataset. (Images courtesy of the University of Chicago.)

size. It is easy to increase any two but at the cost of the third. For example, one can increase the volume size by sending scan lines that are farther apart from each other; of course image resolution drops with this maneuver. Alternatively, one can increase frame rate by transmitting fewer lines that are wider apart but again resolution will suffer. Resolution is increased by firing more and increasingly dense scan

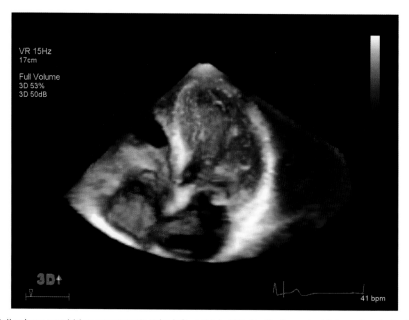

Figure 2.4 Full-volume acquisition encompassing the left ventricle (LV). Depth-dependent "dynamic colorization" has been used to code hue according to depth perspective of the viewer. This adds visual cues to increase the "3D sense."

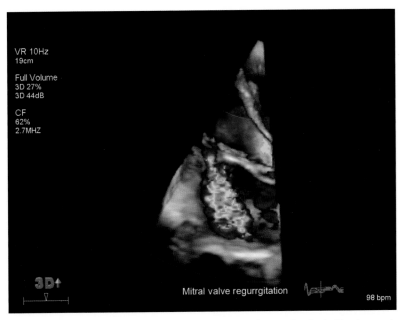

Figure 2.5 Gated 3D color acquisition. A 3D jet of mitral regurgitation is shown. The classic 2D color map has been adapted to render color voxels showing the 3D nature of the jet.

lines. This can easily be done by allowing frame rate to decrease. Enough time must be allowed for a scan line to propagate and return to the system before the next scan line is fired. A balanced approach to system settings should be ensured to the appropriate clinical question. Larger, lower temporal rate volumes are reasonable when the clinical question involves ascertaining global left ventricle (LV) function. Smaller, quicker volumes should be used for quickly moving structures such as assessing valvular function or regional myocardial deformation.

Display of 3D information

2D computer displays consist of rows and blocks of pixels (picture elements) that comprise a 2D image. A 3D dataset consists of "bricks" of pixels called volume elements or "voxels." Since the computer screen is only 2D in nature, a perspective is used to simulate the appearance of 3D depth as an object virtually "deeper" or farther away from the viewing screen. Essentially the 3D dataset, i.e., collection of voxels, can be rotated with respect to the computer screen. Moreover, a process known as "cropping" can be used to cut away into the volume and make some voxels invisible; e.g., one can cut away the left

atrium to see the mitral valve (MV). After rotation and cropping, the remaining voxels are ready to be projected onto pixels in the same way as 3D objects in a room are projected onto the retina in 2D.

3D datasets of voxels are turned into 2D images in a process known as *volume rendering*. The 2D image appears in "3D" because of perspective. There are several different algorithms to accomplish this conversion (e.g., ray casting, shear-warp), but they essentially cast a "light beam" through the collection of voxels. Either the light beam hits enough tissue so as to render it opaque (e.g., tissue) or it keeps shining through transparent voxels so as to render it transparent (e.g., blood pool). Tissue surfaces derived from voxel datasets are sometimes termed *surface rendering*, but this is inaccurate terminology. Additional algorithms can be used to increase the perception of depth by applying different hues on the front (near the screen) of the dataset as opposed to voxels far from the screen.

Quantification in 3D

While visualization of anatomy in its true 3D state is important, many physicians believe that the most significant value 3D echocardiography has for adult

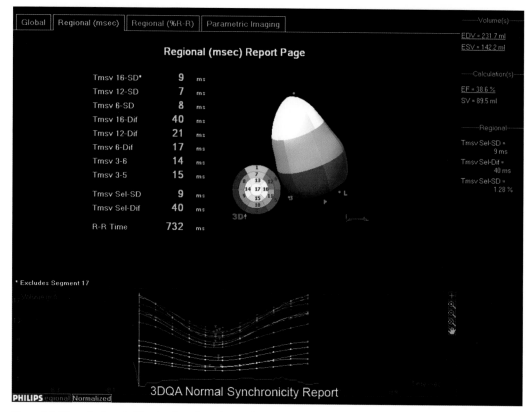

Figure 2.6 3D semiautomated border detection using surface rendering of the LV "shell" to display its 3D nature in QLAB. Each segment has been analyzed for regional ejection, and segmental function is shown by the waveforms.

echocardiography is quantification. True myocardial motion occurs in 3D and traditional 2D scanning planes do not capture the entire motion or else move or "slip" while scanning. Quantifying implies *segmenting* structures of interest from the 3D voxel set. While the voxels themselves can be tagged, e.g., coloring the right ventricle (RV) voxels separately from the LV, computer vision techniques frequently employ methods that define an interface, e.g., the LV endocardial border. This interface is typically constructed as a mesh of points and lines and displayed in a process known as surface rendering (Figure 2.6). Automobiles and building and engineering parts are rendered as meshes by surface rendering in computer-aided design tools.

The 3D quantification of the LV typically employs a surface-rendered mesh. This allows accurate computation of volume, regional wall motion, as well as regional synchrony. Since the entire extent of the LV is taken into account, no foreshortening errors or

assumption of LV volume are generated [1,3]. Technically, a 3D deformable is used to find the LV endocardial surface in three dimensions. This is the most accurate way to quantify LV volumes. Moreover, 3D LV remodeling can be parametrically displayed using differential geometry techniques (Figure 2.7). Bi- and triplane methods help avoid foreshortening errors, but if an aneurysmal dilatation occurs between planes, the computed LV volumes will have some interpolation error. The quantification of LV synchrony is possible in 3D as well [4]. The required frame rate depends on the questions being asked. Frame rate of 30 Hz (33 ms between frames) are inadequate to quantify intramyocardial motion; these are better suited to be studied by tissue Doppler or speckle tracking techniques. However, regional synchrony *can* be measured by 3D because it assesses blood ejection not tissue motion. Since the ejection curve is naturally smooth, it requires less frame rate (has a lower band limit). Moreover, the Nyquist

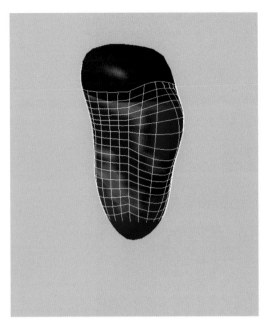

cated analyses of the nonplanar shape of the mitral annulus [5,6]. These 3D measurements include:

- Annular diameters
- Annular nonplanarity
- Commissural lengths
- Leaflet surface areas
- Aortic-to-mitral annular orientation

Other areas subject to 3D quantification include quantifying volumes of all chambers of the heart (i.e., the left and right atria and RV). The quantification of 3D color flow is an active area of research [7]. One of the limitations for color flow quantification includes measuring unsteady flow (as in an intermittent jet of mitral regurgitation) that may not be adequately sampled by gated 3D color Doppler methods.

What to use when

As 3D technology increases in sophistication, so do the new physiologic parameters that can be measured [8]. It is important to begin with anatomic or physiologic questions and turn to 3D as needed to answer these questions with accuracy. The single-most requested measurement for any indication for an echo exam is the assessment of LV function and size. This should be measured by 3D, and techniques to assess LV endocardial volume, mass, and regional function are readily available [9–11]. 3D techniques are more accurate than multiplane techniques, which are, in turn, more accurate than single-plane methods. For example, local changes in LV remodeling can be appreciated by segmenting the entire LV and looking for regional geometric changes (see Figure 2.6). Echo contrast can be used to increase volume accuracy in patients with poor acoustic windows [12]. Stress echo exams can benefit from 3D or triplane methods [13,14]. This is because single-plane scanning does not assure with quantitative certainty that the true apex of the heart is within the scanning volume. "One-beat" LV acquisition techniques are an excellent choice, especially in patients with irregular cardiac rhythms. At this point, the application of 3D technology depends on the referring question.

Patients who undergo MV repair should have intraoperative transesophageal echo as part of their care. 3D methods now allow leaflet anatomy to

Figure 2.7 3D surface-rendered mesh from QLAB has been analyzed using principal curvature analysis. An aneurysmal portion of the anterior basal segment is shown in red. Note that the apex is normally red due to its high degree of curvature. In addition, a set of white grid lines applying geodesic computation shows the "bulge" at the aneurysmal segment.

theorem is frequently misrepresented in this area. Some investigators argue that a 20-millisecond phenomenon (e.g., regional phase differences in peak ejection at different segments) cannot be quantified at 33-millisecond frame intervals. This is an incomplete statement. In fact, if the waveform's upper natural frequency limit reaches its maximum at 15 Hz (half the sampling frame rate), *the waveform is fully determined*. Thus, increasing the frame rate to 100 Hz (10-millisecond intervals) would yield no additional information if the wave was already fully sampled at 30 Hz. This appears to be the case for many dyssynchrony patients and that is why 3D echocardiography stratifies dyssynchrony successfully.

Newer 3D electronically steered transesophageal transducers are yielding ultrasound images never seen before on the beating MV (Figure 2.8). This also allows the mitral apparatus to be segmented at end-systole with great accuracy. The true 3D nature of the mitral annulus, leaflets, and chordal apparatus can be measured. This further allows sophisti-

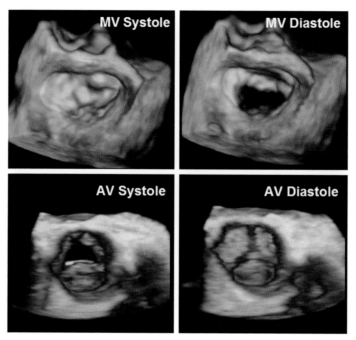

Figure 2.8 3D matrix TEE acquisitions of the aortic (AV) and mitral valves (MV). (Images courtesy of the University of Chicago.)

be displayed functionally with resolution that was not possible before. While conventional 2D echo is likely sufficient for the detection of thrombus and vegetations, 3D echocardiography allows visualization and quantification of the mitral and tricuspid apparatus in its living 3D state [15,16]. Live 3DTEE is especially useful in delineating areas of leaflet prolapse as in patients with Barlow's disease. Moreover, 3D echocardiography is useful in assessing the degree of leaflet restriction within the apparatus as well as annular changes [17,18] (Figure 2.9). Sophisticated changes in LV remodeling can be assessed in ischemic mitral regurgitation [19,20]. Changes in mitral leaflet systolic anterior motion can be assessed in hypertrophic cardiomyopathy [21].

3D visualization is especially useful in identifying intracardiac problems such as atrial septal defects (ASDs). This is especially useful in identifying and characterizing congenital defects for both children and the growing population of adults with congenital heart disease.

The future of 3D echocardiography looks bright. Advances in technology will allow larger scanning volumes as well as more sophisticated methods of quantification such as 3D speckle tracking and analysis of LV torsion and mechanics. Quantification techniques that encompass more automation in

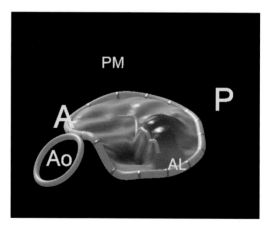

Figure 2.9 3D mitral valve quantification from matrix TEE images (QLAB). The mitral annulus in relation to the aortic annulus is shown. In addition, coaptation from commissure to commissure is shown. Leaflet segmentation allows computation of leaflet restriction and billow area. The abnormal segment is shown near P1 and P2. The green box displays the nonplanarity of the mitral annulus in 3D space. A, anterior; AL, anterior mitral leaflet; Ao, aorta; P, posterior; PM, posterior mitral leaflet.

order to speed clinical workflow and improve inter-observer variability will progress. One of the most exciting areas includes the use of 3D echocardiography to guide intracardiac procedures without the need for cardiopulmonary bypass [22,23]. Placement of ASD devices and percutaneous valve therapies will likely benefit from the live nature of 3DTEE imaging and broaden not only the diagnostic uses of 3D echocardiography but those used for therapy as well.

Acknowledgments

This work was supported in part by NIH grant RO1 HL073647. The author gratefully acknowledges the support and friendship of Bernard Savord and Karl Thiele in preparation of this manuscript.

References

1. Salgo IS. Three-dimensional echocardiography [review]. *J Cardiothorac Vasc Anesth* 1997;11(4):506–16.

2. Ivan Salgo. Three-dimensional echocardiography. *Cardiol Clin* 2007;25(2):231–239.

3. Gerard O, Billon AC, Rouet JM, *et al.* Efficient model-based quantification of left ventricular function in 3-D echocardiography. *IEEE Trans Med Imaging* 2002;21(9):1059–68.

4. Kapetanakis S, Kearney MT, Siva A, *et al.* Real-time three-dimensional echocardiography: a novel technique to quantify global left ventricular mechanical dyssynchrony. *Circulation* 2005;112(7):992–1000.

5. Salgo IS, Gorman JH, III, Gorman RC, *et al.* Effect of annular shape on leaflet curvature in reducing mitral leaflet stress. *Circulation* 2002;106(6):711–17.

6. Watanabe N, Ogasawara Y, Yamaura Y, *et al.* Mitral annulus flattens in ischemic mitral regurgitation: geometric differences between inferior and anterior myocardial infarction: a real-time 3-dimensional echocardiographic study. *Circulation* 2005;112(9,Suppl):I458–62.

7. Pemberton J, Ge S, Thiele K, *et al.* Real-time three-dimensional color Doppler echocardiography overcomes the inaccuracies of spectral Doppler for stroke volume calculation [review]. *J Am Soc Echocardiogr* 2006;19(11):1403–10.

8. Lang RM, Mor-Avi V, Sugeng L, *et al.* Three-dimensional echocardiography: the benefits of the additional dimension [review]. *J Am Coll Cardiol* 2006;48(10):2053–69.

9. Thomas JD, Popovi ZB, Thomas JD, Popovi ZB. Assessment of left ventricular function by cardiac ultrasound [review]. *J Am Coll Cardiol* 2006;48(10):2012–25.

10. Mor-Avi V, Sugeng L, Weinert L, *et al.* Fast measurement of left ventricular mass with real-time three-dimensional echocardiography: comparison with magnetic resonance imaging. *Circulation* 2004;110(13):1814–18.

11. Sugeng L, Mor-Avi V, Weinert L, *et al.* Quantitative assessment of left ventricular size and function: side-by-side comparison of real-time three-dimensional echocardiography and computed tomography with magnetic resonance reference. *Circulation* 2006;114(7):654–61.

12. Corsi C, Coon P, Goonewardena S, *et al.* Quantification of regional left ventricular wall motion from real-time 3-dimensional echocardiography in patients with poor acoustic windows: effects of contrast enhancement tested against cardiac magnetic resonance. *J Am Soc Echocardiogr* 2006;19(7):886–93.

13. Malm S, Frigstad S, Sagberg E, *et al.* Real-time simultaneous triplane contrast echocardiography gives rapid, accurate, and reproducible assessment of left ventricular volumes and ejection fraction: a comparison with magnetic resonance imaging. *J Am Soc Echocardiogr* 2006;19(12):1494–501.

14. Yang HS, Pellikka PA, McCully RB, *et al.* Role of biplane and biplane echocardiographically guided 3-dimensional echocardiography during dobutamine stress echocardiography. *J Am Soc Echocardiogr* 2006;19(9):1136–43.

15. Garcia-Orta R, Moreno E, Vidal M, *et al.* Three-dimensional versus two-dimensional transesophageal echocardiography in mitral valve repair. *J Am Soc Echocardiogr* 2007;20(1):4–12.

16. Ton-Nu TT, Levine RA, Handschumacher MD, *et al.* Geometric determinants of functional tricuspid regurgitation: insights from 3-dimensional echocardiography. *Circulation* 2006;114(2):143–19.

17. Watanabe N, Ogasawara Y, Yamaura Y, *et al.* Quantitation of mitral valve tenting in ischemic mitral regurgitation by transthoracic real-time three-dimensional echocardiography. *J Am Coll Cardiol* 2005;45(5):763–9.

18. Yamaura Y, Watanabe N, Ogasawara Y, *et al.* Geometric change of mitral valve leaflets and annulus after reconstructive surgery for ischemic mitral regurgitation: real-time 3-dimensional echocardiographic study. *J Thorac Cardiovasc Surg* 2005;130(5):1459–61.

19. Hung J, Guerrero JL, Handschumacher MD, *et al.* Reverse ventricular remodeling reduces ischemic mitral regurgitation: echo-guided device application in the beating heart. *Circulation* 2002;106(20):2594–600.

20. Messas E, Yosefy C, Chaput M, *et al.* Chordal cutting does not adversely affect left ventricle contractile function. *Circulation* 2006;114(1, Suppl):I524–8.

21. Song JM, Fukuda S, Lever HM, *et al.* Asymmetry of systolic anterior motion of the mitral valve in patients with hypertrophic obstructive cardiomyopathy: a real-time three-dimensional echocardiographic study. *J Am Soc Echocardiogr* 2006;19(9):1129–35.

22. Cannon JW, Stoll JA, Salgo IS, *et al.* Real-time three-dimensional ultrasound for guiding surgical tasks. *Comput Aided Surg* 2003;8(2):82–90.

23. Suematsu Y, Takamoto S, Kaneko Y, *et al.* Beating atrial septal defect closure monitored by epicardial real-time three-dimensional echocardiography without cardiopulmonary bypass. *Circulation* 2003;107(5):785–90.

CHAPTER 3

How to do a 3D Echocardiogram: Examination Protocol and Normal Anatomy

Live/real time 3D echocardiography is a breakthrough in cardiac imaging that allows us to see the heart in a more realistic display than standard 2D echocardiography. Just as 2D echocardiography, and before it M-mode, revolutionized the practice of cardiology, it is expected that 3D echocardiography will transform the field in a yet unprecedented fashion. The advent of the full matrix array transducer has permitted the live acquisition of a 3D pyramidal dataset that can be cropped in any desired plane. Using this technology, one can evaluate the various cardiac structures, chamber dimensions, and the structure and function of the valves. As we will examine at length in the chapters of this book, 3D echocardiography has already established its clinical validity in various cardiovascular conditions.

3D imaging

Current 3D transducers consist of broadband 4 MHz matrix phased array systems containing up to 6400 elements connected to 10,000 channels and over 150 mini-circuit boards. This allows instantaneous 3D volume-rendered, color-Doppler, and harmonic capabilities. The transducer's piezoelectric crystal is cut by laser into the minute equal-sized elements that form the element matrix (see Figure 1.1) [1]. In order to generate 3D images, the transducer generates ultrasonic beams in a phased

Live/Real Time 3D Echocardiography, 1st edition.
By Navin C. Nanda, Ming Chon Hsiung, Andrew P. Miller, and Fadi G. Hage. Published 2010 by Blackwell Publishing Ltd.

array manner. The ultrasound beam generates 2D sector images in the usual manner employed for 2D echocardiography, but in addition travels along the Z-axis to produce the pyramidal 3D image dataset in which the scanning direction is perpendicular to each other at the X-, Y-, and Z-axes (Figure 3.1). Using the transducer, the echocardiographer can image the heart in narrow sectors in real time (Figure 3.2), or alternatively by combining four sectors together. A wide sector scan consisting of 60° along both the Y- and Z-axes is generated (the so-called "live" imaging; Figure 3.3). This last display mode has been termed the "full-volume scan" or the "pyramidal dataset," and has the advantage of covering a wider region of interest without moving the transducer. In fact in pediatric subjects, it is not unusual for the pyramidal dataset to include the entire heart. This image is usually taken over several heartbeats (5–8 s), preferably with the patients holding their breath in order to decrease respiratory artifact. Imaging in this manner allows for the examination of normal cardiac anatomy in a fashion not imaginable with 2D echocardiography in addition to better visualization of abnormal cardiac morphology.

3D examination protocol

Since the 3D images obtained from live 3D echocardiography correspond closely to actual anatomy, the user is able to manipulate the images more naturally and to derive clinical information from that manipulation that cannot be obtained from the standard 2D images. However, the images need

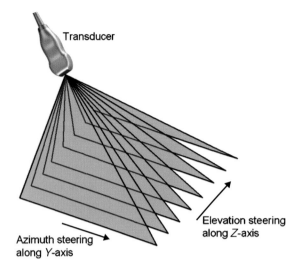

Figure 3.1 The scanning beam performs azimuth steering along the Y-axis in a phased array manner and produces 2D sector images. The 2D sector image performs elevation steering along Z-axis and finally produces a pyramidal 3D dataset (courtesy of Philips Medical Systems, Bothell, WA). (Reproduced from Wang et al. [1], with permission). Movie clip 3.1.

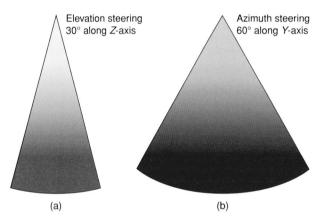

Figure 3.2 (a) 30° elevation steering along the Z-axis; (b) 60° azimuth steering along the Y-axis. (Reproduced from Wang et al. [1], with permission)

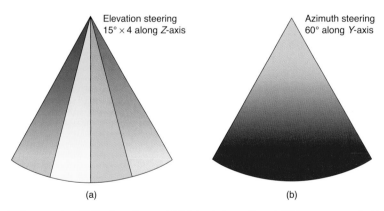

Figure 3.3 In order to generate a "full-volume" pyramidal dataset, four adjacent 15° images generated by elevation steering along the Z-axis are combined to produce 60° images (a) and the image with 60° azimuth steering along the Y-axis (b). (Reproduced from Wang et al. [1], with permission)

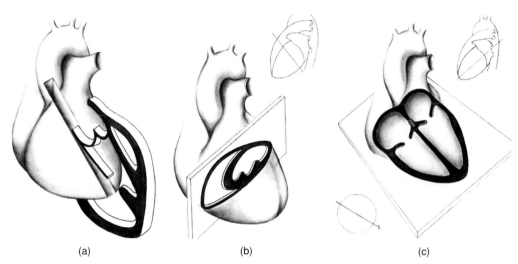

(a)   (b)   (c)

Figure 3.4 Some of the standard 2D echocardiographic imaging planes. (a) Parasternal long-axis plane; (b) parasternal short-axis plane; (c) apical four-chamber plane. Note that the planes are described in relation to the left ventricle of the heart rather than to the anatomic orientation of the patient. (Reproduced from Nanda NC, Gramiak R. *Clinical Echocardiography*. St. Louis: C.V. Mosby; 1978:371, 393, 408, with permission.)

to be displayed in a consistent manner to simplify the visualization of the images and to facilitate the interpretation of the examination [2]. This is routinely done by taking advantage of the standard 2D transthoracic echocardiographic (2DTTE) imaging views familiar to echocardiographers and anatomic orientation standards.

In standard 2DTTE, the images are displayed in relation to the left ventricle of the heart rather than to the standard anatomic orientation of the patient

that is commonly used by other radiographic imaging such as computed tomography or magnetic resonance imaging (Figure 3.4). In the 3D examination, the echocardiographer uses the standard acquisition windows of 2D echocardiography (left parasternal, apical, subcostal, suprasternal, right/left supraclavicular, and right parasternal), but the images can be displayed in reference to the heart itself and not the body axis (Figures 3.5 and 3.6). This anatomic orientation assumes that the

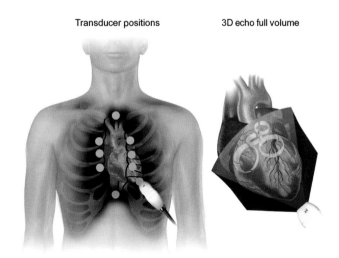

Transducer positions   3D echo full volume

Figure 3.5 Transducer positions for live 3D echocardiography standard examination used to acquire a full-volume dataset of the heart. (Reproduced from Nanda *et al.* [2], with permission.)

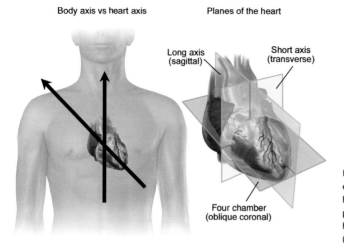

Figure 3.6 Cropping planes used for 3D echocardiography. The long axis of the heart is at an angle to the body axis. The planes of the heart are in reference to the heart itself and not the body axis. (Reproduced from Nanda *et al.* [2], with permission.)

patient is standing upright, facing the observer with the arms hanging on the sides.

After obtaining the full-volume pyramidal dataset, the echocardiographer can use cropping planes to study the 3D images from different perspectives using a 2D display (Figure 3.7). The dissection of the heart using these cropping planes can be performed on the spot or off-line at a later time. The most frequently utilized planes are the sagittal (left-to-right or lateral control; when used in relation to the heart, it divides it into right and left portions similar to long axis), coronal (top-to-bottom or elevation control; divides the heart into anterior and posterior portions similar to apical

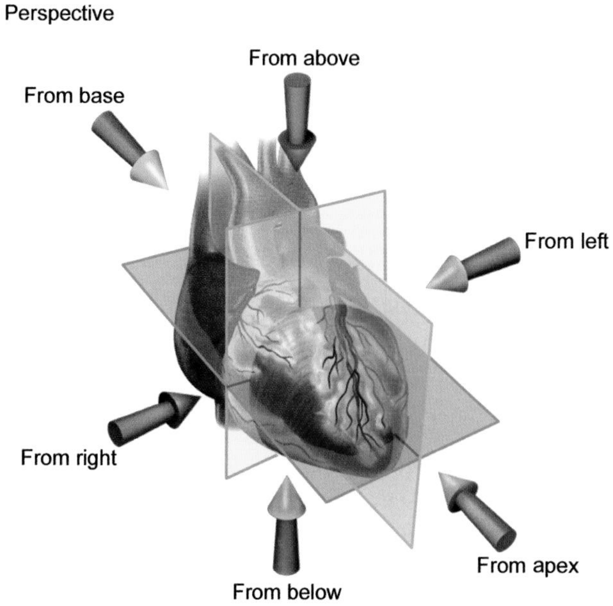

Figure 3.7 The use of anatomic planes to describe live 3D echocardiographic images results in six different cardiac perspectives for any cardiac structure. These may be described using two descriptive terms: the plane and the viewing perspective. (Reproduced from Nanda *et al.* [2], with permission.)

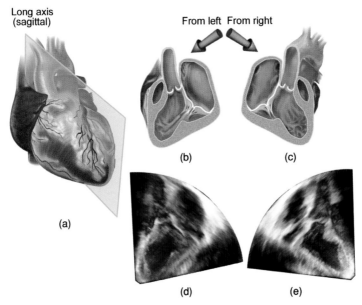

Figure 3.8 (a–e) Sagittal (long-axis or longitudinal) section—viewed from left side or right side—as used in live 3D echocardiography. (Reproduced from Nanda *et al.* [2], with permission.)

four-chamber view), and transverse (front-to-back or depth control; divides the heart into superior and inferior portions similar to short axis) planes (Figures 3.8–3.10, respectively). Therefore, 3D images allow echocardiographers to view the heart in the standard views they are accustomed to, but also open the opportunity to view the various cardiac structures from *any* orientation, which can

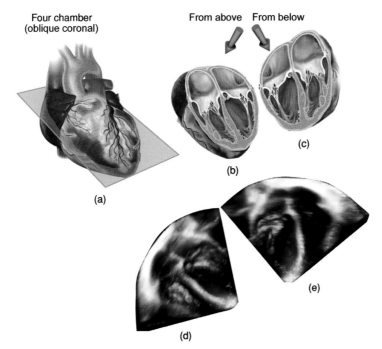

Figure 3.9 (a–e) Oblique coronal (frontal) section—viewed from above and below—as used in live 3D echocardiography. (Reproduced from Nanda *et al.* [2], —, with permission.)

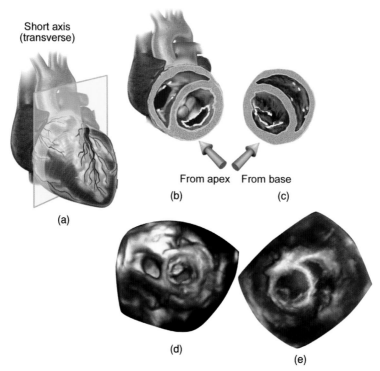

Short axis
(transverse)

From apex From base
(b)   (c)

(a)

(d)

(e)

Figure 3.10 (a–e) Transverse (short-axis) section—viewed from base or apex—as used in live 3D echocardiography. (Reproduced from Nanda *et al.* [2], —, with permission.)

prove useful in particular clinical scenarios. Due to the versatility of the cropping planes, any cardiac structure can be viewed from six different perspectives, as shown in Figure 3.7. Using the cropping planes, the heart can thus be sectioned anatomically with the sections displayed consecutively like pages of a book. To do so, the heart is first displayed with the apex down on the screen and sectioned systematically using the following planes to get a comprehensive examination:

1 *Sagittal cropping:* (Long-axis or longitudinal sectioning) with the images displayed from left side or the right side (Figure 3.8).

2 *Coronal cropping:* (Frontal sectioning) with the images displayed from above or below (Figure 3.9).

3 *Transverse cropping:* (Short-axis sectioning) with the images displayed from base or apex (Figure 3.10).

4 *Oblique cropping:* Nonstandard sectioning planes can be used for the best visualization of structures not seen well on the standard cropping planes.

Using these cropping planes with the standard anatomic orientation helps in the proper identification of various cardiac structures and normal and abnormal pathology, as described below.

Left parasternal approach (Figure 3.11–3.21)

The echocardiographer who is familiar with the left parasternal approach from 2D echocardiography can obtain a wealth of information with regard to various cardiac structures by sectioning the 3D datasets, as explained above [1]. This approach can therefore be very useful to identify normal structures and differentiate them from pathological entities. For example, we have utilized 3DTTE to identify the structure seen as an echo-free space posterior to the proximal ascending aorta in the left parasternal long-axis view [3]. This has been traditionally described as the right pulmonary artery

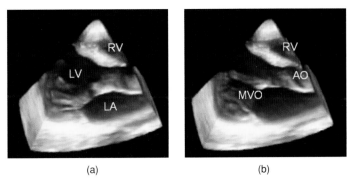

(a)   (b)

Figure 3.11 Live 3D echocardiographic images of a long-axis view of the normal left heart. (a) A long-axis view of the left heart. Left ventricle (LV), left atrium (LA), right ventricle (RV), and aorta (AO) are displayed clearly. During systole, the mitral orifice (MVO) is closed. (b) The same live 3D image in diastole with the MVO open. (Reproduced from Wang *et al.* [1], —, with permission.)

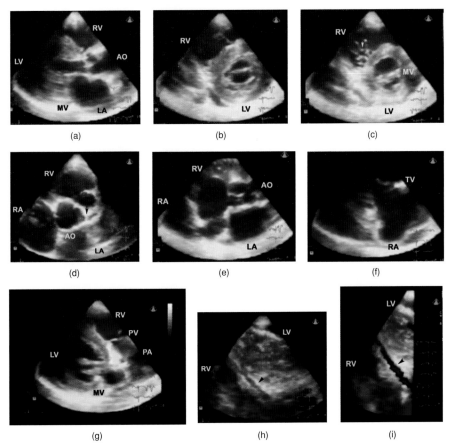

(a)   (b)   (c)

(d)   (e)   (f)

(g)   (h)   (i)

Figure 3.12 Live/real time 3D transthoracic echocardiograpy. Parasternal examination. (a–g) Multiple sections showing various anatomic structures obtained by cropping a single parasternal long-axis dataset. The arrow in (c) points to the tricuspid valve (TV). The arrow in (d) shows the left main coronary artery. AO, aorta; LA, left atrium; LV, left ventricle; MV, mitral valve; PA, pulmonary artery; PV, pulmonary valve; RA, right atrium; RV, right ventricle. (h, i) Cropping of another parasternal dataset from the same patient shows a long segment of the left anterior descending coronary artery (arrow) in B mode (h) and with color Doppler (i). Short-axis views of this artery are also visualized in the accompanying Movie clip 3.12. LV, left ventricle; RV, right ventricle.

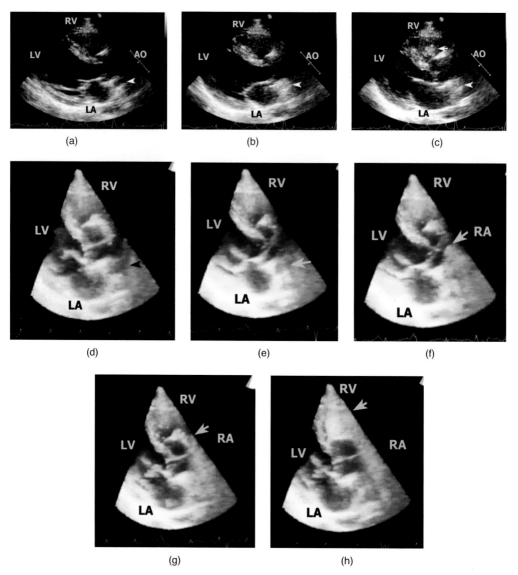

(a)   (b)   (c)

(d)   (e)   (f)

(g)   (h)

Figure 3.13 2D and live/real time 3D transthoracic echocardiographic (3DTTE) identification of the superior vena cava (SVC) and right pulmonary artery behind the aorta imaged in parasternal long-axis view. Bounded echo-free space behind the aorta imaged in parasternal long-axis view. (a–c) 2D transthoracic echocardiographic (2DTTE) bubble study. Intravenous injection of agitated normal saline shows contrast echoes first appearing in the bounded echo-free space (arrowhead in (b)) and then in the right ventricle (RV; arrow in (c)). This suggests that the echo-free space represents the SVC. Movie clip shows biplane imaging with bubble study. (d–h) Real time 3DTTE bubble study. Intravenous injection of agitated normal saline shows contrast echoes appearing first in the bounded echo-free space (arrow in (e)) and then sequentially moving into the right atrium (RA; arrow in (f)) and RV (arrow in (g) and (h)). This suggests that the bounded space is the SVC. The 3DTTE image was tilted to demonstrate the progression of contrast echoes into the RA and RV. AO, aorta; LA, left atrium; LV, left ventricle. (Reproduced from Burri et al. [3], with permission) Movie clips 3.13 A–C and 3.13 D–H.

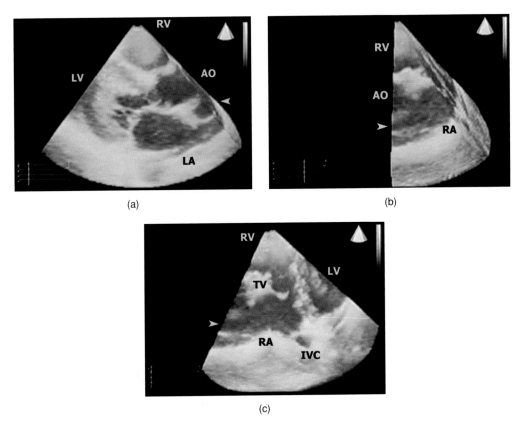

(a)

(b)

(c)

Figure 3.14 2D and live/real time 3D transthoracic echocardiographic (3DTTE) identification of the superior vena cava (SVC) and right pulmonary artery behind the aorta imaged in parasternal long-axis view. Bounded echo-free space behind the aorta imaged in parasternal long-axis view. Live 3DTTE. (a–c) Tilting of the full-volume 3D dataset shows the bounded echo-free space (arrowhead) to be continuous with the right atrium (RA). This is consistent with SVC. AO, aorta; IVC, inferior vena cava; LA, left atrium; LV, left ventricle; RV, right ventricle; TV, tricuspid valve. (Reproduced from Burri *et al.* [3], with permission.) Movie clip 3.14.

but could also represent an aortic dissection/intimal hematoma, aortic pseudoaneurysm, sinus of Valsalva aneurysm, pericardial fluid in the transverse sinus, an abscess cavity, or the superior vena cava (SVC). In order to clarify this issue, we used contrast echocardiography with agitated saline and 3DTTE in a series of patients in whom this space was seen on 2DTTE. In the majority of patients (almost 80%), this space was confirmed to represent the SVC. In these patients, this space can be shown to be in continuity with the right atrium with 3DTTE. In another 12% of patients, two echo-free spaces were seen that represented the SVC and the right pulmonary artery. Only in a minority of patients (8%) did the space represent right pulmonary artery alone [3]. Therefore, 3DTTE provides an opportunity to confirm the echo-free space seen behind the aorta in the parasternal long-axis view as the SVC or a pulmonary artery. The transducer has to be angled superiorly and to the right in order to view the proximal ascending aorta and then tilted posteriorly, in order to optimally image the SVC [3]. Images from this view are ideal for the visualization of the mitral valve, the left atrium, and the interventricular septum, and are therefore helpful in the assessment of mitral stenosis and ventricular septal defects, including the visualization of patches used for their repair [1].

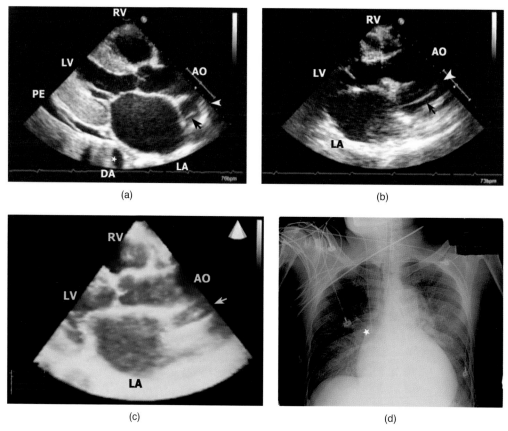

(a)

(b)

(c)

(d)

Figure 3.15 2D and live/real time 3D transthoracic echocardiographic (3DTTE) identification of the superior vena cava (SVC) and right pulmonary artery behind the aorta imaged in parasternal long-axis view. Bounded echo-free space behind the aorta imaged in parasternal long-axis view. 2DTTE and 3DTTE. (a–c) The arrow points to the central line in the bounded echo-free space imaged behind the aorta (AO) by 2DTTE in (a) and (b), and by 3DTTE in (c). The asterisk in (a) points to the dissection flap in the descending thoracic aorta (DA). (d) Chest X-ray (posteroanterior view) shows the tip of the central line (asterisk) located at the SVC–RA (right atrium) junction. The above findings indicate that the bounded echo-free space is the SVC. LA, left atrium; LV, left ventricle; RV, right ventricle; PE, pericardial effusion. (Reproduced from Burri *et al.* [3], with permission) Movie clips 3.15 A, 3.15 B and 3.15 C.

Apical approach (Figures 3.22 and 3.23)

From the apical approach, the entire left ventricle can be visualized, and using appropriate software, its volumes can be accurately measured [1]. This view can thus be very helpful in the measurement of end-systolic and end-diastolic volumes, which are required for the calculation of left ventricular ejection fraction. Cropping the four-chamber apical dataset can also provide apical five-chamber, apical two-chamber, and apical three-chamber views.

Cropping of the apical dataset also permits the echocardiographer to view all four cardiac valves simultaneously, in a manner that is not possible with 2D imaging and which allows for a better appreciation of the anatomical relationship of the valves [1].

Subcostal approach (Figure 3.24)

The subcostal approach can be valuable for the visualization of multiple cardiac structures,

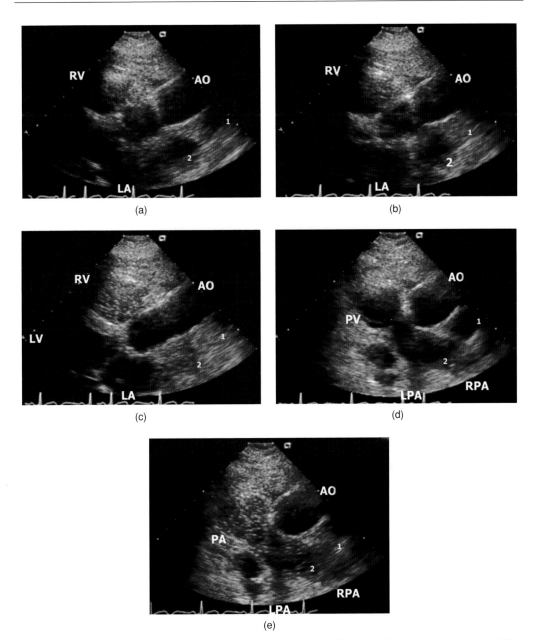

(a)

(b)

(c)

(d)

(e)

Figure 3.16 2D and live/real time 3D transthoracic echocardiographic (3DTTE) identification of the superior vena cava (SVC) and right pulmonary artery behind the aorta imaged in parasternal long-axis view. Two bounded echo-free spaces behind the aorta imaged in parasternal long-axis view in a patient with primary pulmonary hypertension. 2DTTE bubble study. (a–e) Intravenous injection of agitated normal saline resulted in the appearance of contrast echoes initially in the superior space (#1 in (b)) and then in the more inferior space (#2 in (c)). The superior space therefore represents the SVC. The inferior space is the right pulmonary artery and its continuity with the main pulmonary artery (PA) is clearly shown in (d) and (e). AO, aorta; LA, left atrium; LPA, left pulmonary artery; LV, left ventricle; PV, pulmonary valve; RPA, right pulmonary artery; RV, right ventricle. (Reproduced from Burri et al. [3], with permission.) Movie clips 3.16 A–C and 3.16 D–E.

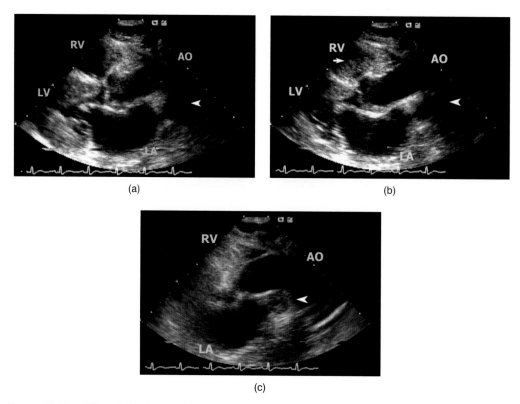

(a)

(b)

(c)

Figure 3.17 2D and live/real time 3D transthoracic echocardiographic (3DTTE) identification of the superior vena cava (SVC) and right pulmonary artery behind the aorta imaged in parasternal long-axis view. Bounded echo-free space behind the aorta imaged in parasternal long-axis view in a patient with systemic hypertension and no obvious pulmonary hypertension. 2DTTE bubble study. (a–c) Intravenous injection of agitated normal saline resulted in contrast echoes first appearing in the right ventricle (RV) (arrow in (b)) and then in the bounded echo-free space (arrowhead in (c)). This suggests that the bounded echo-free space represents a pulmonary artery and not the SVC. AO, aorta; LA, left atrium; LV, left ventricle; RV, right ventricle (Reproduced from Burri et al. [3], with permission) Movie clip 3.17.

especially with suboptimal acoustic windows from the parasternal and apical approaches. Not unlike the 2DTTE examination, the subcostal approach can be the only window that provides significant information on patients with chronic obstructive pulmonary disease.

Suprasternal approach
(Figure 3.25)

The suprasternal approach provides the best images for the visualization of the ascending aorta, aortic arch, and proximal descending aorta. From this window, the echocardiographer can also image the vessels arising from the aortic arch, the pulmonary arteries, and various venous structures such as the innominate veins.

Supraclavicular approach
(Figure 3.26)

In addition to the usual acoustic windows (left parasternal, apical, subcostal, and suprasternal) utilized in 2DTTE, the supraclavicular and right parasternal approaches have been shown to be useful in particular circumstances [4,5]. Using the

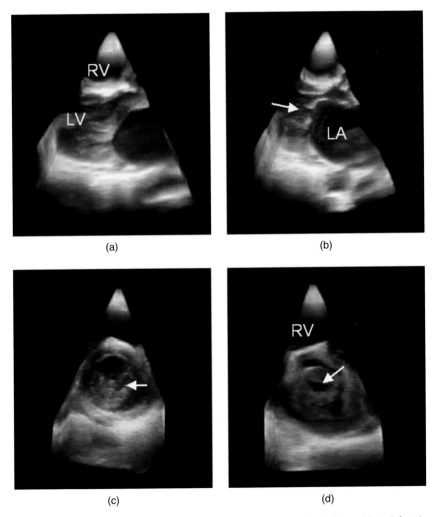

(a)

(b)

(c)

(d)

Figure 3.18 Live 3D echocardiography in mitral stenosis. (a) A live 3D image from the long-axis view of the left heart. The left atrium (LA) is enlarged, and in systole, the mitral orifice is closed with good coaptation between anterior and posterior leaflets. (b) The same live 3D image in diastole, with restricted opening of the mitral orifice (arrow). (c) View from left ventricle to left atrium, with the mitral valve closed in systole (arrow). (d) The same image in diastole. The mitral orifice is an elliptical small opening (arrow). LV, left ventricle; RV, right ventricle. (Reproduced from Wang *et al.* [1], with permission)

supraclavicular window, we were able to visualize the entire length of the SVC and the junction of the IVC (inferior vena cava) with the right atrium as well as their tributaries. The aortic arch and the major arteries were also well seen from this window, and by complementing the examination with the suprasternal views, even longer segments of the aortic arch branch vessels and the adjacent veins were seen [6].

Right parasternal approach (Figures 3.27–3.29)

The right parasternal window is even more revealing in the presence of particular conditions that tend to push the right lung away from the sternum such as pericardial effusion, right heart enlargement, or ascending aortic dilatation. We have recently examined the usefulness of these windows using a

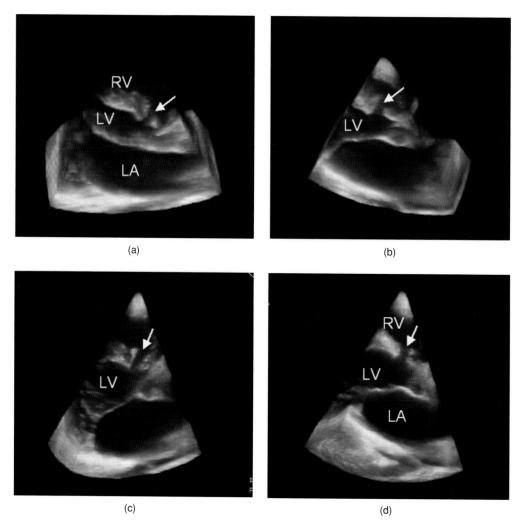

(a)

(b)

(c)

(d)

Figure 3.19 Live 3D echocardiography using narrow-angle display in a patient with a ventricular septal defect. (a–d) Images are obtained from frontal, posterior, inferior, or superior direction and the defect is visualized (arrows) clearly. LA, left atrium; LV, left ventricle; RV, right ventricle. (Reproduced from Wang *et al.* [1], with permission)

Philips Sonos 7500 (Philips Medical Systems, Inc., Andover, MA) ultrasound system and both B mode and color Doppler live 3D datasets [6]. By cropping the 3D datasets we were able to visualize the SVC and IVC and the coronary sinus entering the right atrium as well as the pulmonary veins entering the left atrium. The entire atrial septum could be seen *en face*, resulting in a more confident diagnosis or exclusion of an atrial septal defect. Also, in the presence of an atrial septal defect, *en face* evaluation of its rim and its relation to adjacent structures can be very helpful for the assessment of transcatheter closure. Structures that are difficult to evaluate with 2DTTE, such as the right atrial appendage and the three leaflets of the tricuspid valve, were well seen on 3DTTE. The ascending aorta and the origin and proximal portion of the left main coronary artery in addition to the pulmonary valve and main pulmonary artery with its branches as well as other structures could be well seen.

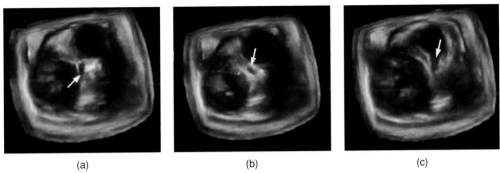

(a)   (b)   (c)

Figure 3.20 These are the wide-angle pyramidal display images (60° 60°). The echo of the chest wall on top of the live 3D echocardiography was removed and the wide-angle square images of intracardiac structures are shown clearly. A ventricular septal defect was visualized (arrows). The tubular defect from left ventricle into right ventricle is seen in images(a), (b), and (c). (Reproduced from Wang *et al.* [1], with permission)

Last, it is important to appreciate the limitations of 3DTTE. Since the acoustic windows are essentially the same in 3DTTE as those in 2DTTE, if the echocardiographer finds that the acoustic windows are poor and the 2D images are suboptimal in quality, the 3DTTE images will also be poor and inadequate. In general, 3DTTE images are even poorer in quality than 2DTTE images. The rule of thumb is, therefore, that 2DTTE images have to be of reasonable quality to obtain a good 3DTTE examination. In clinical practice, the 3DTTE examination should be focused, looking for whatever incremental value the examiner thinks it will provide, and act as a supplement rather than a replacement of the 2DTTE examination.

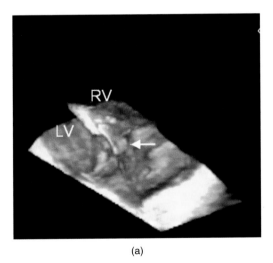

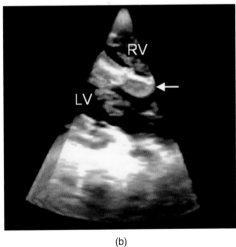

(a)   (b)

Figure 3.21 Live/real time 3D transthoracic echocardiographic (3DTTE) images of a patient with interventricular septal defect which was repaired with a patch (arrow). (a) Long-axis view of the left heart viewed from the superior aspect. The echo of the chest wall was removed and the patch appears separating the right (RV) and left (LV) ventricles. (b) Long-axis view of the left heart viewed from the inferior aspect. (Reproduced from Wang *et al.* [1], with permission.)

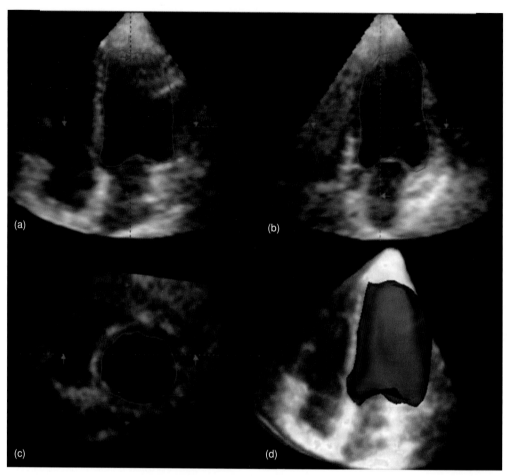

Figure 3.22 Live/real time 3DTTE. Apical examination. (a) Apical four-chamber view and endocardial margin of the left ventricle. (b) Two-chamber view and endocardial margin of the left ventricle. (c) Short-axis view of the ventricles and their endocardial margin. (d) Reconstructed 3D volume of the left ventricle. (Reproduced from Wang *et al.* [1], with permission.) Other apical views such as apical five-chamber, apical two-chamber, and apical three-chamber can be obtained by suitable cropping of the apical four-chamber dataset (Movie clip 3.22 Part 1). Short-axis views of the left ventricle at various levels such as apex, papillary muscles, and mitral valve can also be obtained from the same dataset. Movie clips 3.22 Part 1 and 3.22 Part 2.

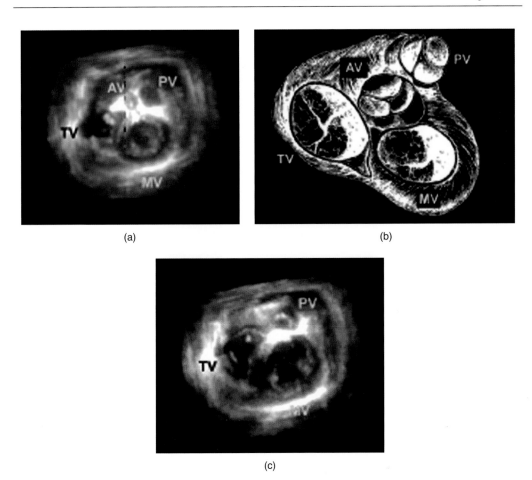

(a)   (b)

(c)

Figure 3.23 Live/real time 3D transthoracic echocardiography. Apical examination. (a) Cropping of the apical 3D dataset permits viewing of all four cardiac valves simultaneously. This is not possible using standard 2D echocardiography. Also see Figure 11.51c and accompanying movie clip in Chapter 11. (b) Anatomic schematic showing the relationship of the four cardiac valves. Note the striking resemblance of the live 3D echo image to actual anatomy. (c) Another live 3D echo view from the same patient, showing the relationship of three cardiac valves. AV, aortic valve; MV, mitral valve; PV, pulmonary valve; TV, tricuspid valve. (a, c) Reproduced from Nanda NC: Live 3D Echo Delivering Real-Time benefits to Cardiologists. World Medical Association Report on Cardiac Health. Business Briefing (Extract): Global Healthcare 2003;2–4, with permission; (b) reproduced from a modified figure from Gray H. *Anatomy of the Human Body*. (30th ed.) C.D. Clemente (ed.); 1985:632, with permission of Williams & Wilkins). Movie clip 3.23 Part 1 shows cropping of the apical dataset from both ventricular and atrial aspects to view all four cardiac valves. Oblique cropping was also used to view the ventricular septum (VS) *en face* from the right side. The asterisk points to a few trabeculations in the left ventricular cavity resulting from the cropping plane cutting through the apical portion of the VS. A pacing lead is also noted in the right atrium (RA) and right ventricle (RV). Oblique cropping was also used from the left side to view the left ventricle (LV) more comprehensively. MV, mitral valve; PV, pulmonary valve; TV, tricuspid valve. Movie clip 3.23 Part 2. Apical dataset has been cropped to view the attachment (arrow) of the anterolateral papillary muscle in the LV. A small papillary muscle is also visualized in the RV. Short-axis cropping using the same dataset views both anterolateral and posteromedial papillary muscles (arrows). Movie clip 3.23 Part 3 shows cropping of the right heart to display the entrance of the coronary sinus into the RA. The anterior and septal leaflets of the tricuspid valve are well seen. Movie clips 3.23 Parts 1–3.

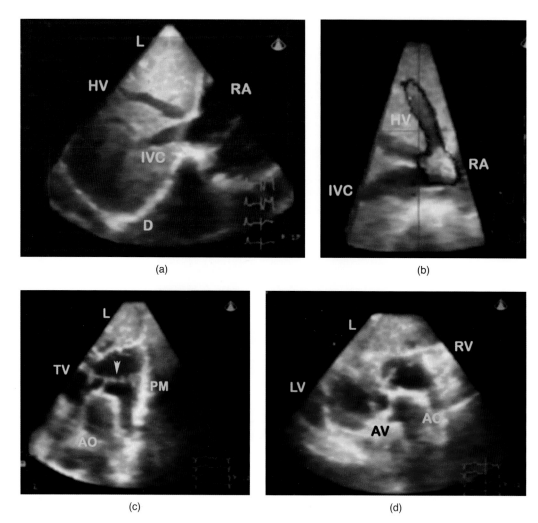

(a)

(b)

(c)

(d)

Figure 3.24 (a–h) Live/real time 3D transthoracic echocardiography. Subcostal examination. Demonstrates several anatomic structures in B mode and with color Doppler obtained from cropping of subcostally acquired 3D datasets. The arrow in (c) points to the tricuspid subvalvular apparatus. The arrow in (g) denotes the right ventricular apex. AO, aorta; AS, interatrial septum; AV, aortic valve; D, diaphragm; HV, hepatic vein; IVC, inferior vena cava; L, liver; LA, left atrium; LPA, left pulmonary artery; LV, left ventricle; PA, pulmonary artery; PM, papillary muscle; PV, pulmonary valve; RA, right atrium; RPA, right pulmonary artery; RV, right ventricle; TV, tricuspid valve.

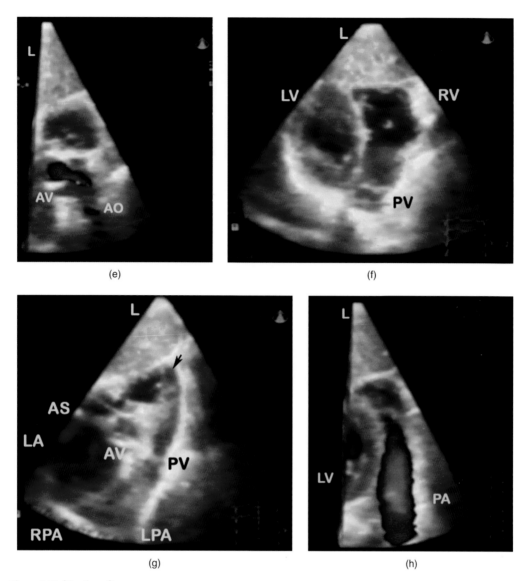

(e)

(f)

(g)

(h)

Figure 3.24 (*Continued*)

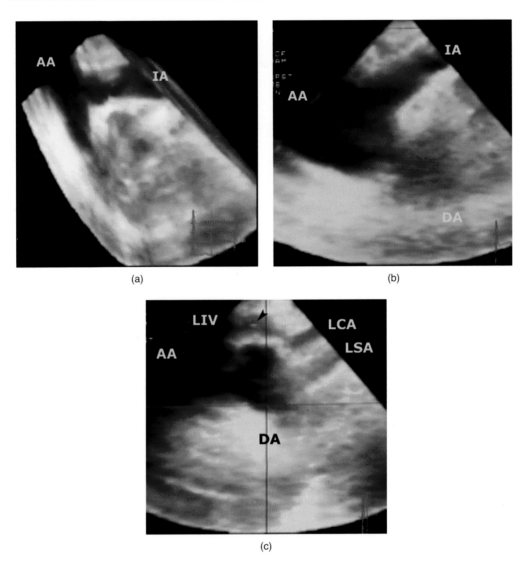

(a)

(b)

(c)

Figure 3.25 Live 3D suprasternal echocardiographic examination. (a, b) Demonstrate a long segment of innominate artery (IA). (c) The arrowhead points to a venous valve in left innominate vein (LIV). Left common carotid artery (LCA), left subclavian artery (LSA), and descending thoracic aorta (DA) are shown. AA, ascending aorta. (Reproduced from Patel *et al.* [6], with permission.)

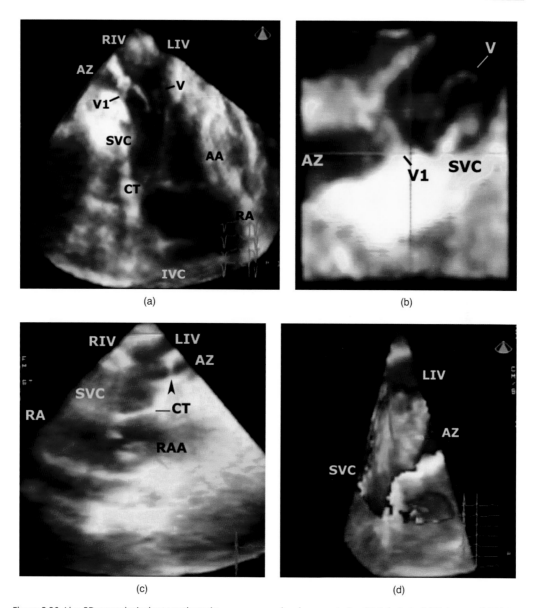

(a)

(b)

(c)

(d)

Figure 3.26 Live 3D supraclavicular transthoracic echocardiographic examination. (a) Foreshortened image demonstrates both right (RIV) and left (LIV) innominate veins joining to form the superior vena cava (SVC), which then enters into right atrium (RA). A venous valve (V) is seen at the entrance of SVC. Another venous valve (V1) is imaged at the junction of azygos vein (AZ) and SVC. IVC is also shown entering RA inferiorly. (b) Entrance of AZ into SVC from the postero-right aspect. (c) Another patient showing AZ entering the SVC from the left instead of from the usual postero-right aspect. The arrowhead points to a venous valve in AZ. (d) Color Doppler examination shows flow signals in the SVC and AZ. (*Continued on next page*)

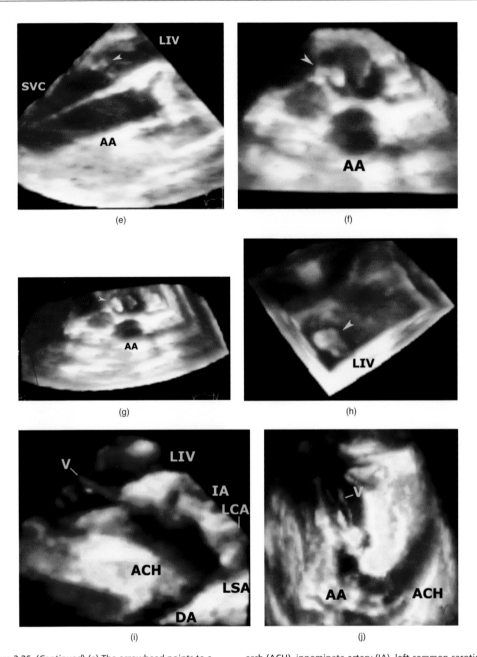

Figure 3.26 (*Continued*) (e) The arrowhead points to a venous valve at the junction of LIV with SVC. (f, g) The arrowhead points to a venous valve at the entrance of SVC. Note thickening of one of the leaflets of the venous valve. (h) The arrowhead points to a closed venous valve in LIV viewed from top. (i) LIV (with a venous valve, V), aortic arch (ACH), innominate artery (IA), left common carotid artery (LCA), left subclavian artery (LSA), and descending thoracic aorta (DA). (j) AA and ACH viewed from below. A venous valve is also imaged. (Reproduced from Patel *et al.* [6], with permission.) Movie clip 3.26.

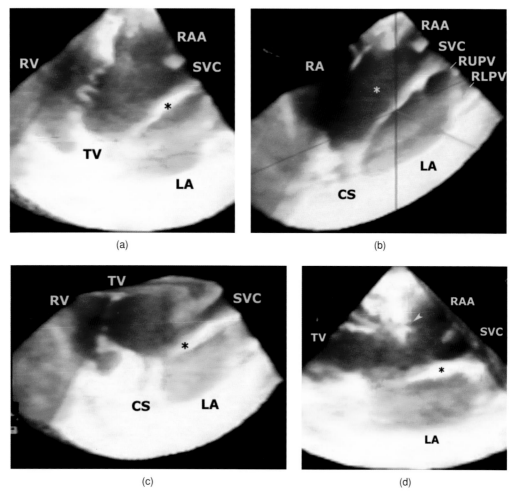

(a)

(b)

(c)

(d)

Figure 3.27 Live 3D right parasternal transthoracic echocardiographic examination of atrial septum and superior and inferior vena cavae. (a) The atrial septum (*), the entrance of superior vena cava (SVC) into the right atrium, the base of the right atrial appendage (RAA), tricuspid valve (TV), and left atrium (LA) are shown. RV, right ventricle. (b) The previous image has been tilted to view the atrial septum (*) *en face* and to more clearly demonstrate the entrance of both right upper (RUPV) and right lower (RLPV) pulmonary veins into LA. (c) The entrance of coronary sinus (CS) into right atrium is shown. A longer segment of SVC is demonstrated. (d) The arrowhead points to the right coronary artery located in the right atrioventricular groove. Movie clips 3.27 A–B, 3.27PQ. (*Continued on next page*)

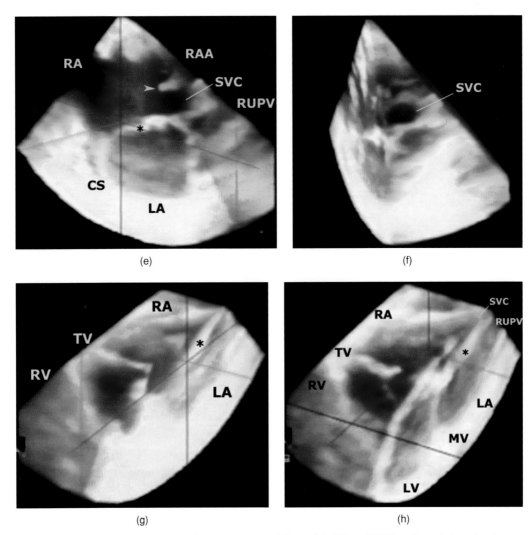

(e)

(f)

(g)

(h)

Figure 3.27 (*Continued*) (e) The arrowhead points to crista terminalis. RA, right atrium. (f) SVC viewed in short axis. (g) RA, RV, and TV viewed from top. (h) Mitral valve (MV), left ventricle (LV), and RUVP are brought into view by further cropping. (*Continued on next page*)

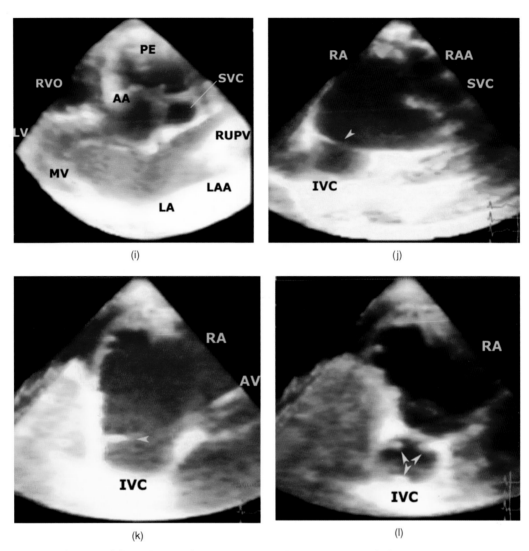

(i)

(j)

(k)

(l)

Figure 3.27 (*Continued*) (i) Another view demonstrating SVC in short axis, long segment of RUPV, LA appendage (LAA), MV, LV, and ascending aorta (AA). PE, pericardial effusion. (j–m) The arrowheads demonstrate Eustachian valve at the entrance of inferior vena cava (IVC) into RA in long-axis (j, k) and short-axis (l, m) views. Aortic valve (AV) is also imaged in (k). (*Continued on next page*)

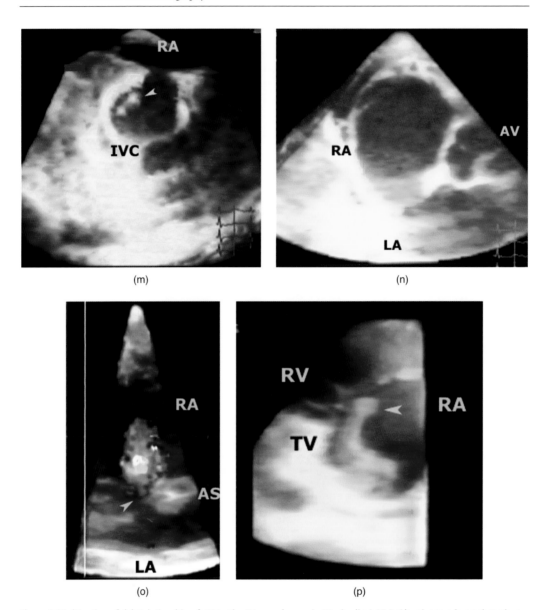

(m)

(n)

(o)

(p)

Figure 3.27 (*Continued*) (n) Relationship of AV to the RA and LA. (o) Color Doppler examination showing flow signals moving into RA through a secundum atrial septal (AS) defect in a different patient. (p, q) The arrowheads (arrow in Movie clip 3.27 P–Q) point to a large thrombus lodged in RA adjacent to atrial septum (*) in another patient. (*Continued on next page*)

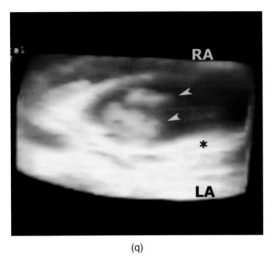

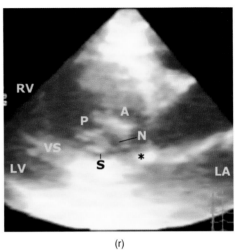

(q)   (r)

Figure 3.27 (*Continued*) (r) A large area of non-coaptation (N) is shown during tricuspid valve closure in systole in a patient with an infected tricuspid valve and torrential tricuspid regurgitation. The anterior leaflet (A) was predominantly involved and appears echogenic. P, posterior or inferior tricuspid leaflet; S, septal tricuspid leaflet; VS, ventricular septum. (Reproduced from Patel *et al.* [6], with permission.)

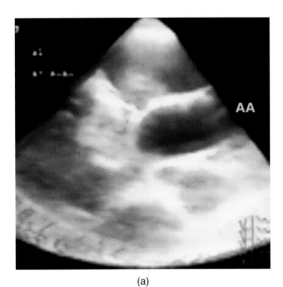

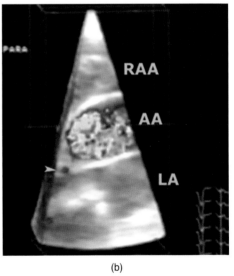

(a)   (b)

Figure 3.28 Live 3D right parasternal transthoracic echocardiographic examination of ascending aorta and right atrial appendage (RAA). (a, b) Normal ascending aorta (AA). The arrowhead in (b) points to left main coronary artery. (c) Enlarged AA. (d–h) RAA and its relationship to superior vena cava (SVC) are demonstrated. The arrowhead in (e) points to contrast signals in RAA, following an intravenous bubble study. A small portion of AA is imaged between RAA and SVC. Color Doppler examination (f) shows flow signals in SVC and RAA. The arrowhead in (g) points to the right coronary artery. AV, atrium; LA, left atrium; PE, pericardial effusion; RPA, right pulmonary artery. RAA is viewed from top in (h). (i) Relationship of RAA to both AA and pulmonary valve (PV) is shown. PA, pulmonary artery. (j) RAA viewed from the back. (k) Relationship of RAA to SVC, AA, and PA. (Reproduced from Patel *et al.* [6], with permission.) Movie clips 3.28 Part 1 and 3.28 Part 2.

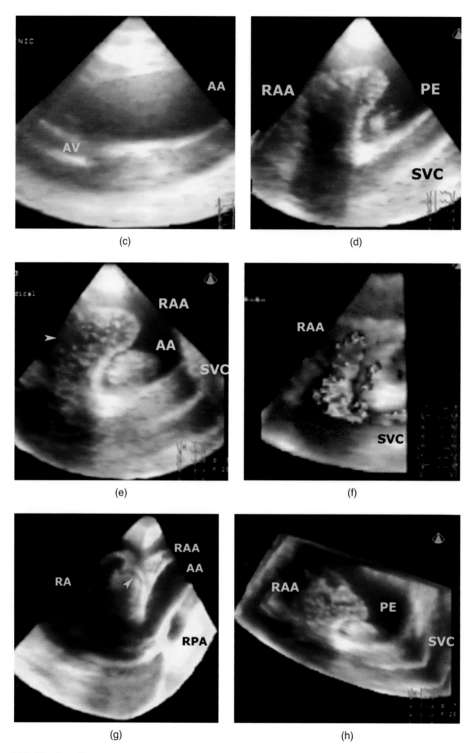

Figure 3.28 (*Continued*)

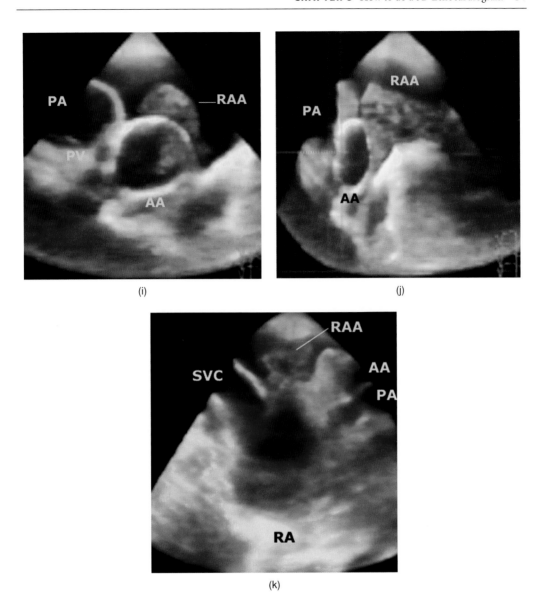

(i)

(j)

(k)

Figure 3.28 (*Continued*)

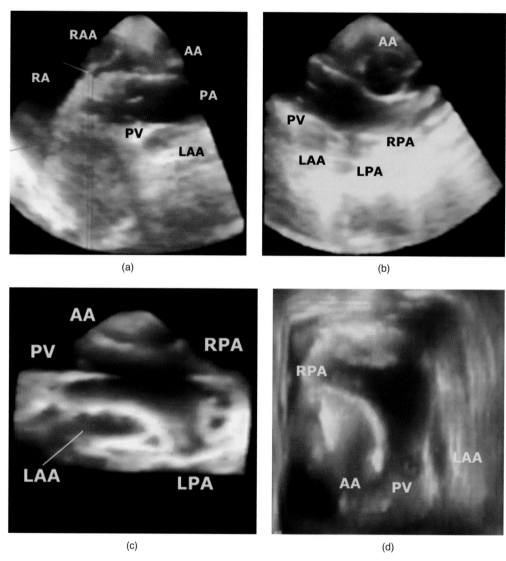

(a)

(b)

(c)

(d)

Figure 3.29 Live 3D right parasternal transthoracic echocardiographic examination of pulmonary valve, main pulmonary artery, pulmonary artery branches, and left atrium. (a–d) Pulmonary valve (PV), main pulmonary artery (PA), proximal right pulmonary artery (RPA), left pulmonary artery (LPA) branches, and left atrium appendage (LAA). (e–g) PA viewed in short-axis adjacent to atrial appendage (AA), mitral valve (MV), left ventricle (LV), left atrium (LA), and left atrium appendage (LAA). Descending thoracic aorta (DA) is also imaged. (Reproduced from Patel et al. [6], with permission.) Movie clip 3.29.

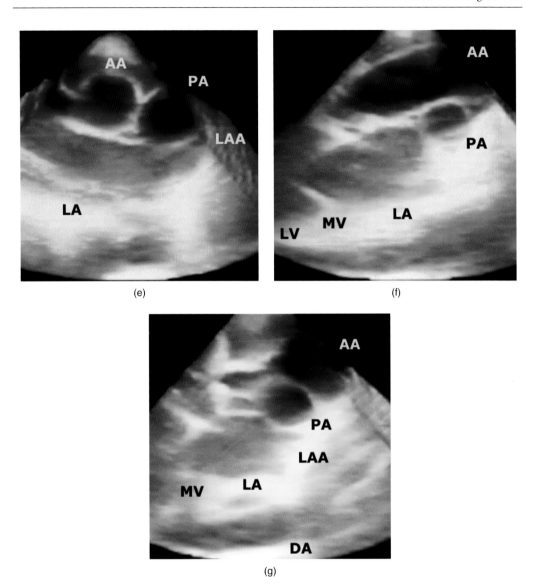

Figure 3.29 (*Continued*)

References

1. Wang XF, Deng YB, Nanda NC, Deng J, Miller AP, Xie MX. Live three-dimensional echocardiography: imaging principles and clinical application. *Echocardiography* 2003; 20:593–604.

2. Nanda NC, Kisslo J, Lang R, *et al.* Examination protocol for three-dimensional echocardiography. *Echocardiography* 2004;21:763–8.

3. Burri MV, Mahan EF, III, Nanda NC, *et al.* Superior vena cava, right pulmonary artery or both: real time two- and three-dimensional transthoracic contrast echocardiographic identification of the echo-free space posterior to the ascending aorta. *Echocardiography* 2007;24:875–82.

4. Marcella CP, Johnson LE. Right parasternal imaging: an underutilized echocardiographic technique. *J Am Soc Echocardiogr* 1993;6:453–66.

5. McDonald RW, Rice MJ, Reller MD, Marcella CP, Sahn DJ. Echocardiographic imaging techniques with subcostal and right parasternal longitudinal views in detecting sinus venous atrial septal defects. *J Am Soc Echocardiogr* 1996;9:195–8.

6. Patel V, Nanda NC, Upendram S, *et al.* Live three-dimensional right parasternal and supraclavicular transthoracic echocardiographic examination. *Echocardiography* 2005;22:349–60.

4

CHAPTER 4

Mitral Valve

Introduction

Evaluation of the mitral valve (MV) requires appreciation of its complex geometry. In vertical space, the mitral annulus takes the shape of a saddle or ski-slope, with the anteroseptal portion being more cephalad [1,2]. In pathologic conditions, this geometry is perturbed; e.g., the annulus flattens when stretched in conditions such as dilated cardiomyopathies [3]. When viewed *en face*, the MV is composed of an anterior leaflet that can be artificially divided into three segments (A1, A2, and A3 = anterolateral, middle, and posteromedial segments of the anterior mitral leaflet) and a posterior leaflet composed of three scallops (P1, P2, and P3 = anterolateral, middle, and posteromedial scallops of the posterior mitral leaflet) [4]. In order to accurately guide surgical interventions and describe pathology, familiarity with this nomenclature and orientation of the valve in 3D space is necessary. For this reason, 3D transthoracic echocardiography (3DTTE) is an immense improvement over the cumbersome mental reconstruction required by 2DTTE or 2D transesophageal echocardiography (2DTEE).

In the common clinical conditions of mitral stenosis (MS), regurgitation, and prolapse, 3D imaging of the MV *en face* or parallel to its orifice, with orientation in vertical space, significantly improves diagnostic accuracy and permits quantification of these lesions. This chapter reviews quantitative 3DTTE techniques for assessing (1) MS, (2) mitral regurgitation (MR), and (3) MV prolapse, in comparison to other time-honored techniques.

Live/Real Time 3D Echocardiography, 1st edition.
By Navin C. Nanda, Ming Chon Hsiung, Andrew P. Miller, and Fadi G. Hage. Published 2010 by Blackwell Publishing Ltd.

Mitral stenosis

Conventional Doppler and 2DTTE are routinely employed to evaluate severity of MS and to characterize valve anatomy as potentially suitable for balloon valvuloplasty. Doppler assessment using the pressure half-time method is an indirect measure fraught with inaccuracies, even in the best hands [5–7]. The most robust 2D measurement is planimetry of the mitral orifice at the level of the tips of the leaflets. This technique does suffer pitfalls though, such as an oblique, and not parallel-oriented, short-axis plane may provide an inaccurate estimate of orifice area. 3DTTE offers incremental value in this assessment because of its ability to orient imaging planes exactly parallel to the MV orifice at the leaflet tips to precisely determine the flow-limiting orifice [8]. Further analysis of a full pyramidal dataset containing the MV and its subvalvular apparatus affords a comprehensive assessment that can guide decisions for interventions.

In the first report by Singh *et al.*, we reported our early experience in six individuals with severe MS [8]. Using a Philips Sonos 7500 (Philips Medical Systems, Inc., Andover, MA) ultrasound system equipped with a 4 matrix transducer, grayscale and color Doppler flow full-volume 3D images were acquired from the apical and left parasternal positions. Systematic cropping using the X, Y, and Z cutting planes was performed to orient a short-axis image at the tips of the mitral leaflets. This image was analyzed offline using a Tom Tec Cardio view-RT (TomTec, Inc., Munich, Germany) to calibrate and planimeter mitral orifice area. Currently, these measurements are accomplished much quicker using the online QLAB software package. Since the plane of imaging can be positioned exactly perpendicular to the mitral orifice, we were able to obtain an accurate estimation of the orifice area at the flow-limiting tip of the funnel-shaped MV in these patients. In addition, since the chordal apparatus and the papillary muscles can be viewed in 3D imaging, we were able to estimate chordal and papillary muscle shortening as well as chordal fusion and matting, and therefore evaluate for the presence and severity of chordal stenosis. This report demonstrated other advantages of 3DTTE, including evaluation of the subvalvular apparatus for calcification and pliability, thin slice imaging, and assessment of the left atrial appendage. This latter observation supported an important role for 3DTTE, since systematic cropping of the left atrial appendage and left atrium ruled out thrombus in all patients with MS in this study, a finding that was confirmed by transesophageal or intracardiac echocardiography. We have expanded this effort in our laboratory and have found that cropping of the 3D dataset in patients with acceptable images is capable of evaluating fully the left atrial appendage lobes for the presence of thrombi, and can thus obviate a TEE exam in many patients, an observation that is supported by others [9].

In addition, four patients underwent percutaneous balloon valvotomy in this series. Due to changes in loading conditions, Doppler measures of MS are particularly misleading in this situation [10]. Direct planimetry with 3DTTE in this early report agreed closely with catheter measures after valvotomy (Table 4.1) [8]. Further, color flow volumes demonstrated leaflet noncoaptation and significant MR after valvotomy in one patient.

Later reports have confirmed our experience in other centers [11–13]. Zamorano et al. evaluated 80 patients with rheumatic MS with 3DTTE planimetry [11]. Compared with the invasively determined MV area, 3DTTE had better agreement than all other echo-Doppler methods. In a separate report, Zamorano et al. compared invasively determined MV areas in pre- and post percutaneous mitral valvotomy with 2D and 3DTTE methods [12]. In the 29 patients studied, 3DTTE planimetry outperformed 2DTTE techniques in the pre- and immediate postvalvotomy periods. In addition, Sugeng et al. evaluated 11 patients with MS in a case series [13]. They were able to adequately measure mitral orifice area in nine of these, and similarly assessed the adequacy of balloon valvotomy. They found that in 150 consecutive 3DTTE exams, the mitral orifice was well seen in 69% of all patients studied. This report highlights the remaining challenge of measuring mitral orifice area in patients with difficult acoustic windows (Figures 4.1–4.7).

Mitral regurgitation

Accurate grading of MR severity using qualitative and quantitative color Doppler 2DTTE techniques has been challenging [14]. The most commonly employed measure is the ratio of the regurgitant jet area to left atrial area (RJA/LAA), but this is really a semiquantitative or qualitative technique. Techniques utilizing volumetric approaches or the proximal flow convergence do provide quantitative assessment, but are limited by being time-consuming and involve calculations based on assumptions that introduce inaccuracies [15,16]. Measurement of vena contracta width (VCW) by 2DTTE has been validated against regurgitant fraction and angiography [17,18]; however, grading criteria assume a circular or elliptical shape that may not represent the true geometric appearance of the vena contracta [19]. For these reasons, we evaluated 3DTTE measurements of vena contracta area (VCA), with comparisons to 2DTTE measures of RJA/LAA and VCW and to angiographic grading by left ventriculography [20].

Using a Philips Sonos 7500 (Philips Medical Systems, Inc., Andover, MA) ultrasound system equipped with a 4 matrix transducer, B-mode and color Doppler 3D datasets were acquired from the apical and parasternal long-axis views. Color Doppler gain was set at 70% and the Nyquist limit was set between 43 and 69 cm/s, since VCA measurements remained relatively constant in this range. Most cropping was performed from the apical views. First, the best vena contracta image was obtained in long axis by anterior-to-posterior cropping. Second, by cropping from the top of the dataset, an imaging plane was placed at the level of the vena contracta, at or just below the MV leaflet tips in a plane that was parallel to the orifice. The image was then rotated to view the vena contracta en face, and the previously cropped anterior portion was added back to obtain the maximum VCA. This procedure was recorded in its entirety on a VHS tape. Measurements of VCA were obtained by:

Table 4.1 Clinical, echocardiographic, and cardiac catheterization findings.

Case no.	Clinical presentation	2DTTE MVA by planimetry	2DTTE MVA by PHT method	Live 3DTTE MVA by planimetry	Cath. MVA	Outcome
1. 46-year-old female	DOE, previous valvotomy in 1994	1.2 cm^2	1.2 cm^2	1.0 cm^2	Not done	Not yet scheduled for valvotomy
2. 34-year-old female	DOE, pulmonary edema after delivery	Pre = 0.9 cm^2 Post = 1.4 cm^2 Δ = 0.5 cm^2	Pre = 1.15 cm^2 Post = Not done	Pre = 0.9 cm^2 Post =1.6 cm^2 Δ = 0.7 cm^2	Pre = 0.6 cm^2 Post = 1.3 cm^2 Δ = 0.7 cm^2	Mild MR increased from mild to moderate
3. 32-year-old female	DOE, palpitations	Pre = 0.5 cm^2 Post = 1.2 cm^2 Δ = 0.7 cm^2	Pre = 0.9 cm^2 Post = 1.1 cm^2 Δ = 0.3 cm^2	Pre = 0.6 cm^2 Post = 1.3 cm^2 Δ = 0.7 cm^2	Pre = 0.7 cm^2 Post = 1.5 cm^2 Δ = 0.8 cm^2	No change in mild-to-moderate MR
4. 62-year-old female	DOE	Not done due to suboptimal images	Pre = 1.65 cm^2 Post = 1.5 cm^2 Δ = −0.15 cm^2	Pre = 0.9 cm^2 Post = 3.3 cm^2 Δ = 2.4 cm^2	Pre = 1.26 cm^2 Post = 3.5 cm^2 Δ = 2.24 cm^2	Increase in MR severity from mild to moderate
5. 46-year-old female	DOE, previous valvotomy in 1992	Pre = 0.6 cm^2 Post = 1.2 cm^2	Pre = 1.09 cm^2 Post = 1.6 cm^2	Pre = Not done Post = 1.2 cm^2	Pre = 0.7 cm^2 Post = 1.3 cm^2	Trivial MR increased from mild to moderate
6. 47-year-old female	DOE, orthopnea	0.9 cm^2	2 cm^2	0.7 cm^2	1.2 cm^2	Severe MS by surgeon, mitral valve replacement

Cath, cardiac catheterization; DOE, dyspnea on exertion; MR, mitral regurgitation; MS, mitral stenosis; MVA, mitral valve area; PHT, pressure half-time method; Pre, before valvotomy; Post, after valvotomy; 2DTTE, 2D transthoracic echocardiography; 3DTTE, 3D transthoracic echocardiography; Δ, change in mitral valve area.
Reproduced from Singh et al. [8], with permission.

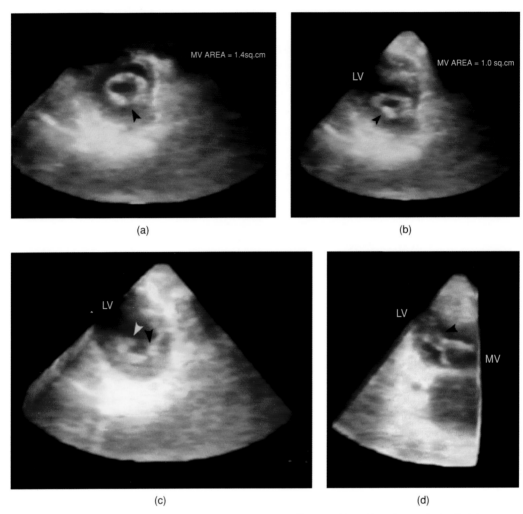

(a)

(b)

(c)

(d)

Figure 4.1 Live/real time 3D transthoracic echocardiography in mitral stenosis. (a) Section taken at the base of the mitral valve showing a large mitral orifice (arrowhead) measuring 1.4 cm^2 in area. (b) Section taken at the tip of the mitral valve demonstrating the flow-limiting mitral orifice (arrowhead), which measured 1.0 cm^2 in area. (c) Section taken at the level of the papillary muscles (arrowheads). All three sections could be taken perpendicular to the mitral orifice. (d) Chordal thickening (arrowhead) viewed in long axis. LV, left ventricle; MV, mitral valve. (Reproduced from Singh *et al.* [8], with permission.)

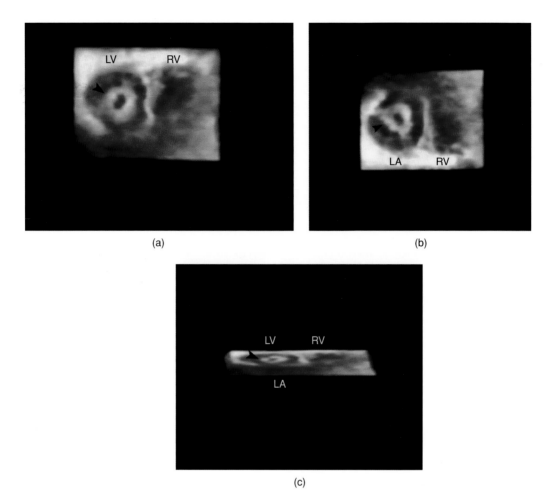

(a)   (b)

(c)

Figure 4.2 Live/real time 3D transthoracic echocardiography in mitral stenosis. By flipping a thin slice taken at the tip of the mitral valve, the mitral orifice (arrowhead) can be viewed in short axis from both the ventricular (a) and atrial (b) sides. (c) Shows the slice being flipped. LA, left atrium; LV, left ventricle; RV, right ventricle. (Reproduced from Singh *et al.* [8], with permission.)

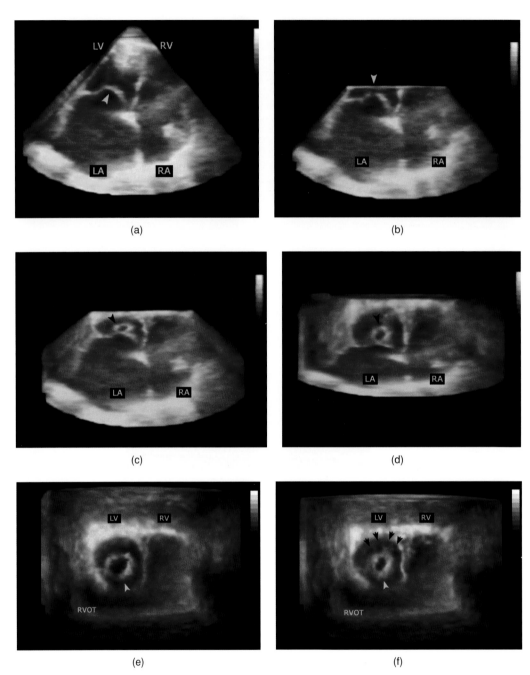

(a)

(b)

(c)

(d)

(e)

(f)

Figure 4.3 Live/real time 3D transthoracic echocardiography in mitral stenosis. (a–d) A useful and easy technique is to crop an apical four-chamber section at the tip of the mitral valve and tilt or rotate the image toward the examiner to view the flow-limiting mitral orifice (arrowhead) in short axis. (e) Section taken at the base of the mitral valve (using apical four-chamber view) shows a much larger orifice. (f) Demonstrates subvalvular chordal stenosis. The arrows point to multiple small openings produced by chordal fusion. The cumulative area of the openings measured 0.5 cm^2, indicative of severe chordal stenosis. Movie clip 4.3 is from another patient with severe mitral stenosis. The apical four-chamber dataset was cropped to view the mitral valve *en face*. The mitral leaflets are thickened and the orifice is small, but there is no evidence of commissural calcification. For a description of the tricuspid valve seen in this clip, see movie clip and legend 6.2A, Part 2. LA, left atrium; LV, left ventricle; RA, right atrium; RV, right ventricle; RVOT, right ventricular outflow tract. (Reproduced from Singh *et al.* [8], with permission.)

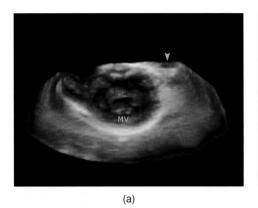 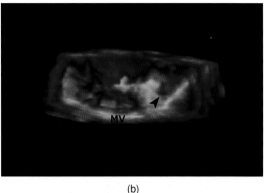

(a) (b)

Figure 4.4 Live/real time 3D transthoracic echocardiography in mitral stenosis. (a, b) In addition to conventional aortic short-axis and apical views, the left atrial appendage can be assessed by cropping a short-axis section of the mitral valve from the top, and tilting the image toward the examiner. The left atrial appendage (arrowhead) shows no evidence of clot in this patient. MV, mitral valve. (Reproduced from Singh *et al.* [8], with permission.)

(1) direct video planimetry (using the VCR function on the ultrasound system to play back the recorded cropping, the depth markers viewable in the initial image were used for calibration, and then the VCA was traced), and (2) offline computer analysis (using a Tom Tec Cardio view-RT, TomTec, Inc., Munich, Germany). Our subsequent experience with the QLAB software suggests that measurements with this software package may slightly underestimate those performed in our original publication.

Using this technique, we assessed MR by measurements of VCA with 3DTTE and other standard 2DTTE measurements in 44 patients who underwent left ventriculography [20]. Results revealed close agreement for 3DTTE VCA measurements and angiographic grading, with discernment between angiographic grades using the following diagnostic criteria: <0.2 cm^2 for mild (grade I), 0.2–0.4 cm^2 for moderate (grade II), and >0.4 cm^2 for severe (grade III) MR. Direct video planimetry and offline computer analysis agreed well, and inter- and intra-observer variability was low (sum of residuals, $r^2 = 0.99$ and 0.97, respectively) for this parameter. 3DTTE measurements of VCA performed better against the angiographic standard than did the traditional 2DTTE measurements of RJA/LAA, RJA, VCW, and calculated VCA. We have found this technique robust as a clinical tool for diagnosing and following patients with MR, since

3DTTE VCA offers a quantifiable indirect measure of the "hole" in the MV that is not considered load-dependent.

In addition to quantifying MR, the 3DTTE dataset is useful in assessing anatomy responsible for valvular insufficiency. Leaflet geometry can be assessed with available software packages, and may be useful in surgical decision-making [21,22]. Chordae rupture and flail leaflets can be seen, improving diagnostic confidence in patients with acute MR and often obviating the need for a TEE exam. In addition, we have found 3DTTE particularly useful in evaluating patients with endocarditis. *En face* views permit correct characterization of valvular perforations, and systematic cropping is useful in excluding abscess formation. The 3D dataset can be cropped to accurately describe and measure vegetations. The presence and extent of vegetations can be clearly visualized with 3DTTE and, when the leaflets are imaged *en face*, perforations can be seen and their area measured. The assessment of vegetation volume in this way is a more accurate representation of the burden of endocarditis rather than measurements of dimensions, and since the size of vegetations has been shown in previous studies to be a strong prognostic indicator in patients with infective endocarditis, this information may be prognostically valuable [23–25]. Since the 3D dataset contains the entire MV apparatus, comprehensive evaluation

62   Live/Real Time 3D Echocardiography

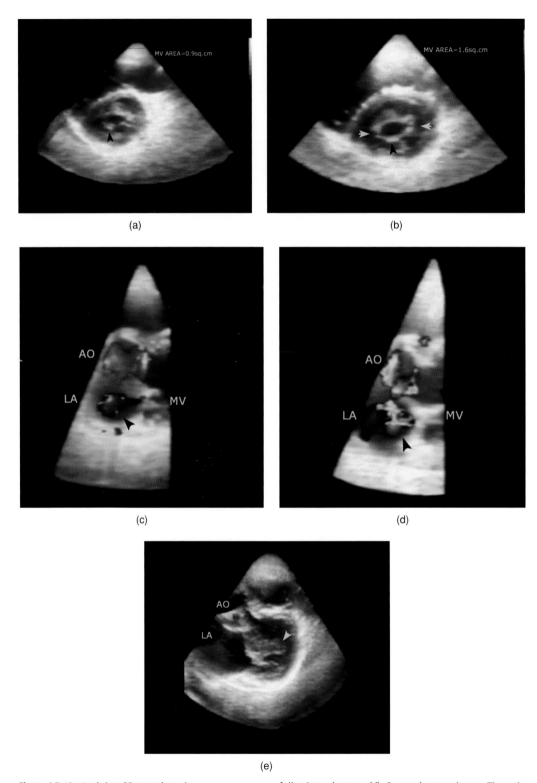

Figure 4.5 Live/real time 3D transthoracic echocardiography in mitral stenosis. (a) The arrowhead points to a severely stenotic mitral valve with an orifice area of 0.9 cm². (b) Postvalvotomy, the area of the mitral orifice (arrowhead) increased to 1.6 cm². The arrows show the valvotomy. (c) 3D color Doppler flow imaging. Note the increase in mitral regurgitation (arrowhead) severity following valvotomy (d). C, prevalvotomy image. The ratio of volume of mitral regurgitation color Doppler signals to the left atrial volume increased from 0.2 prevalvotomy to 0.3 postvalvotomy. (e) Prevalvotomy long-axis view rotated to show the entire surface of the anterior mitral leaflet (arrowhead). AO, aorta; LA, left atrium; MV, mitral valve. (Reproduced from Singh *et al.* [8], with permission.)

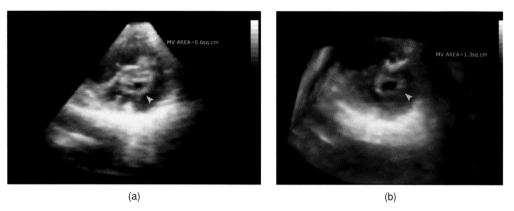

(a)   (b)

Figure 4.6 Live/real time 3D transthoracic echocardiography in mitral stenosis. (a) The arrowhead points to severe mitral stenosis with an orifice area of 0.6 cm². (b) Postvalvotomy, the orifice area increased to 1.3 cm²; MV, mitral valve. (Reproduced from Singh *et al.* [8], with permission.)

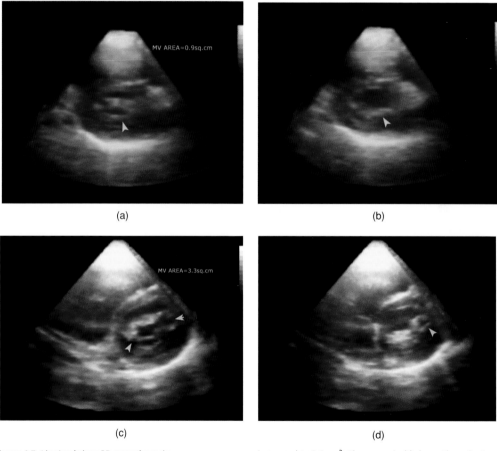

(a)   (b)

(c)   (d)

Figure 4.7 Live/real time 3D transthoracic echocardiography in mitral stenosis. (a) The arrowhead points to severe mitral stenosis with an orifice area measuring 0.9 cm². (b) Systolic frame showing full coaptation of the mitral leaflets (arrowhead). (c, d) Postvalvotomy, the area of the mitral orifice (arrowhead) increased to 3.3 cm². The arrow in (c) shows the valvotomy. However, in systole (d), a large area of leaflet noncoaptation (arrowhead) is noted laterally consistent with development of significant mitral regurgitation. MV, mitral valve. (Reproduced from Singh *et al.* [8], with permission.)

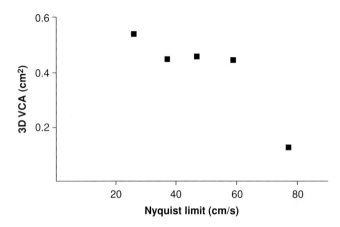

Figure 4.8 Mitral regurgitation vena contracta area by live 3D color Doppler transthoracic echocardiography (3D VCA) measured at different Nyquist limits in a patient with mitral regurgitation. Note marked changes in 3D VCA size at the lowest and the highest Nyquist limits. (Reproduced from Khanna et al. [20], with permission.)

with 3DTTE is possible in a time-efficient manner (Figures 4.8–4.15).

Mitral valve prolapse

Since MV repair is always preferable to replacement for mitral valve prolapse (MVP) [26–28], preoperative evaluation of the MV for suitability for repair and precise identification of the prolapsing segment/scallop is necessary [29]. 2DTTE and 2DTEE have been primarily used to delineate and localize MVP, as well as evaluate chordae integrity, the subvalvular apparatus, annular calcification, and left ventricular size and function. Determining which segment/scallop is prolapsing is difficult by 2D echocardiography, however, and we and others have found utility in 3D assessment [4,13,30–38].

We evaluated 34 patients in whom surgical intervention was undertaken for severe mitral insufficiency due to MVP [30]. Parasternal and apically acquired 3D datasets were analyzed using the QLAB 4.1 software package. By cropping from the left atrial side to just above the mitral annulus, a short-axis view was obtained. Individual prolapsing parts of segments or scallops were identified by their increased echogenicity from this view. To view all parts of the saddle-shaped MV, two or three oblique planes were used. This procedure was performed using the apically acquired dataset and the dataset from the parasternal window. Segments/scallops were identified based on their anterior (closer to the aorta) or posterior (deeper in the left atrium) and medial (closer to the ventricular septum),

middle, or lateral positions as: A3 and P3, A2 and P2, A1 and P1 for posteromedial, middle, and anterolateral segments/scallops of the MV, respectively. In this report, we accurately determined MVP location when compared with surgical findings with 95% sensitivity and 87% specificity, and with low inter- and intra-observer variability. We now routinely perform 3DTTE exams on all patients the day before surgery to help guide, and hopefully improve the likelihood of, MV repair (Figures 4.16 and 4.17 and Tables 4.2 and 4.3).

Summary

Taken together, assessment of MR may play the leading role in the current echocardiography lab as an indication for a 3DTTE exam. In this role, 3DTTE offers incremental value over 2D techniques by providing a quantifiable measure of MR for accurate diagnostic grading and for reproducible longitudinal follow-up. In addition, the ability to prospectively locate and quantify pathological changes provides guidance for surgical interventions, making preferable valve repair more likely. Assessment of MS is, likewise, robust by 3DTTE techniques, permitting confident measurements of the true flow-limiting orifice. Since these direct measurements of valve area and insufficiency are load independent, time-efficient, and do not involve calculations based on assumptions, 3DTTE assessment of the MV is an important addition to the echocardiography armamentarium.

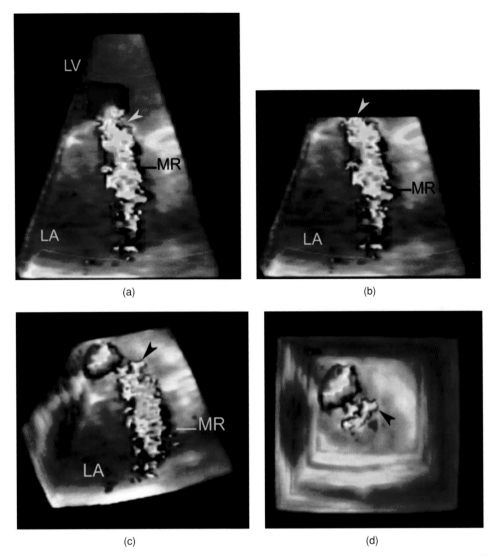

(a)

(b)

(c)

(d)

Figure 4.9 Live/real time 3D color Doppler transthoracic echocardiographic technique for assessment of vena contracta area. 3D color Doppler dataset showing mitral regurgitation (MR, a) is cropped from top to the level of the vena contracta (arrowhead, b) and tilted to view it *en face* (c, d). The vena contracta is then planimetered by copying onto a videotape. The vena contracta may also be planimetered using the QLAB. Movie clip 4.9, from another patient, shows cropping of the apical four-chamber dataset using an oblique plane to align it parallel to the flow-limiting tips of the mitral leaflets. The posterior leaflet is calcified at the tip and shows restricted mobility. *En face* view shows an oval-shaped stenotic orifice (arrow) with calcification involving only the posterior leaflet. The commissures are free of calcification. This patient also had significant MR on the 2D study, and hence another apical four-chamber dataset was acquired using color Doppler flow imaging. This was cropped to view the MR vena contracta *en face* (arrow). The blue laminar signals adjacent to the vena contracta represent flow in the left ventricular outflow tract. LA, left atrium; LV, left ventricle. (Reproduced from Khanna *et al.* [20], with permission.)

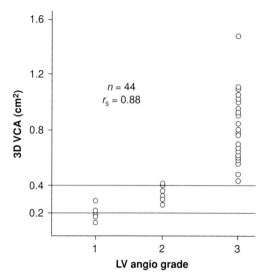

Figure 4.10 Mitral regurgitation vena contracta area by live/real time 3D color Doppler transthoracic echocardiography (3D VCA) correlated with left ventricular angiographic (LV angio) assessment. (Reproduced from Khanna *et al.* [20], with permission.)

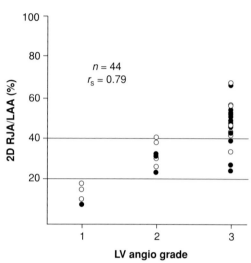

Figure 4.12 2D color Doppler transthoracic echocardiographic ratio of mitral regurgitation jet area (RJA) to left atrial area (LAA) correlated with left ventricular angiographic (LV angio) assessment. Open circles represent patients with central mitral regurgitation jets and closed circles eccentric jets. (Reproduced from Khanna *et al.* [20], with permission.)

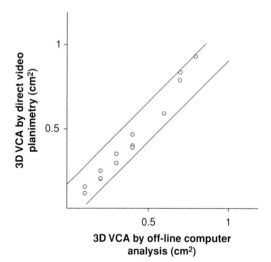

Figure 4.11 Mitral regurgitation vena contracta area by live/real time 3D color Doppler transthoracic echocardiography (3D VCA) measured by direct video planimetry correlated with offline TomTec computer measurements. 95% confidence limits are as shown. (Reproduced from Khanna *et al.* [20], with permission.)

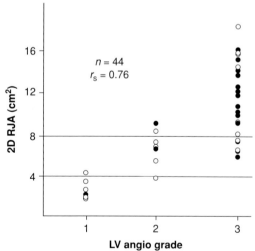

Figure 4.13 2D color Doppler transthoracic echocardiographic mitral regurgitation area (RJA) correlated with left ventricular angiographic (LV angio) assessment. Open circles represent patients with central mitral regurgitation jets and closed circles eccentric jets. (Reproduced from Khanna *et al.* [20], with permission.)

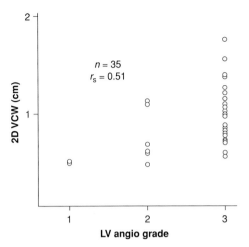

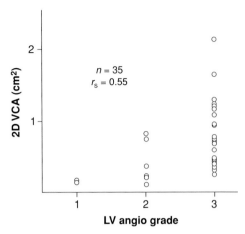

Figure 4.14 2D color Doppler transthoracic echocardiographic mitral regurgitation vena contracta width (2D VCW) correlated with left ventricular angiographic (LV angio) assessment. (Reproduced from Khanna *et al.* [20], with permission.)

Figure 4.15 2D color Doppler transthoracic echocardiographic mitral regurgitation vena contracta area (2D VCA) correlated with left ventricular angiographic (LV angio) assessment. (Reproduced from Khanna *et al.* [20], with permission.)

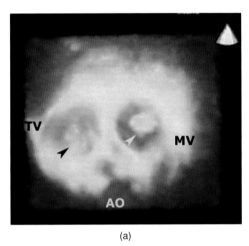

(a)

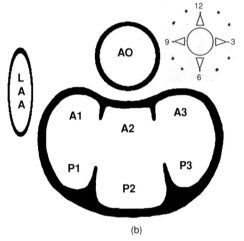

(b)

Figure 4.16 Live/real time 3D transthoracic echocardiography in the assessment of mitral valve prolapse. (a) Apically acquired four-chamber dataset was cropped from bottom to the level of mitral valve and tilted to view both mitral (MV) and tricuspid (TV) valves *en face*. Yellow arrowhead shows prominent and echogenic prolapse of P2 scallop. Black arrowhead points to prolapse of the middle segment of septal TV leaflet. AO, aorta. (b) Schematic diagram of the segmental classification used to describe MVP, as viewed by the surgeon. A1, A2, and A3, anterolateral, middle, and posteromedial segments of anterior MV leaflet; AO, aorta; LAA, left atrial appendage; P1, P2, and P3, anterolateral, middle, and posteromedial scallops of posterior MV leaflet. Movie clips 4.16A Part 1–4, from another patient, show cropping of the apical four-chamber dataset from the bottom (atrial aspect) to view the MV (arrowhead) *en face*. Prominent echogenic bulging of A2 and A3 segments and P2 and P3 scallops are noted. Movie clip 4.16 B, from a different patient, begins with a 2D study showing prolapse of both mitral leaflets. The arrow points to a clear left atrial appendage which is well visualized in the apical two-chamber view. This is followed by 3D apical acquisition which also shows prolapse of both MV leaflets (arrow). Cropping of the dataset from bottom shows prominent prolapse of A1, A2, and A3 segments and P2 scallop. Prolapse of A2 and P2 is more extensive than A1 and A3. Subsequently, the apical dataset was cropped from the side to identify sites of chordae rupture (arrows). Finally, the dataset was cropped from the top (ventricular aspect) to view the MV and chordae *en face*. Movie clips 4.16A Parts 1–4: Reproduced from Patel *et al.* [30], with permission. Movie clip 4.16B: Reproduced from Ahmed *et al.* [4], with permission.

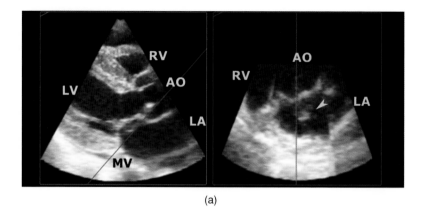

(a)

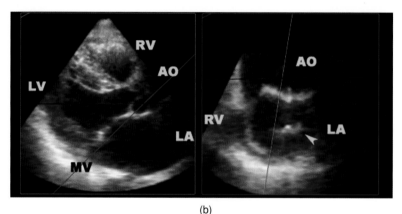

(b)

Figure 4.17 Live/real time 3D transthoracic echocardiography in the assessment of mitral valve prolapse using parasternally acquired datasets and an offline QLAB 4.1 software. (a, b) The cropping plane (red) was placed at the level of mitral valve (MV) annulus in parasternal long-axis view (left panels in (a) and (b)) and the prolapsing segment identified in the corresponding short-axis view (right panels in (a) and (b)). The position of aorta (AO) and the right ventricle (RV) was used for anatomical orientation. Anterior MV leaflet prolapse will appear in the left atrium anteriorly (adjacent to aorta) while posterior leaflet prolapse will be located more posteriorly. Depending on whether prolapsing MV leaflet tissue is located medially toward the ventricular septum, in the middle, or laterally, posteromedial (A3/P3), middle (A2/P2), and anterolateral (A1/P1) segment/scallop prolapse can be identified. The arrowheads (arrows in the movie clips) show A2 prolapse in (a) and P2 prolapse in (b). Movie clip 4.17 C. MV vegetation. The arrowhead points to

a 1.8   0.4 cm vegetation on the MV on the 2D transesophageal study done on February 27, 2007. A follow-up transesophageal study done on March 13, 2007, showed increase in the size of vegetation to 1.8   0.9 cm as well as a new second vegetation measuring 1.4   0.5 cm. A standard 2D transthoracic examination on the same day shows the vegetations to be smaller than the transesophageal study (1.7   0.7 cm and 1.0   0.5 cm). Live/real time 3D transthoracic study performed on the same patient on both days permitted assessment of the volumes of vegetations, which increased from 1.7 to 3.2 mL. Assessment of volumes of vegetations by the 3D technique would be expected to be more reliable than measurement of dimensions by 2D transthoracic or transesophageal examination. LA, left atrium; LV, left ventricle. (Reproduced from Patel *et al.* [30], with permission.) Movie clips 4.17 A (Left), 4.17 A (Right), 4.17 B (Left), 4.17 B (Right), 4.17 C.

Table 4.2 Live/real time 3D transthoracic assessment of MV scallop/segment prolapse using QLAB.

Surgical findings (34 patients)	3D Echocardiographic findings (34 patients)
A1, A2 (4 pts)	A1, A2 (1 pt)
	A2, A3 (1 pt)
	A2, P2 (1 pt)
	A1, A2, P2 (1 pt)
A1, A2, A3 (1 pt)	A2, A3, mild P3 (1 pt)
A1, A2, A3, P1, P2, P3 (2 pts)	A1, A2, A3, P1, P2, P3 (2 pts)
A1, P2 (1 pt)	A1, mild A2, P2 (1 pt)
A2 (3 pts)	A2 (2 pts)
	A2, mild A3 (1 pt)
A2, A3 (2 pts)	A2, A3 (2 pts)
A2, P2 (3 pts)	A2, P2 (1 pt)
	A2, mild A3, P2, mild P3 (1 pt)
	A2, mild A3, P2 (1 pt)
A3 (1 pt)	A3 (1 pt)
P1, P2 (2 pts)	Mild A2, P1, P2 (1 pt)
	P1, P2, mild P3 (1 pt)
P2, P3 (1 pt)	Mild A2, P2, P3 (1 pt)
P2 (11 pts)	P2 (7 pts)
	P2, mild P3 (1 pt)
	Mild A2, mild A3, P2 (1 pt)
	Mild A2, P2 (1 pt)
	Mild P1, P2 (1 pt)
P3 (2 pts)	P3 (1 pt)
	Mild P2, P3 (1 pt)
A2, P2, P3 (1 pt)	A2, P2, P3 (1 pt)

A1, A2, and A3, anterolateral, middle, and posteromedial segments of anterior mitral valve leaflet; P1, P2, and P3, anterolateral, middle, and posteromedial scallops of posterior mitral valve leaflet; pt(s), patient(s).
Reproduced from Patel *et al.* [30], with permission.

Table 4.3 Live/real time 3D transthoracic assessment of MV scallop/segment prolapse without using QLAB.

Surgical findings (23 patients)	3D Echocardiographic findings (23 patients)
A1, A2 (4 pts)	A1, A2 (4 pts)
A1, P2 (1 pt)	P2 (1 pt)
A2 (2 pts)	A2 (2 pts)
A3 (1 pt)	A3 (1 pt)
A2, A3 (2 pts)	A2, A3 (2 pts)
A2, P2 (2 pts)	A2, P2 (1 pt)
	A2, P2, mild A3 (1 pt)
P1, P2 (1 pt)	A2, A3, P2 (1 pt)
P2 (7 pts)	P2 (4 pts)
	Mild A2, P2 (2 pts)
	Mild A3, P2 (1 pt)
P3 (2 pts)	P3 (1 pt)
	Mild P2, P3 (1 pt)
A2, P2, P3 (1 pt)	Mild A1, mild P1, P2, P3 (1 pt)

A1, A2, and A3, anterolateral, middle, and posteromedial segments of anterior mitral valve leaflet; P1, P2, and P3, anterolateral, middle, and posteromedial scallops of posterior mitral valve leaflet; pt(s), patient(s).
Reproduced from Patel *et al.* [30], with permission.

References

1. Pai RG, Tanimoto M, Jintapakorn W, Azevedo J, Pandian NG, Shah PM. Volume-rendered three-dimensional dynamic anatomy of the mitral annulus using a transesophageal echocardiographic technique. *J Heart Valve Dis* 1995;4(6):623–7.

2. Flachskampf FA, Chandra S, Gaddipatti A, *et al.* Analysis of shape and motion of the mitral annulus in subjects with and without cardiomyopathy by echocardiographic 3-dimensional reconstruction. *J Am Soc Echocardiogr* 2000;13(4):277–87.

3. Kwan J, Qin JX, Popovic ZB, Agler DA, Thomas JD, Shiota T. Geometric changes of mitral annulus assessed by real-time 3-dimensional echocardiography: becoming enlarged and less nonplanar in the anteroposterior direction during systole in proportion to global left ventricular systolic function. *J Am Soc Echocardiogr* 2004;17(11):1179–84.

4. Ahmed S, Nanda NC, Miller AP, *et al.* Usefulness of transesophageal three-dimensional echocardiography in the identification of individual segment/scallop prolapse of the mitral valve. *Echocardiography.* 2003;20(2):203–9.

5. Karp K, Teien D, Bjerle P, Eriksson P. Reassessment of valve area determinations in mitral stenosis by the pressure half-time method: impact of left ventricular stiffness and peak diastolic pressure difference. *J Am Coll Cardiol* 1989;13(3):594–9.

6. Flachskampf FA, Weyman AE, Gillam L, Liu CM, Abascal VM, Thomas JD. Aortic regurgitation shortens Doppler pressure half-time in mitral stenosis: clinical evidence, in vitro simulation and theoretic analysis. *J Am Coll Cardiol* 1990;16(2):396–404.

7. Wisenbaugh T, Berk M, Essop R, Middlemost S, Sareli P. Effect of mitral regurgitation and volume loading on pressure half-time before and after balloon valvotomy in mitral stenosis. *Am J Cardiol* 1991;67(2):162–8.

8. Singh V, Nanda NC, Agrawal G, *et al.* Live three-dimensional echocardiographic assessment of mitral stenosis. *Echocardiography* 2003;20(8):743–50.

9. Agoston I, Xie T, Tiller FL, Rahman AM, Ahmad M. Assessment of left atrial appendage by live three-dimensional echocardiography: early experience and comparison with transesophageal echocardiography. *Echocardiography* 2006;23(2):127–32.

10. Reid CL, Rahimtoola SH. The role of echocardiography/Doppler in catheter balloon treatment of adults with aortic and mitral stenosis. *Circulation* 1991;84(3, Suppl):I240–249.

11. Zamorano J, Cordeiro P, Sugeng L, *et al.* Real-time three-dimensional echocardiography for rheumatic mitral valve stenosis evaluation: an accurate and novel approach. *J Am Coll Cardiol* 2004;43(11):2091–6.

12. Zamorano J, Perez de Isla L, Sugeng L, *et al.* Non-invasive assessment of mitral valve area during percutaneous balloon mitral valvuloplasty: role of real-time 3D echocardiography. *Eur Heart J* 2004;25(23):2086–91.

13. Sugeng L, Coon P, Weinert L, *et al.* Use of real-time 3-dimensional transthoracic echocardiography in the evaluation of mitral valve disease. *J Am Soc Echocardiogr* 2006;19(4):413–21.

14. Khanna D, Miller AP, Nanda NC, Ahmed S, Lloyd SG. Transthoracic and transesophageal echocardiographic assessment of mitral regurgitation severity: usefulness of qualitative and semiquantitative techniques. *Echocardiography* 2005;22(9):748–69.

15. Grossmann G, Giesler M, Stein M, Kochs M, Hoher M, Hombach V. Quantification of mitral and tricuspid regurgitation by the proximal flow convergence method using two-dimensional color Doppler and color Doppler M-mode: influence of the mechanism of regurgitation. *Int J Cardiol* 1998;66(3):299–307.

16. Enriquez-Sarano M, Bailey KR, Seward JB, Tajik AJ, Krohn MJ, Mays JM. Quantitative Doppler assessment of valvular regurgitation. *Circulation* 1993;87(3):841–8.

17. Fehske W, Omran H, Manz M, Kohler J, Hagendorff A, Luderitz B. Color-coded Doppler imaging of the vena contracta as a basis for quantification of pure mitral regurgitation. *Am J Cardiol* 1994;73(4):268–74.

18. Hall SA, Brickner ME, Willett DL, Irani WN, Afridi I, Grayburn PA. Assessment of mitral regurgitation severity by Doppler color flow mapping of the vena contracta. *Circulation* 1997;95(3):636–42.

19. Velayudhan DE, Brown TM, Nanda NC, *et al.* Quantification of tricuspid regurgitation by live three-dimensional transthoracic echocardiographic measurements of vena contracta area. *Echocardiography* 2006;23(9):793–800.

20. Khanna D, Vengala S, Miller AP, *et al.* Quantification of mitral regurgitation by live three-dimensional transthoracic echocardiographic measurements of vena contracta area. *Echocardiography* 2004;21(8):737–43.

21. Watanabe N, Ogasawara Y, Yamaura Y, *et al.* Geometric differences of the mitral valve tenting between anterior and inferior myocardial infarction with significant ischemic mitral regurgitation: quantitation by novel software system with transthoracic real-time three-dimensional echocardiography. *J Am Soc Echocardiogr* 2006;19(1):71–5.

22. Watanabe N, Ogasawara Y, Yamaura Y, *et al.* Quantitation of mitral valve tenting in ischemic mitral regurgitation by transthoracic real-time three-dimensional

echocardiography. *J Am Coll Cardiol* 2005;45(5): 763–9.

23. Vilacosta I, Graupner C, San Roman JA, *et al*. Risk of embolization after institution of antibiotic therapy for infective endocarditis. *J Am Coll Cardiol* 2002;39(9):1489–95.

24. Tischler MD, Vaitkus PT. The ability of vegetation size on echocardiography to predict clinical complications: a meta-analysis. *J Am Soc Echocardiogr* 1997;10(5):562–8.

25. Mugge A, Daniel WG, Frank G, Lichtlen PR. Echocardiography in infective endocarditis: reassessment of prognostic implications of vegetation size determined by the transthoracic and the transesophageal approach. *J Am Coll Cardiol* 1989;14(3):631–8.

26. Carpentier A, Chauvaud S, Fabiani JN, *et al*. Reconstructive surgery of mitral valve incompetence: ten-year appraisal. *J Thorac Cardiovasc Surg* 1980;79(3):338–48.

27. Galloway AC, Colvin SB, Baumann FG, *et al*. A comparison of mitral valve reconstruction with mitral valve replacement: intermediate-term results. *Ann Thorac Surg* 1989;47(5):655–62.

28. Sand ME, Naftel DC, Blackstone EH, Kirklin JW, Karp RB. A comparison of repair and replacement for mitral valve incompetence. *J Thorac Cardiovasc Surg* 1987;94(2):208–19.

29. Hellemans IM, Pieper EG, Ravelli AC, *et al*. Prediction of surgical strategy in mitral valve regurgitation based on echocardiography. Interuniversity Cardiology Institute of The Netherlands. *Am J Cardiol* 1997;79(3):334–8.

30. Patel V, Hsiung MC, Nanda NC, *et al*. Usefulness of live/real time three-dimensional transthoracic echocardiography in the identification of individual segment/scallop prolapse of the mitral valve. *Echocardiography* 2006;23(6):513–18.

31. Fabricius AM, Walther T, Falk V, Mohr FW. Three-dimensional echocardiography for planning of mitral valve surgery: current applicability? *Ann Thorac Surg* 2004;78(2):575–8.

32. Delabays A, Jeanrenaud X, Chassot PG, Von Segesser LK, Kappenberger L. Localization and quantification of mitral valve prolapse using three-dimensional echocardiography. *Eur J Echocardiogr* 2004;5(6):422–9.

33. Hozumi T, Yoshikawa J, Yoshida K, Akasaka T, Takagi T, Yamamuro A. Assessment of flail mitral leaflets by dynamic three-dimensional echocardiographic imaging. *Am J Cardiol* 1997;79(2):223–5.

34. De Castro S, Salandin V, Cartoni D, *et al*. Qualitative and quantitative evaluation of mitral valve morphology by intraoperative volume-rendered three-dimensional echocardiography. *J Heart Valve Dis* 2002;11(2):173–80.

35. Chauvel C, Bogino E, Clerc P, *et al*. Usefulness of three-dimensional echocardiography for the evaluation of mitral valve prolapse: an intraoperative study. *J Heart Valve Dis* 2000;9(3):341–9.

36. Levine RA, Handschumacher MD, Sanfilippo AJ, *et al*. Three-dimensional echocardiographic reconstruction of the mitral valve, with implications for the diagnosis of mitral valve prolapse. *Circulation* 1989;80(3):589–98.

37. Chung R, Pepper J, Henein M. Images in cardiology: mitral valve anterior leaflet prolapse by real time three dimensional transthoracic echocardiography. *Heart (Brit Cardiac Soc)* 2005;91(9):e55.

38. Pepi M, Tamborini G, Maltagliati A, *et al*. Head-to-head comparison of two- and three-dimensional transthoracic and transesophageal echocardiography in the localization of mitral valve prolapse. *J Am Coll Cardiol* 2006;48(12):2524–30.

CHAPTER 5

Aortic Valve and Aorta

Aortic valve (AV) pathologies are very common and are only expected to become more frequent as the population ages [1]. Evaluating pathologies that affect the AV require a basic understanding of its anatomy and the structural and hemodynamic derangements imposed by its malfunctioning as well as the impact of these changes on left ventricular (LV) size and function. The normal AV is composed of three crescent-shaped thin leaflets that are positioned at the end of the LV outflow tract (OT), between the heart and the aorta [2]. The leaflets are symmetrically arranged by attaching laterally to the margin between the LVOT and the aorta, thus forming a central orifice. Normally the cusps open in systole to form an aperture that measures 3–4 cm^2 and close in diastole to prevent backflow of blood to the heart from the aorta. The left and right coronary arteries originate from the sinuses behind the left and the right coronary leaflets. The noncoronary leaflet is anatomically identified on echocardiography to be adjacent to the interatrial septum. The AV is located anterior in the chest in an ideal position for interrogation by transthoracic and transesophageal echocardiography. It is precisely due to this anatomic advantage that 3D transthoracic echocardiography (3DTTE) has been utilized for the evaluation of aortic pathologies early on in its development [3]. This allowed for better visualization of the morphology of the valve in 3D space and the ability to directly measure the aortic valve orifice using planimetry for the assessment of aortic stenosis (AS) without the use of Doppler. The advancements in 3DTTE technologies have only made its applications for the evaluation of the AV

more time-efficient and clinically applicable. The full-volume 3D dataset obtained during 3DTTE can encompass the whole aortic root, which can then be sectioned using cropping planes at any level and angulation, allowing for a comprehensive assessment of the valve structure [4]. 3DTTE has since shown incremental value on top of 2DTTE and 2D transesophageal echocardiography (2DTEE) for the evaluation of AS, aortic regurgitation (AR), as well as endocarditis and other pathologies afflicting the AV. Beyond the AV itself, evaluation of the aorta by 2DTTE is somewhat limited since it usually can image only about 5 cm of the ascending aorta and a small portion of the descending aorta. Therefore, although 2DTTE can still be helpful in identifying Stanford type A aortic dissection, 2DTEE has largely replaced 2DTTE for most aortic pathologies [5]. However, since it is able to capture a wide pyramidal dataset, 3DTTE has proven itself helpful in establishing the diagnosis, especially in unstable patients.

Aortic stenosis and supravalvular stenosis

Recommendations for AV replacement in AS are based on the development of symptoms and the severity of AS [1]. The evaluation of AS severity is most commonly done by echocardiography, and more specifically 2DTTE [6]. Standard measurements include Doppler evaluation of the velocity of blood as it traverses the aortic orifice, and using the Bernoulli and the continuity equations, calculating the pressure gradient and the effective aortic valve orifice area. However, these measurements are susceptible to error that could lead to significant discrepancy from invasive measurements [7,8]. This discrepancy can be attributed to the variation of hemodynamics when the tests are nonsimultaneous

Live/Real Time 3D Echocardiography, 1st edition.
By Navin C. Nanda, Ming Chon Hsiung, Andrew P. Miller, and Fadi G. Hage. Published 2010 by Blackwell Publishing Ltd.

and to measurement variability of both the invasive and noninvasive data. Doppler assessment of the pressure gradient can underestimate the severity of AS if the Doppler beam is not parallel to the jet velocity, or overestimate the severity of stenosis due to the phenomenon of pressure recovery [9–11]. The calculation of the aortic valve orifice area is further limited by the dependence of the continuity equation on the measurement of the LVOT diameter, and since this measurement is squared in the equation, even minor errors will lead to large variations in the area [6]. Direct measurement of aortic valve orifice area by planimetry could be performed by 2DTTE, but the superior image quality of 2DTEE allows for more reliable and accurate measurements [12,13]. However, 2DTEE measurements are complicated by the inability to ensure that the 2D plane is through the actual flow-limiting orifice, and, in some patients, it is technically not feasible to align the 2D imaging plane to be exactly parallel to the AO due to the fixed relationship of the esophagus to the ascending aorta and the AV. When the imaging plane is slanted, the aortic valve orifice area could be overestimated, and severe AS could be missed. Bernard *et al.*, e.g., reported that multiplane 2DTEE planimetry is inaccurate in assessing AS severity [14]. Invasive assessment of AS using the Gorlin formula is itself not free from error, especially in low-flow states [15–17]. Besides these limitations, both 2DTTE and left heart catheterization are invasive procedures that carry inherent risk and discomfort to the patient.

The evaluation of the AV in 3D space by a noninvasive method is appealing and desirable. Our group was the first to utilize 3D echocardiography for the quantitative assessment of normal and stenotic AVs [3]. The development of live 3DTTE and the full matrix-array transducer transformed the cumbersome process of 3D imaging into a time-efficient, cost-feasible, and clinically viable technique. It, thus, provided improved spatial orientation over 2D imaging, and since one can crop the 3D dataset in any 2D plane, it provided the unique opportunity to measure the aortic valve orifice precisely and accurately by aligning the imaging plane exactly parallel to the aortic valve orifice in the short-axis view. Using these techniques, the orifice can be planimetered with confidence and the accuracy of the results, and the severity of AS can

be gauged without the use of Doppler. Therefore, 3DTTE provides a completely noninvasive alternative to 2DTTE and 2DTEE that avoids the criticisms of the use of Doppler for assessment of the severity of stenosis and at the same time provides a reliable method for the precise quantification of the anatomic stenotic orifice in the required imaging plane. Using a Philips Sonos 7500 (Philips Medical Systems, Inc., Andover, MA) ultrasound system and a 4-MHz 4 matrix transducer capable of providing real time B-mode and color Doppler 3D images, we evaluated 11 patients for AS severity [18]. From the 3D pyramidal dataset cropping planes aligned exactly parallel to the flow-limiting orifice, viewed in both long- and short axes, were used to obtain a 3D image of the aortic valve orifice. The orifice area was subsequently measured by planimetry using an offline Tom Tec Scan 4D View-RT (TomTec, Inc., Munich, Germany). All these patients subsequently underwent surgery for AV replacement and the orifice area was evaluated using planimetry by intraoperative multiplane 2DTEE and 3DTEE reconstruction [3,12,13,19]. Areas measured by live 3DTTE were compared with 2DTTE/Doppler-derived areas using the continuity equation, intraoperative 2DTEE and 3DTEE reconstruction measurements using planimetry as well as surgical estimation of AS severity. In this study, live 3DTTE was able to visualize the aortic valve orifice in all patients studied and it correctly estimated the severity of AS in all 10 patients in whom AS severity could be evaluated at surgery (Table 5.1). Measurements of the AV area by 3DTTE correlated well with intraoperative 3DTEE reconstruction measurements ($r = 0.85$), but not as well with 2DTTE/Doppler ($r = 0.46$) or with 2DTEE measurements ($r = 0.64$). Altogether four patients (Cases # 5, 8, 9, and 10 in Table 5.1) with severe AS by live 3DTTE and subsequently confirmed at surgery were misdiagnosed as having moderate AS by 2DTTE [18]. 2DTTE, 2DTEE, and even cardiac catheterization have limitations in the quantification of AS severity and can lead to misdiagnosis (Table 5.2). Therefore, 3DTTE is useful as a complimentary tool for the assessment of AS severity. The capability of visualizing the aortic valve orifice in 3D and using any desired plane and angulation can be especially useful in domed valves and angulated orifices. The additive value of 3DTTE over 2DTTE has now been demonstrated

Table 5.1 Live 3D transthoracic echocardiographic assessment of aortic valve orifice area.

	Patient	2DTTE AVO area (cm²)	Cardiac catheterization AVO area (cm²)	2DTEE AVO area (cm²)	3DTEE AVO area (cm²)	Live 3DTTE AVO area (cm²)	Surgery
1.	71 yr male*	0.71	Mild stenosis	0.85	0.80 (Tricuspid)	0.83 (Tricuspid)	Heavily calcified trileaflet AV. Severity could not be assessed.
2.	75 yr female	0.60	0.87	0.60	0.60 (Bicuspid)	0.70 (Bicuspid)	Heavily calcified, severely stenotic bicuspid AV.
3.	78 yr male	Severe stenosis. AVO area N/A	0.8–1.0	1.0	0.70 (Tricuspid)	0.70 (Tricuspid)	Heavily calcified, severely stenotic trileaflet AV.
4.	71 yr female	N/A	0.80	0.50	0.60 (Tricuspid)	0.70 (Tricuspid)	Hypertrophic cardiomyopathy. Heavily calcified, severely stenotic trileaflet AV.
5.	75 yr male	0.93	Mean gradient 33 mmHg. AVO N/A	0.46	0.40 (Bicuspid)	0.45 (Bicuspid)	Heavily calcified, very severely stenotic bicuspid AV.
6.	68 yr female	Peak gradient 69 mmHg. AVO area N/A	Peak gradient 68 mmHg. AVO area N/A	0.69	0.70 (Tricuspid)	0.70 (Tricuspid)	Heavily calcified, very severely stenotic trileaflet AV.
7.	70 yr female	0.76	N/A	0.41	0.80 (Bicuspid)	1.1 (Bicuspid)	Rheumatic with commissural fusion. Moderately stenotic AV.
8.	77 yr male	1.0	Moderate-to-severe stenosis. AVO area N/A	1.0	0.80 (Bicuspid)	0.70 (Bicuspid)	Heavily calcified, severely stenotic bicuspid AV.
9.	82 yr female	1.0	N/A	0.40	0.50 (Tricuspid)	0.60 (Tricuspid)	Heavily calcified, severely stenotic trileaflet AV.
10.	52 yr female	0.9	N/A	0.70	0.60 (Tricuspid)	0.70 (Tricuspid)	Heavily calcified, severely stenotic trileaflet AV.
11.	48 yr female	Peak gradient 76 mmHg. AVO area N/A	N/A	0.50	0.70 (Tricuspid)	1.1 (Tricuspid)	Hypertrophic cardiomyopathy. Moderately stenotic trileaflet AV.

*Left ventricular ejection fraction 20%.
Done at an outside institution.

AV, aortic valve; AVO, aortic valve orifice area; N/A, not available; 2DTEE, 2D transesophageal echocardiography; 2DTTE, 2D transthoracic echocardiography; 3DTEE, 3D transesophageal echocardiographic reconstruction; 3DTTE, 3D transthoracic echocardiography.
Reproduced from Vengala et al., [18], with permission.

Table 5.2 Limitations of various methods currently employed in the assessment of aortic valve stenosis severity.

TTE/Doppler	1. Continuity equation provides only indirect estimation of AVO area. 2. Difficulty in measuring LVOT diameter due to poor acoustic window or calcification of the mitral or aortic annulus. 3. Difficulty in differentiating LVOT velocity by pulsed wave Doppler from the significantly higher flow acceleration velocity. 4. Poor acoustic window may preclude accurate estimation of AV gradient. 5. Doppler cursor may not be in the jet core even with color Doppler guidance, resulting in AS severity underestimation. 6. Inability to properly align the Doppler cursor when the jet is eccentric. 7. Pressure recovery phenomenon may result in AS severity overestimation* 8. Contamination of AS jet with MR jet. High velocity MR jet may be misinterpreted as AS. 9. Left ventricular dysfunction/low cardiac output states may result in underestimation of AS severity. 10. Inability to accurately assess AS severity by Doppler in the presence of subaortic or supra-aortic stenosis.
TEE	1. Semi-invasive, entails patient discomfort, and not completely without risk to the patient. 2. Depending on the anatomic relation of the esophagus to the aortic valve, 2D-echo plane may not be aligned parallel to the flow-limiting aortic valve orifice, which in case of aortic valve doming, is located at the apex of the domed valve. 3. Significant calcification limits direct planimetry. 4. Effective stenotic orifice may differ from measured anatomic orifice.
Cardiac catheterization	1. Invasive. 2. Retrograde entry into the left ventricle difficult/impossible and risky with heavily calcified valve. 3. Inability to stabilize the catheter tip close to aortic valve orifice. 4. Cardiac output estimation by thermodilution has many limitations. 5. Fluid-filled catheters, which are widely used, are not as accurate as manometer tip catheters. 6. Catheter "fling" could result in false measurements. 7. Limitations of Gorlin formula: • Associated significant AR results in overestimation of AS severity. • Constant of 1 used for coefficient is empirically derived. • Low output states may result in underestimation of AS severity.

Pressure recovery phenomenon: At the level of stenosis, pressure (potential energy) is converted to velocity (kinetic energy). Distally, the energy that is not "wasted" in friction, turbulence, heat generation, and eddy currents is converted back to pressure. This is pressure recovery. While Doppler measures the actual maximal pressure drop at the vena contracta, catheterization estimates the distal pressure some distance away from the AS jet after "pressure recovery" has occurred. Arguably, although Doppler estimates the correct gradient, left ventricular load correlates more with distal perfusion pressure, and thus catheterization may be more physiologic. This Doppler "overestimation" is generally significant with tubular rather than discrete stenosis, domed aortic valves, small ascending aorta (<3 cm width just beyond sinotubular junction), and narrow LVOT (<2 cm).

AS, aortic stenosis; AV, aortic valve; AR, aortic regurgitation; LVOT, left ventricular outflow tract; MR, mitral regurgitation; TEE, transesophageal echocardiography; TTE, transthoracic echocardiography.

Reproduced from Vengala *et al.* [18], with permission.

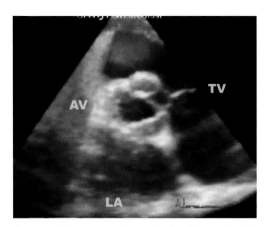

Figure 5.1 Short-axis cropping at the tip of the aortic valve (AV) obtained from a parasternal long-axis dataset shows a large aortic orifice (arrowhead in Movie clip 5.1) with no evidence of stenosis. The AV leaflets are mildly thickened consistent with sclerosis. LA, left atrium; TV, tricuspid valve.

by multiple investigators [20,21] (Figures 5.1–5.3).

Another advantage of 3DTTE over 2DTTE/Doppler measurements is its ability to accurately measure the flow-limiting area in patients with serial flow-limiting lesions such as hypertrophic cardiomyopathy (Cases # 4 and 11 in Table 5.1) or combined valvular and supravalvular AS (Figure 5.4) [18,22]. A similar limitation to 2DTTE/Doppler is its inability to reliably localize the site of high velocity flow when continuous wave Doppler is used. Therefore, patients with fixed anatomic discrete obstruction of their LVOT secondary to a focal membranous structure or a diffuse tunnel-type lesion (subaortic membranous stenosis) [23] have been misdiagnosed as hypertrophic obstructive cardiomyopathy (with a dynamic subvalvular obstruction secondary to the systolic anterior motion of the mitral valve and mitral-septal contact) or as aortic valvular stenosis [24,25]. Even invasive pressure measurements might miss the diagnosis in some patients [25]. Traditionally, 2DTEE has been used to help with the diagnosis in difficult cases [26], but more recently, 3D reconstruction of 2DTEE images has enabled a more comprehensive assessment of this lesion by virtue of the ease of cropping above and below the AV and identifying the true site of stenosis [27–29]. Live 3DTTE can also be used to identify the exact site and full extent of the subaortic membrane as well as to measure the

narrow opening within the membrane to quantify the severity of stenosis [30]. Using these anatomic measurements, which require no assumptions or estimations, might be more accurate than Doppler-derived gradients [31].

Aortic regurgitation

2DTEE usually reveals clues to the presence of AR, including an abnormal morphology of the valve leaflets (e.g., prolapse and endocarditis), aortic root (e.g., aneurysm and dissection), and the LV (eccentric hypertrophy). However, direct assessment of the presence and severity of AR requires the utilization of Doppler ultrasound. Unlike mitral regurgitation, the area of the LV that is filled by the regurgitant jet on color Doppler is not closely associated with the severity of AR. On the other hand, the width of the jet, as measured by the vena contracta, is. The vena contracta is the narrowest diameter of the regurgitant jet located at the intersection of the proximal flow convergence region in the aorta and the full-blown regurgitant jet in the LV. It is important to note that the vena contracta does not anatomically correspond with the aortic valve orifice, but nevertheless its width is directly proportional to the severity of regurgitation (vena contracta >0.6 cm suggests severe regurgitation) and has good correlation with angiographic grading and regurgitant orifice area [32–34]. Therefore, the most common assessment of AR currently includes either a measure of the vena contracta or a ratio of the vena contracta to the inner width of the LVOT [35]. More quantitative evaluations such as the regurgitant volume can be estimated using approaches such as the proximal isovelocity surface area method (PISA) or by subtracting the flow of blood across the mitral valve (stroke volume in the absence of significant mitral regurgitation) from the flow across the AV (stroke volume + regurgitant volume). Other measures for quantitating AR have also been used such as the effective orifice regurgitant area [35]. However, these quantitative measures are inaccurate and require assumptions that are often invalid. The guidelines, therefore, stress the importance of an integrative approach using several of the above measures, depending on the clinical scenario rather than depending on a single approach.

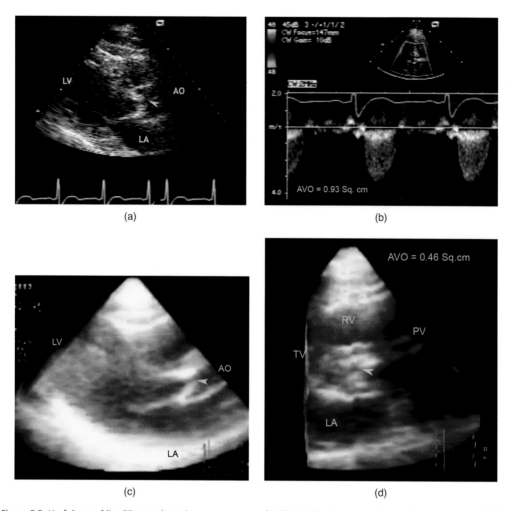

(a)

(b)

(c)

(d)

Figure 5.2 Usefulness of live 3D transthoracic echocardiography in aortic valve (AV) stenosis evaluation. (a, b) 2D transthoracic echocardiography. The arrowhead points to the calcified AV with restricted motion consistent with stenosis. Color Doppler-guided continuous wave Doppler examination of the AV (b) showed peak and mean gradients of 56 and 32 mmHg, respectively. AV orifice (AVO) area by the continuity equation was estimated to be 0.93 cm^2, indicative of moderate stenosis. (c, d) Live 3D transthoracic echocardiography. The arrowhead in (c) points to calcified AV with restricted motion, viewed in long axis. The arrowhead in (d) points to AVO viewed in short axis. AVO area measured 0.46 cm^2, an indication of severe stenosis. (*Continued on next page*)

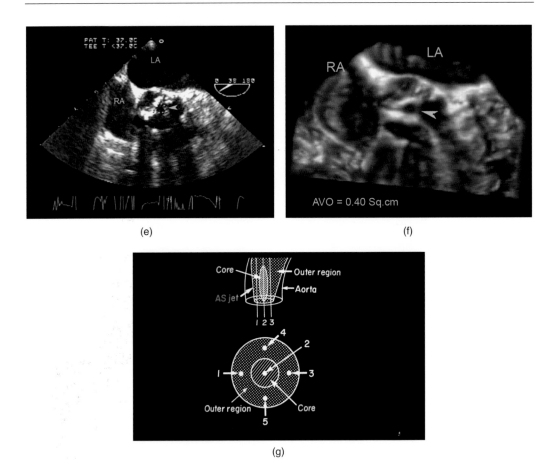

(e)

(f)

(g)

Figure 5.2 *(Continued)* (e) Intraoperative 2D transesophageal echocardiography. The arrowhead points to AVO which measured 0.46 cm^2 by planimetry consistent with severe stenosis. (f) Intraoperative 3D transesophageal echocardiographic reconstruction. The arrowhead points to AVO which measured 0.40 cm^2 consistent with severe stenosis. In this patient, severe AV stenosis was missed by 2D transthoracic echocardiography/Doppler, but correctly diagnosed by both live 3D transthoracic echocardiography and subsequently confirmed by intraoperative 2D- and 3D-transesophageal echocardiography, and at surgery. Movie clip 5.2 Part 1 shows the 3D nature of the aortic stenosis jet. Even though the color Doppler-guided continuous wave Doppler beam may appear to be aligned parallel to the stenotic jet, it may still be outside the jet core (numbered 2) where the gradient is highest, and thus miss severe stenosis. The gradients are much lower in the outer region (numbered 1, 3, 4, and 5). Movie clip 5.2 Part 2 shows another adult patient with severe AV stenosis (arrowhead) studied using QLAB. The diagnosis could be made easily, despite the presence of a motion artifact. AO, aorta; LA, left atrium; LV, left ventricle; PV, pulmonary valve; RA, right atrium; RV, right ventricle; TV, tricuspid valve. ((a–f) Reproduced from Vengala *et al.* [18], with permission; (g) Reproduced from Nanda NC. *Atlas of Color Doppler Echocardiography*. Philadelphia: Lea & Febiger; 1989:112, with permission.)

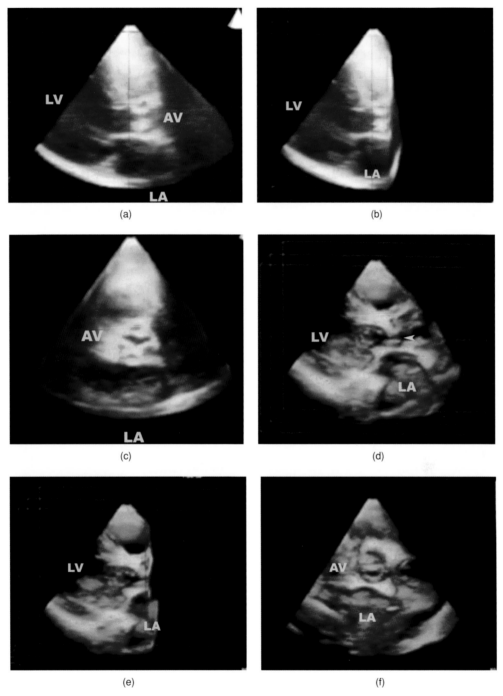

(a)

(b)

(c)

(d)

(e)

(f)

Figure 5.3 Live/real time 3D transthoracic echocardiography in aortic valve (AV) stenosis. (a–c) Careful cropping of the parasternal long-axis dataset at the flow-limiting tips of the AV leaflets demonstrated a bicuspid morphology and severe stenosis. (d–f) Another adult patient with AV stenosis. The arrow in (d) points to thickened AV leaflets with restricted opening motion viewed in parasternal long axis. Short-axis cropping at the AV tip demonstrates a severely stenotic bicuspid valve. QLAB cropping in another adult patient shows a small orifice consistent with significant AV stenosis. Despite the presence of motion artifact, it was possible to assess the orifice size in this patient. LA, left atrium; LV, left ventricle. Movie clips 5.3 A–C Part 1, 5.3 A–C Part 2, 5.3 A–C Part 3, 5.3 A–C Part 4, 5.3 D–F Part 1, 5.3 D–F Part 2, 5.3 D–F Part 3, 5.3 D–F Part 4.

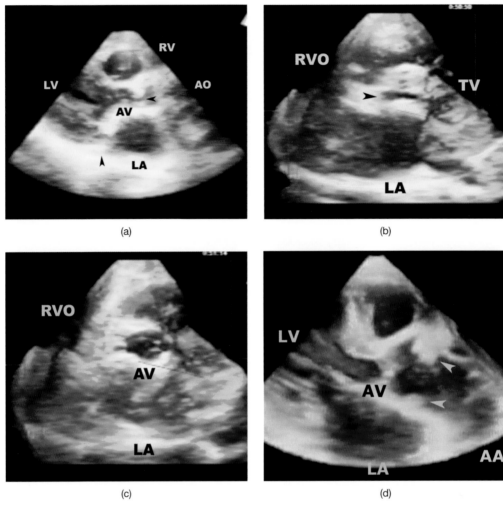

(a)

(b)

(c)

(d)

Figure 5.4 Live/real time 3D transthoracic echocardiographic assessment of combined valvular and supravalvular aortic stenosis. (a–c) Images from a 74-year-old female presenting with progressive shortness of breath on exertion who had undergone cobalt irradiation for breast cancer in the past. Supravalvular stenosis in this patient was presumably due to age-related and radiation-induced degenerative changes. (a) The horizontal arrowhead points to supravalvular aortic stenosis produced by calcification at the sinotubular junction. The vertical arrowhead shows heavy mitral annular calcification. (b) Supravalvular stenotic orifice viewed in short axis (arrowhead). It shows severe stenosis with the orifice measuring 0.83 cm^2 in area. (c) Short-axis view at the level of the aortic valve leaflets demonstrating mild valvular stenosis. Aortic valve orifice measured 1.5 cm^2 in area. (d–e) Another patient with calcification at the sinotubular junction without significant supravalvular stenosis. (d) The arrowheads point to prominent calcification at the sinotubular junction viewed in long axis. (e) Short-axis view at the sinotubular junction shows a large orifice (arrowhead) which measured 2.5 cm^2. (f) Short-axis view at the level of the aortic valve (left) and immediately above it (right). The aortic valve orifice measured 1.7 cm^2 by planimetry consistent with very mild aortic stenosis. The arrowhead in the right panel points to sinotubular calcification protruding into the aortic lumen imaged just beyond aortic valve leaflets. AA, ascending aorta; AO, aortic root; AV, aortic valve; LA, left atrium, LV, left ventricle; PA, pulmonary artery; RA, right atrium; RV, right ventricle; RVO, right ventricular outflow tract; TV, tricuspid valve. Movie clip 5.4 A–C. (Reproduced from Rajdev *et al.* [45], with permission.)

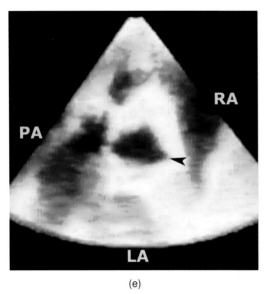

(e)

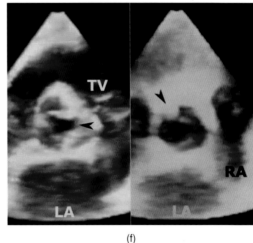

(f)

Figure 5.4 *(Continued)*

A better assessment of regurgitant volume can be derived by multiplying the area of the vena contracta (VCA) with the velocity time integral (VTI) of the continuous wave Doppler waveform of the AR jet. Since only one dimension of the vena contracta can be seen on the parasternal long axis and apical five chamber views, to do so with 2D imaging would require geometrical assumptions that are often incorrect [36]. It is possible to see the vena contracta *en face* from the short-axis parasternal view at the level of the AV, but it is difficult to be confident that the imaging plane is exactly parallel to the vena contracta and that the imaging plane is not farther downstream from the vena contracta where the jet is wider [32]. Both these problems are easily addressed by 3DTTE since after obtaining the 3D dataset of the aortic jet, one can crop offline with an imaging plane that is exactly parallel to the vena contracta and be certain that the plane is at the narrowest diameter of the regurgitant jet (Figure 5.5). To verify this concept, we studied 56 patients (36 females, aged 58.3 16.6 years) referred to echocardiography for evaluation of AR who subsequently underwent cardiac catheterization with aortography and/or cardiac surgery within 72 hours of the echocardiogram, which included standard 2DTTE with Doppler as well as 3DTTE [37].

Measures of the VCA by 3DTTE and width by 2DTTE showed strong correlation with angiographic grading, with less overlap evident between grades of AR by 3DTTE than by 2DTTE (Figures 5.6 and 5.7). Furthermore, the grading by 3DTTE was not affected by whether the regurgitant jet was central or eccentric, and measurements were reproducible with low interobserver and intraobserver ($r = 0.95$ and $r = 0.95$) variability. Furthermore, 3DTTE proved helpful in identifying mechanisms of AR that closely matched the surgical findings [37]. Thus, 3DTTE is able to dissect the complex geometry of the regurgitant jet and to overcome the shortcomings of 2DTTE for the quantitative assessment of AR. We have also found 3DTTE superior to 2DTTE in accurately assessing the size of vegetations and in detecting abscesses, leaflet perforations, and mycotic aneurysms (Figures 5.8–5.11). These aneurysms that result from infective aortitis account for a minority of all aortic aneurysms but are fatal if not diagnosed early [38]. Current treatment consists of antibiotic administration and early surgery to avoid rupture [38]. Although CT and 2DTEE are the most commonly used diagnostic tests, 3DTTE can establish the diagnosis with certainty by systemic and comprehensive cropping of the 3D dataset [39]

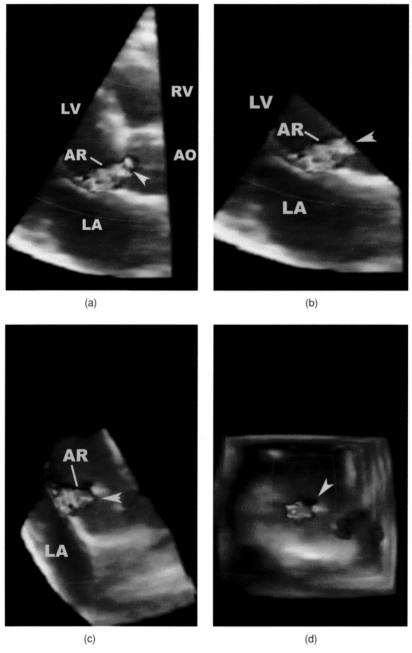

(a)

(b)

(c)

(d)

Figure 5.5 Live 3D color Doppler transthoracic echocardiographic technique for assessment of aortic regurgitation (AR) vena contracta. The 3D color Doppler dataset showing AR. (a) is cropped using an oblique plane to the level of the vena contracta (arrowhead, (b)) and tilted to view it *en face* (c, d). The vena contracta is then planimetered. AO, aorta; LA, left atrium; LV, left ventricle; RV, right ventricle. Movie clip 5.5. (Reproduced from Fang *et al.* [37], with permission.)

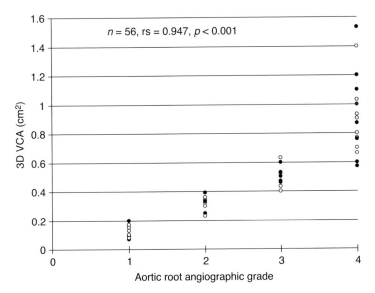

Figure 5.6 Shows the correlation between live 3D transthoracic color Doppler echocardiographic measurements of aortic regurgitation vena contracta (3D VCA) and aortic root angiographic grading. Open circles denote patients with eccentric aortic regurgitant jets; closed circles denote central jets. (Reproduced from Fang *et al.* [37], with permission.)

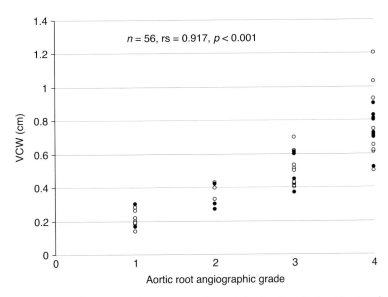

Figure 5.7 Shows the correlation between aortic regurgitation vena contracta widths (VCW) measured by 2D transthoracic color Doppler echocardiography and aortic root angiographic grades of aortic regurgitation. Open circles denote patients with eccentric aortic regurgitant jets; closed circles denote central jets. (Reproduced from Fang *et al.* [37], with permission.)

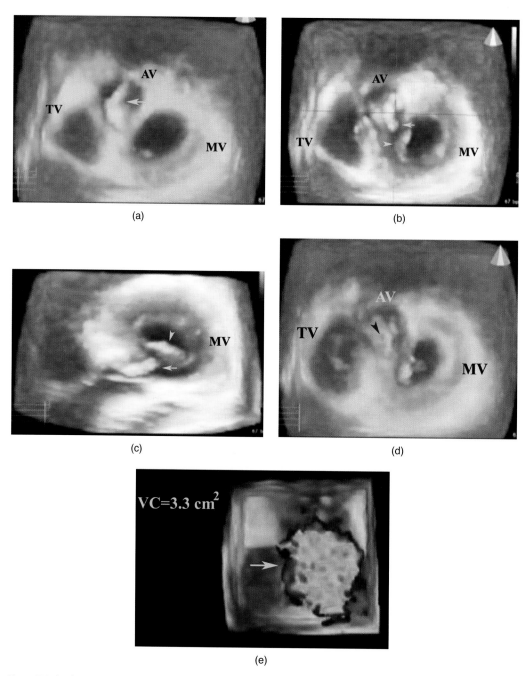

(a)

(b)

(c)

(d)

(e)

Figure 5.8 (a–e) Live/real time 3D transthoracic echocardiography in a patient with aortic valve (AV) endocarditis. The arrow in (a) points to a vegetation involving the AV viewed in short axis. Figures (b) and (c) show the vegetation (arrow) prolapsing into the left ventricular outflow tract and almost in contact with the mitral valve (MV, arrowhead). The black arrowhead in (d) shows a perforation in the AV. (e) Color Doppler examination shows a huge vena contracta measuring 3.3 cm², indicating torrential aortic regurgitation. AV, aortic valve; MV, mitral valve; TV, tricuspid valve; VC, vena contracta. Movie clip 5.8.

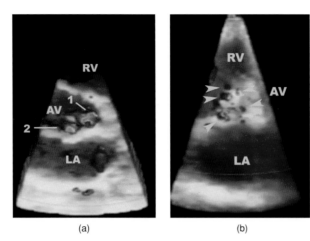

(a)   (b)

Figure 5.9 Live 3D transthoracic echocardiographic assessment of aortic valve perforations in two patients with endocarditis. (a) Two perforations (numbered 1 and 2) demonstrated by cropping of the 3D color Doppler dataset. (b) The arrowheads demonstrate multiple perforations in a patient with almost totally destroyed aortic cusps at surgery. AV, aortic valve; LA, left atrium; RV, right ventricle. (Reproduced from Fang et al. [37], with permission.)

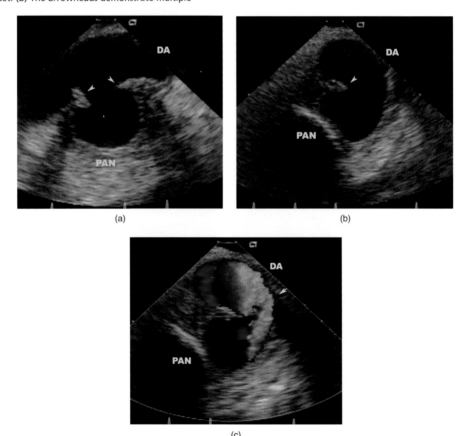

(a)   (b)

(c)

Figure 5.10 2D transesophageal echocardiographic findings. (a, b) The arrowheads point to shaggy-looking echoes at the narrow mouth of the pseudoaneurysm (PAN) consistent with vegetations. Descending aorta (DA) is viewed in long (a) and short (b) axes. (c) The arrow shows color Doppler flow signals moving from DA into PAN. Movie clips 5.10 A and 5.10 C. (Reproduced from Rajdev et al. [45], with permission.)

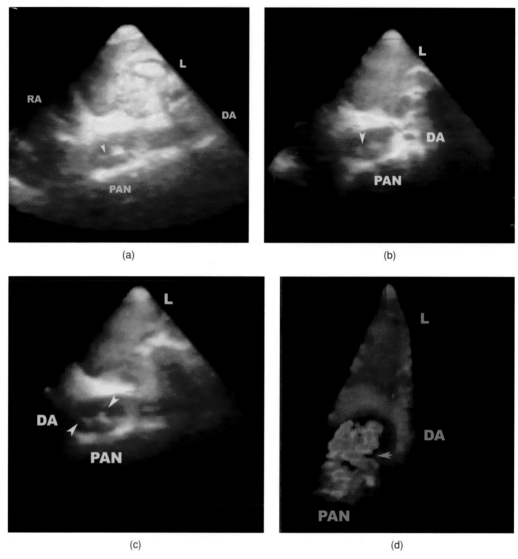

Figure 5.11 Live/real time 3D transthoracic echocardiographic findings of an aortic pseudoaneurysm. (a, b) The arrowhead points to the narrow mouth of pseudoaneurysm (PAN). Descending aorta (DA) is viewed in long (a) and short (b) axes. (c) The arrowheads point to linear echo densities at the mouth of PAN consistent with vegetations. (d) Color Doppler examination shows flow signals in both DA and PAN. L, liver; RA, right atrium. Movie clips 5.11 A and 5.11 C. (Reproduced from Rajdev *et al.* [45], with permission.)

Aortic dissection

Aortic dissection can be classified by the Stanford classification as involving the ascending aorta (type A) or just involving the descending aorta (type B), and this is useful since it generally predicts either a surgical or medical route for care, respectively. Another widely used classification, the DeBakey classification, divides dissection into three groups: I involves the ascending and descending aorta, II is isolated to the ascending aortic arch, and III is isolated to the descending aorta [40]. Although no randomized studies are available to guide the management of acute aortic dissection, rapid and accurate diagnosis with differentiation between ascending and descending aortic dissection is vital. Early detection is crucial since the natural history of acute dissection that is left untreated includes a mortality as high as 2% per hour during the first 48 hours, and therefore, urgent surgical intervention might be warranted [41]. Although electrocardiogram and chest roentgenograms are done on all patients suspected of having aortic dissection, their discriminatory power is low, and therefore they cannot be relied upon to establish or exclude the diagnosis [40]. Most hospitals currently utilize either computed tomography (CT) or 2DTEE, depending on the local availability and expertise and patient-specific factors. CT is rapid and available but cannot be performed at the bedside and requires the introduction of intravascular contrast. Echocardiography, in general, is portable and very useful in unstable patients who cannot be transferred to the CT suite and does not require the use of intravascular contrast. 2DTTE is limited by its inability to view the whole aorta, and therefore, 2DTEE has shown better sensitivity and specificity in making the diagnosis and has virtually replaced 2DTTE in the acute setting. Nevertheless, 2DTEE is semi-invasive and can be challenging to perform in sick patients due to the need for the patients to be cooperative in swallowing the TEE probe and other considerations such as requirement of a fasting state to avoid aspiration [42]. Although 3D reconstruction of 2DTEE can be performed for the diagnosis of aortic dissection, the maneuver is time consuming and could result in delaying the diagnosis and eventual treatment [43]. In patients with adequate acoustic windows, live 3DTTE provides a dataset that is capable of making the diagnosis while being portable, non-invasive, does not require esophageal intubation or intravascular contrast, and at the same time is rapid and cheap. In our original series, we studied 10 patients with acute dissection who underwent 2DTTE and 3DTTE [44]. Although 2DTTE was not capable of establishing the diagnosis in half of the patients, 3DTTE made a definitive diagnosis in all patients. Even in the patients in whom a diagnosis of dissection was made on 2DTTE, live 3DTTE increased the confidence level of the diagnosis since the dissection flap could be seen *en face* in 3D as a sheet of tissue rather than simply a linear echo separating the "true" from the "false" lumen. This is because dissection essentially represents splitting of the aortic wall and 3DTTE is able to visualize it *en face*. Therefore, 3DTTE might be particularly useful when aortic dissection is suspected on 2DTTE, but it cannot be clearly differentiated from reverberation artifacts which are linear in nature [45]. 3DTTE had an additional advantage in its ability to follow the dissection as it extended into branching vessels. Perhaps more importantly, TEE was averted in 4 of the 10 patients based on the visualization of the dissecting flap and the certainty of the diagnosis [44] (Figures 5.12–5.22). Live 3DTTE is also useful in evaluating the size and extent of aortic aneurysms and excluding the presence of dissection by using multiple cropping planes through the 3D dataset (Figure 5.23).

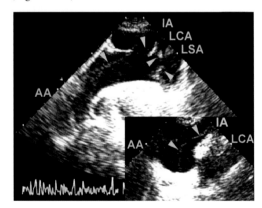

Figure 5.12 2D transthoracic echocardiography in aortic dissection. The arrowheads point to the dissection flap which appears as a linear structure involving the ascending aorta (AA), aortic arch, innominate artery (IA), and the left common carotid artery (LCA). The left subclavian artery (LSA) appears uninvolved. Movie clips 5.12 Part 1 and 5.12 Part 2. (Reproduced from Htay *et al.* [42], with permission.)

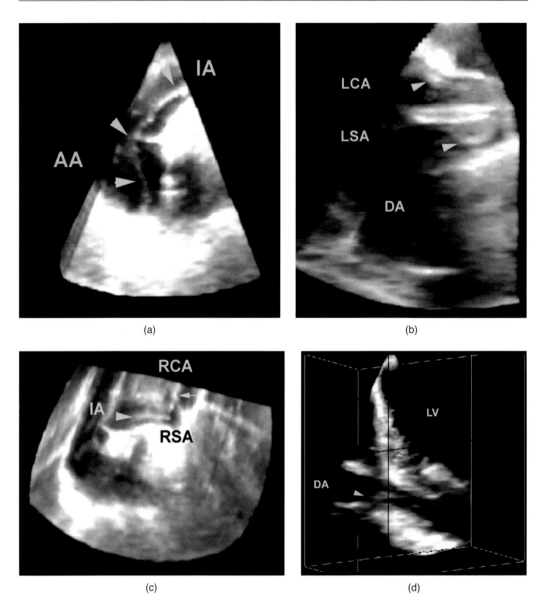

(a) (b)

(c) (d)

Figure 5.13 Live 3D transthoracic echocardiography in aortic dissection (same patient as previous figure). (a) The dissection flap (arrowheads) involving the ascending aorta (AA) and innominate artery (IA) appears as a sheet of tissue and not a linear structure, resulting in a more confident diagnosis. Movie clip 5.13 Part 1. (b) The dissection flap (arrowheads) is clearly seen involving left common carotid artery (LCA) and left subclavian artery (LSA). (c) The dissection flap (arrowhead) is seen to extend from IA into the right common carotid artery (RCA). (d, e) The arrowheads show the dissection flap in the descending thoracic aorta (DA) and abdominal aorta (ABA). (f) Postoperative study shows a clot occupying most of the false lumen (FL) in the aortic arch. B, branch of celiac artery; C, celiac artery; L, liver; RSA, right subclavian artery; TL, true lumen. Movie clips 5.13 Parts 2–4. 13 Part 4 show a clotted false/nonperfusing lumen (NPL, arrowhead) in another patient with ascending aortic dissection. AO, aorta; PL, perfusing lumen. (Reproduced from Htay *et al.* [42], with permission.)

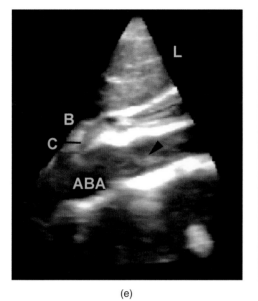

(e)

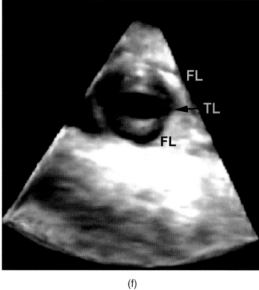

(f)

Figure 5.13 (*Continued*)

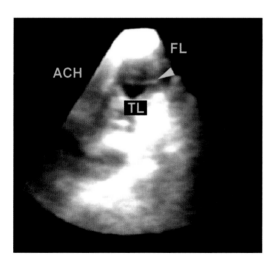

Figure 5.14 Live/real time 3D transthoracic echocardiography in aortic dissection in another patient. The arrowhead shows the dissection flap in the aortic arch (ACH). FL. false lumen; TL, true lumen. (Reproduced from Htay *et al.* [42], with permission.)

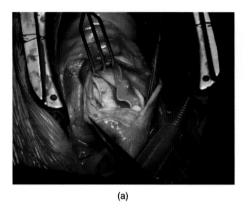
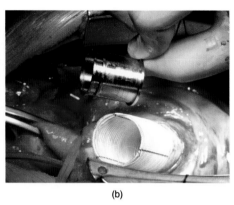

(a)

(b)

Figure 5.15 Live/real time 3D transthoracic echocardiography in another patient with aortic dissection. (a) The dissection flap in the aorta is well visualized in this patient at surgery. (b) Shows graft placement after resection of the ascending aorta. Movie clip 5.15: 2D transthoracic echocardiography shows the flap as a linear echo (arrowhead) while it appears as a sheet of tissue (arrowhead) when examined by 3D transthoracic echocardiography.

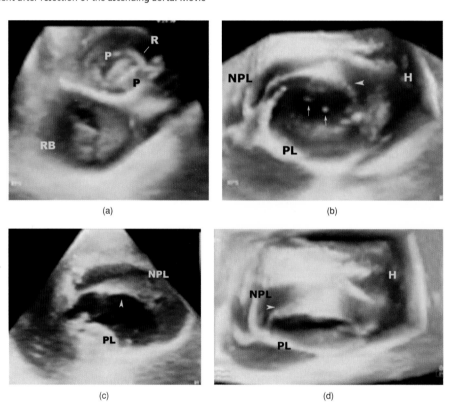

(a)

(b)

(c)

(d)

Figure 5.16 (a–f) Live/real time 3D transthoracic echocardiography in a patient with aortic valve prosthesis and dissection. This patient's aorta was dissected, shortly following by aortic valve replacement with a St. Jude prosthesis. In (a), the two leaflets (P, P) of the normally functioning prosthesis are well visualized. The dissection flap (arrowhead) in the aortic root above the prosthesis is well visualized en face as a sheet of tissue. The arrows in (b) point to spontaneous contrast echoes emanating from the prosthesis. A large hematoma (H) is noted around the prosthesis and aorta. Figures (e) and (f) show extension of dissection into the aortic arch (ACH) and descending thoracic aorta (DA). LSA, left subclavian artery; NPL, nonperfusing lumen; PL, perfusing lumen; R, prosthetic ring; RB, reverberations from the prosthesis. The arrowhead in the Movie clips 5.16 Parts 1–5 points to the dissection flap. R in Part 1 denotes prosthetic valve reverberations. The arrow in Part 4 shows spontaneous contrast echoes originating from the aortic prosthesis (P).

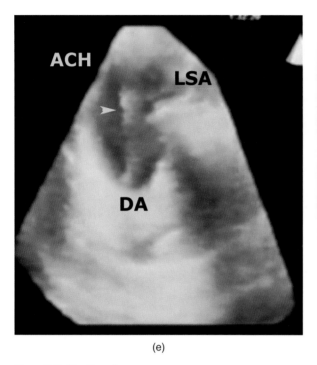

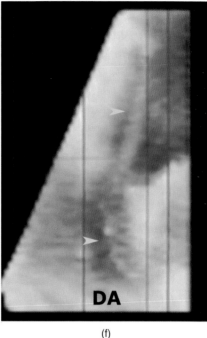

(e)

(f)

Figure 5.16 (*Continued*)

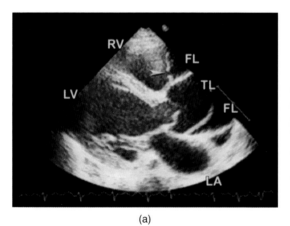

(a)

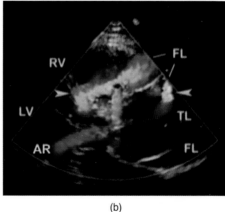

(b)

Figure 5.17 Real time 2D transthoracic echocardiographic assessment of aortic dissection rupture into the right ventricular outflow tract. (a) Parasternal long-axis view. The arrowhead points to the site of rupture of the false lumen (FL) into the right ventricular outflow tract (RVOT). (b) Color Doppler examination. The arrowhead on the right points to a communication between the true lumen (TL) and FL. The arrowhead on the left shows flow signals moving from the FL to the RVOT. Moderate aortic regurgitation (AR) is also displayed. (c) Continuous wave spectral Doppler interrogation of the rupture site showing continuous flow throughout the cardiac cycle. LA, left atrium; LV, left ventricle; RV, right ventricle. Movie clips 5.17 A–5.17 C. (Reproduced from Hansalia *et al.*, *Echocardiography* 2009;26:100–106, with permission from Lippincott, Williams & Wilkins.)

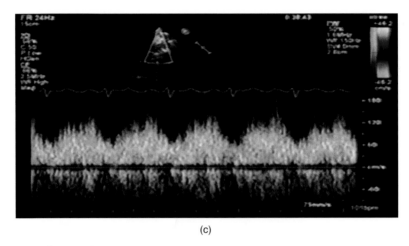

(c)

Figure 5.17 (*Continued*).

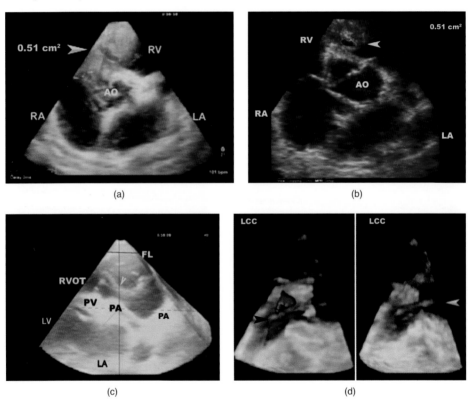

(a)

(b)

(c)

(d)

Figure 5.18 Live/real time 3D transthoracic echocardiographic assessment of aortic dissection rupture into the right ventricle outflow tract. (a) The arrowhead points to the *en face* view of the rupture site upon cropping of the dataset. It is roughly elliptical in shape and measured 0.51 cm^2 in area (A) by planimetry. Movie clip 5.18 A. The cropping plane is advanced to the aortic valve (AV), and then rotated 90° to reveal the AV in short axis, and the rupture site (arrowhead). (b) QLAB image of the same dataset with the orifice (arrowhead) planimeterized.

(c) Compression of the main pulmonary artery (PA) by the false lumen (FL). (d) Extension of the dissection (arrowhead) into the left common carotid artery (LCC) is shown. AO, aorta; LA, left atrium; LV, left ventricle; PV, pulmonary valve; RA, right atrium; RV, right ventricle; RVOT, right ventricular outflow tract. Movie clip 5.18 D. (Reproduced from Hansalia *et al.*, *Echocardiography* 2009;26:100–106, with permission from Lippincott, Williams & Wilkins.)

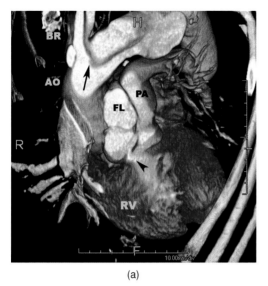

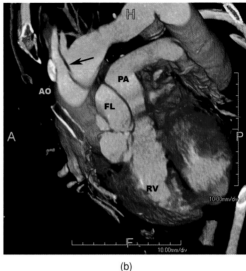

(a)   (b)

Figure 5.19 Computed tomography angiogram assessment of aortic dissection rupture into the right ventricular outflow tract. (a) Left anterior oblique (LAO) view demonstrating the communication (arrowhead) between the false lumen (FL) and right ventricular outflow tract (RVOT). (b) Cut slab volume rendered image in oblique LAO view demonstrating pulmonary artery (PA) compression by the dilated FL. The arrow in (a) and (b) points to the dissection flap extending into the aortic arch and the brachiocephalic artery (BR). A, anterior; AO, aorta; F, foot; H, head; L, left; P, posterior; R, right; RV, right ventricle. Movie clip 5.19. (Reproduced from Hansalia *et al.*, *Echocardiography* 2009;26:110–116, with permission from Lippincott, Williams & Wilkins.)

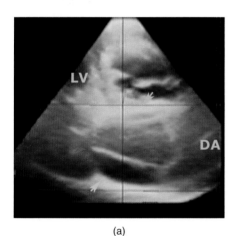

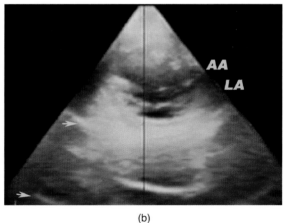

(a)   (b)

Figure 5.20 Definitive diagnosis of descending thoracic aortic dissection by live/real time 3D transthoracic echocardiography. (a) Red arrowhead points to a linear echo in the markedly enlarged descending aorta (DA) consistent with dissection. However, this cannot be differentiated from an artifact commonly seen in this area in the parasternal long-axis view. Yellow arrows point to the walls of the DA. Cropping away the posterior wall of the DA (b), and tilting the 3D pyramidal dataset. (*Continued on next page*)

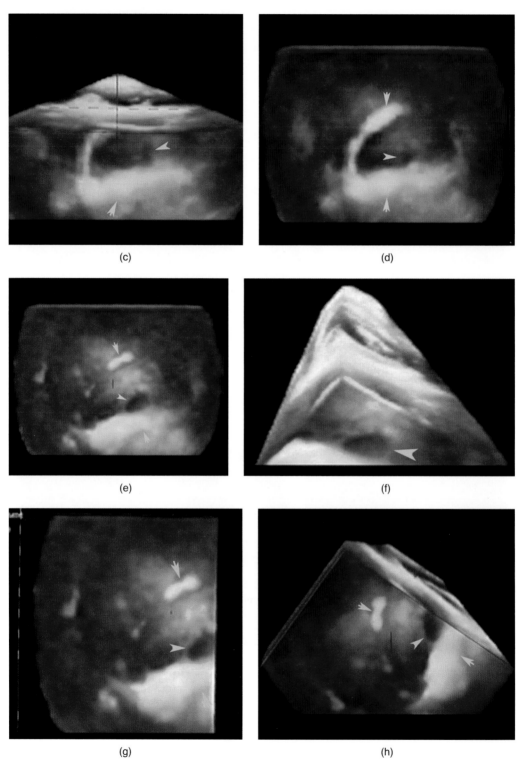

(c)

(d)

(e)

(f)

(g)

(h)

Figure 5.20 (*Continued*) (c–f) views the dissection flap *en face* as a sheet of tissue, resulting in the definitive diagnosis of dissection. In addition, a large rounded communication between the true and false lumen also becomes visible (yellow arrowhead). This was not visualized in (a). (*Continued on next page*)

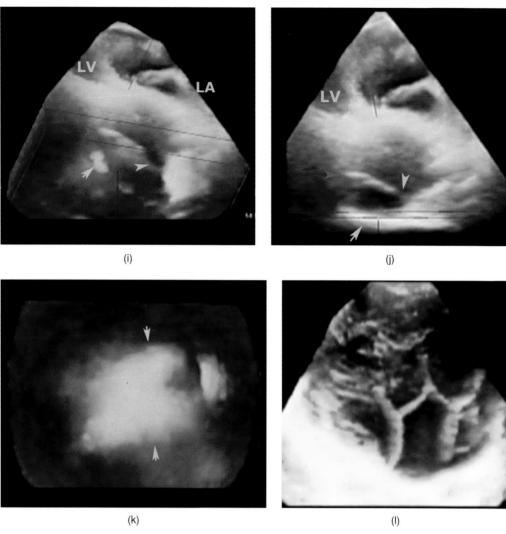

(i)

(j)

(k)

(l)

Figure 5.20 (*Continued*) (g–j) Further cropping of the pyramidal dataset from the side and tilting it shows the dissection flap to be in continuity with the linear echo seen in (a). (k) The 3D dataset has been tilted to view *en face* the uncropped posterior wall of DA. (l) Right polycystic kidney viewed in three dimensions from the subcostal approach in the same patient. AA, ascending aorta; LA, left atrium; LV, left ventricle.Movie clips 5.20 A–E, 5.20 D, E, K, 5.20 E, 5.20 G, H, J, 5.20 L. (Reproduced from Yelamanchili *et al.* [43], with permission.)

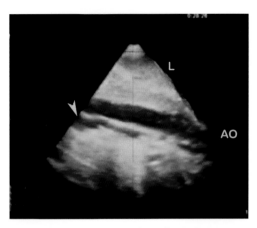

Figure 5.21 Live/real time 3D echocardiography in a patient with abdominal aortic dissection. The arrowhead points to the dissection flap. AO, aorta; L, liver.

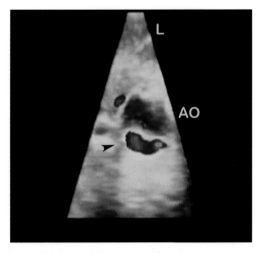

Figure 5.22 Live/real time 3D transthoracic echocardiography in another patient with abdominal aortic dissection. The arrowhead points to the dissection flap which appears as a sheet of tissue when viewed *en face*. AO, abdominal aorta; L, liver.

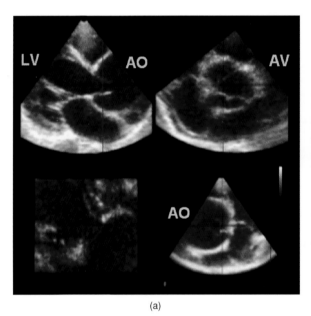

(a)

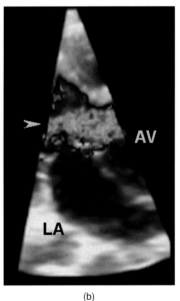

(b)

Figure 5.23 Live/real time 3D transthoracic echocardiography in ascending aortic aneurysm. (a) Ascending aortic aneurysm in a patient with Marfan's syndrome (QLAB examination). Section at the aortic valve (AV) level shows no evidence of dissection. (b) Color Doppler study shows severe aortic regurgitation (arrowhead). AO, aorta; AV, aortic valve; LA, left atrium; LV, left ventricle. Movie clips 5.23 Part 1 and 5.23 Part 2.

With its good spatial orientation and noninvasive nature, 3DTTE has been utilized in other aortic pathologies either as a substitute or, more commonly, to complement 2DTTE and 2DTEE.

References

1. Bonow RO, Carabello BA, Chatterjee K, *et al.* ACC/AHA 2006 guidelines for the management of patients with valvular heart disease: a report of the American College of Cardiology/American Heart Association Task Force on Practice Guidelines (Writing Committee to revise the 1998 guidelines for the management of patients with valvular heart disease) developed in collaboration with the Society of Cardiovascular Anesthesiologists endorsed by the Society for Cardiovascular Angiography and Interventions and the Society of Thoracic Surgeons. *J Am Coll Cardiol* 2006;48:e1–148.

2. Anderson RH. Clinical anatomy of the aortic root. *Heart* 2000;84:670–673.

3. Nanda NC, Roychoudhury D, Chung SM, Kim KS, Ostlund V, Klas B. Quantitative assessment of normal and stenotic aortic valve using transesophageal three-dimensional echocardiography. *Echocardiography* 1994;11:617–25.

4. Burri MV, Nanda NC, Singh A, Panwar SR. Live/real time three-dimensional transthoracic echocardiographic identification of quadricuspid aortic valve. *Echocardiography* 2007;24:653–5.

5. Ince H, Nienaber CA. Diagnosis and management of patients with aortic dissection. *Heart* 2007;93:266–70.

6. Otto CM. Valvular aortic stenosis: disease severity and timing of intervention. *J Am Coll Cardiol* 2006;47:2141–51.

7. Burwash IG, Dickinson A, Teskey RJ, Tam JW, Chan KL. Aortic valve area discrepancy by Gorlin equation and Doppler echocardiography continuity equation: relationship to flow in patients with valvular aortic stenosis. *Can J Cardiol* 2000;16:985–92.

8. Aghassi P, Aurigemma GP, Folland ED, Tighe DA. Catheterization-Doppler discrepancies in nonsimultaneous evaluations of aortic stenosis. *Echocardiography* 2005;22:367–73.

9. Garcia D, Dumesnil JG, Durand LG, Kadem L, Pibarot P. Discrepancies between catheter and Doppler estimates of valve effective orifice area can be predicted from the pressure recovery phenomenon: practical implications with regard to quantification of aortic stenosis severity. *J Am Coll Cardiol* 2003;41:435–42.

10. Levine RA, Jimoh A, Cape EG, McMillan S, Yoganathan AP, Weyman AE. Pressure recovery distal to a stenosis: potential cause of gradient "overestimation" by Doppler echocardiography. *J Am Coll Cardiol* 1989;13:706–15.

11. Baumgartner H, Stefenelli T, Niederberger J, Schima H, Maurer G. "Overestimation" of catheter gradients by Doppler ultrasound in patients with aortic stenosis: a predictable manifestation of pressure recovery. *J Am Coll Cardiol* 1999;33:1655–61.

12. Tribouilloy C, Shen WF, Peltier M, Mirode A, Rey JL, Lesbre JP. Quantitation of aortic valve area in aortic stenosis with multiplane transesophageal echocardiography: comparison with monoplane transesophageal approach. *Am Heart J* 1994;128:526–32.

13. Hoffmann R, Flachskampf FA, Hanrath P. Planimetry of orifice area in aortic stenosis using multiplane transesophageal echocardiography. *J Am Coll Cardiol* 1993;22:529–34.

14. Bernard Y, Meneveau N, Vuillemenot A, *et al.* Planimetry of aortic valve area using multiplane transesophageal echocardiography is not a reliable method for assessing severity of aortic stenosis. *Heart* 1997;78:68–73.

15. Segal J, Lerner DJ, Miller DC, Mitchell RS, Alderman EA, Popp RL. When should Doppler-determined valve area be better than the Gorlin formula?: variation in hydraulic constants in low flow states. *J Am Coll Cardiol* 1987;9:1294–305.

16. Burwash IG, Thomas DD, Sadahiro M, *et al.* Dependence of Gorlin formula and continuity equation valve areas on transvalvular volume flow rate in valvular aortic stenosis. *Circulation* 1994;89:827–35.

17. Cannon SR, Richards KL, Crawford M. Hydraulic estimation of stenotic orifice area: a correction of the Gorlin formula. *Circulation* 1985;71:1170–1178.

18. Vengala S, Nanda NC, Dod HS, *et al.* Images in geriatric cardiology. Usefulness of live three-dimensional transthoracic echocardiography in aortic valve stenosis evaluation. *Am J Geriatr Cardiol* 2004;13:279–84.

19. Kasprzak JD, Salustri A, Roelandt JR, Ten Cate FJ. Three-dimensional echocardiography of the aortic valve: feasibility, clinical potential, and limitations. *Echocardiography* 1998;15:127–38.

20. Gilon D. Three dimensional echocardiography and aortic valve stenosis. *Minerva Cardioangiol* 2003;51:641–5.

21. Goland S, Trento A, Iida K, *et al.* Assessment of aortic stenosis by three-dimensional echocardiography: an accurate and novel approach. *Heart* 2007;93:801–7.

22. Rajdev S, Nanda NC, Patel V, Mehmood F, Singh A, McGiffin DC. Live/real-time three-dimensional transthoracic echocardiographic assessment of combined valvular and supravalvular aortic stenosis. *Am J Geriatr Cardiol* 2006;15:188–90.

23. Aboulhosn J, Child JS. Left ventricular outflow obstruction: subaortic stenosis, bicuspid aortic valve,

supravalvular aortic stenosis, and coarctation of the aorta. *Circulation* 2006;114:2412–22.

24. Bruce CJ, Nishimura RA, Tajik AJ, Schaff HV, Danielson GK. Fixed left ventricular outflow tract obstruction in presumed hypertrophic obstructive cardiomyopathy: implications for therapy. *Ann Thorac Surg* 1999;68:100–104.

25. Hage FG, Zoghbi G, Aqel R, Nanda N. Subaortic stenosis missed by invasive hemodynamic assessment. *Echocardiography* 2008;25:1007–10.

26. Alboliras ET, Gotteiner NL, Berdusis K, Webb CL. Transesophageal echocardiographic imaging for congenital lesions of the left ventricular outflow tract and the aorta. *Echocardiography* 1996;13:439–46.

27. Dall'Agata A, Cromme-Dijkhuis AH, Meijboom FJ, *et al.* Use of three-dimensional echocardiography for analysis of outflow obstruction in congenital heart disease. *Am J Cardiol* 1999;83:921–5.

28. Ge S, Warner JG, Jr., Fowle KM, *et al.* Morphology and dynamic change of discrete subaortic stenosis can be imaged and quantified with three-dimensional transesophageal echocardiography. *J Am Soc Echocardiogr* 1997;10:713–16.

29. Miyamoto K, Nakatani S, Kanzaki H, Tagusari O, Kobayashi J. Detection of discrete subaortic stenosis by 3-dimensional transesophageal echocardiography. *Echocardiography* 2005;22:783–4.

30. Agrawal GG, Nanda NC, Htay T, Dod HS, Gandhari SR. Live three-dimensional transthoracic echocardiographic identification of discrete subaortic membranous stenosis. *Echocardiography* 2003;20:617–19.

31. Bandarupalli N, Faulkner M, Nanda NC, Pothineni KR. Erroneous diagnosis of significant obstruction by Doppler in a patient with discrete subaortic membrane: correct diagnosis by 3D transthoracic echocardiography *Echocardiography* 2005;25:1004–6.

32. Perry GJ, Helmcke F, Nanda NC, Byard C, Soto B. Evaluation of aortic insufficiency by Doppler color flow mapping. *J Am Coll Cardiol* 1987;9:952–9.

33. Tribouilloy CM, Enriquez-Sarano M, Bailey KR, Seward JB, Tajik AJ. Assessment of severity of aortic regurgitation using the width of the vena contracta: a clinical color Doppler imaging study. *Circulation* 2000;102:558–64.

34. Tribouilloy CM, Enriquez-Sarano M, Fett SL, Bailey KR, Seward JB, Tajik AJ. Application of the proximal flow

convergence method to calculate the effective regurgitant orifice area in aortic regurgitation. *J Am Coll Cardiol* 1998;32:1032–9.

35. Zoghbi WA, Enriquez-Sarano M, Foster E, *et al.* Recommendations for evaluation of the severity of native valvular regurgitation with two-dimensional and Doppler echocardiography. *J Am Soc Echocardiogr* 2003;16:777–802.

36. Shiota T, Jones M, Delabays A, *et al.* Direct measurement of three-dimensionally reconstructed flow convergence surface area and regurgitant flow in aortic regurgitation: in vitro and chronic animal model studies. *Circulation* 1997;96:3687–95.

37. Fang L, Hsiung MC, Miller AP, *et al.* Assessment of aortic regurgitation by live three-dimensional transthoracic echocardiographic measurements of vena contracta area: usefulness and validation. *Echocardiography* 2005;22:775–81.

38. Malouf JF, Chandrasekaran K, Orszulak TA. Mycotic aneurysms of the thoracic aorta: a diagnostic challenge. *Am J Med* 2003;115:489–96.

39. Rajdev S, Nanda NC, Patel V, *et al.* Live/real time three-dimensional transthoracic echocardiographic assessment of mycotic pseudoaneurysm involving the descending thoracic aorta. *Echocardiography* 2006;23:340–343.

40. Golledge J, Eagle KA. Acute aortic dissection. *Lancet* 2008;372:55–66.

41. Pretre R, Von Segesser LK. Aortic dissection. *Lancet* 1997;349:1461–4.

42. Nanda NC, Domanski MJ. *Atlas of Transesophageal Echocardiography*. Baltimore: Williams & Wilkins; 1998.

43. Nanda NC, Khatri GK, Samal AK, *et al.* Three-dimensional echocardiographic assessment of aortic dissection. *Echocardiography* 1998;15:745–54.

44. Htay T, Nanda NC, Agrawal G, Ravi BS, Dod HS, McGiffin D. Live three-dimensional transthoracic echocardiographic assessment of aortic dissection. *Echocardiography* 2003;20:573–7.

45. Yelamanchili P, Nanda NC, Patel V, Bogabathina H, Baysan O. Definitive diagnosis of descending thoracic aortic dissection by real time/live three-dimensional transthoracic echocardiography. *Echocardiography* 2006;23:158–61.

CHAPTER 6

Tricuspid and Pulmonary Valves

Introduction

The tricuspid valve represents an important site of confluence between a vast venous system and the right heart, and is an important structure for its own pathology as well as for the insight it can offer to the pulmonary circulation. This trileaflet valve demonstrates complex anatomy, with varying subvalvular chordae and papillary muscle arrangements. The annulus takes a "D" shape, with the straighter portion falling along the septal leaflet [1]. The valve is radially supported within the right ventricle by its subvalvular apparatus, forming a complex that is able to respond to changes in right heart pressures, volume, and architecture. This orientation and complexity of tricuspid valve anatomy leads to difficulties in assessing pathology with 2D planes from the usual transthoracic acoustic windows.

The pulmonic valve, being the most anterior valve, is well seen by transthoracic approaches. This scalloped trileaflet semilunar valve is composed of smooth, thin cusps that form upon the smooth-walled muscular infundibulum. As described in a later chapter, the complex morphogenesis of the conotruncus creates a site for a number of congenital malformations associated with high morbidity and mortality. In this chapter, we will focus on assessment of normal structure affected by degenerative or acquired processes.

Tricuspid stenosis

Stenosis of the tricuspid valve is a rare clinical entity that is caused by rheumatic disease in the far

Live/Real Time 3D Echocardiography, 1st edition.
By Navin C. Nanda, Ming Chon Hsiung, Andrew P. Miller, and Fadi G. Hage. Published 2010 by Blackwell Publishing Ltd.

majority (90%) of cases [2]. Unlike mitral stenosis where careful short-axis inspection can yield a planimetered area, imaging the tricuspid valve in short axis is rarely possible by 2D transthoracic echocardiography (2DTTE). 3DTTE assessment of tricuspid stenosis (TS) has been demonstrated to yield accurate tricuspid valve areas in several case reports [2,3].

We evaluated our experience in assessing tricuspid valve pathology in 29 patients referred to our laboratory and studied with 2D- and 3DTTE using either a Philips 7500 or iE33 (Philips Medical Systems, Inc., Andover, MA) ultrasound system [3]. 3DTTE permitted us to view an *en face* short-axis view of the tricuspid valve, which we confirmed to be almost impossible by 2DTTE (Figure 6.1). The 3DTTE dataset could be cropped to view all three leaflets of the tricuspid valve from both the ventricular and atrial aspects in all patients, including the posterior tricuspid leaflet that is sometimes difficult to characterize with 2DTTE. We were able to perform direct planimetry of the tricuspid valve orifice area in patients with TS. By cropping from the ventricular aspect in a plane that was exactly parallel to the tricuspid valve orifice, a short-axis or *en face* view of the flow-limiting orifice was confidently imaged. Direct planimetry of the orifice area in the maximal systolic frame in two patients yielded measures consistent with mild TS (Figures 6.2a and 6.2b).

Tricuspid regurgitation

Far more common than TS, tricuspid regurgitation (TR) may result from a number of clinical conditions [4]. Valve restriction by rheumatic processes can result in areas of noncoaptation that are visible with *en face* B-mode 3DTTE imaging of the tricuspid valve in systole (Figures 6.2c and 6.2d).

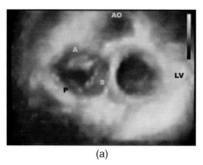

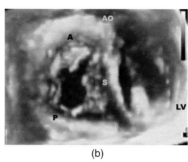

(a)

(b)

Figure 6.1 Live/real time 3D transthoracic echocardiography. Three leaflets of the tricuspid valve. (a, b) *En face* views in two different patients showing all three tricuspid valve leaflets in the open position. In Movie clip TV1 6.1, the septal tricuspid leaflet is adjacent to the ventricular septum. A, anterior leaflet; AO, aorta; LV, left ventricle; P, posterior leaflet; S, septal leaflet. Movie clip 6.1. (Reproduced from Pothineni *et al.* [3], with permission.)

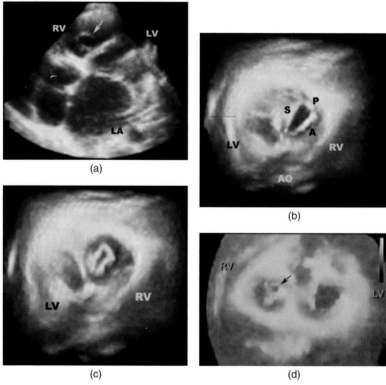

(a)

(b)

(c)

(d)

Figure 6.2 Live/real time 3D transthoracic echocardiography. Rheumatic tricuspid valve stenosis/tricuspid regurgitation. (a) The arrow points to the tricuspid orifice in a patient with tricuspid valve stenosis. The orifice area measured 2.02 cm² in diastole (also shown in Movie clip 6.2 A). (b, c) *En face* views in another patient with mild tricuspid stenosis but severe tricuspid regurgitation. The tricuspid orifice area measured 2.4 cm² in diastole (b). Systolic frame (c) shows noncoaptation of tricuspid valve leaflets. This measured 0.4 cm² in area and resulted in severe tricuspid regurgitation, as assessed by 2D color Doppler. Movie clip 6.2 B–C is from another patient with severe rheumatic mitral stenosis. The tricuspid valve in this patient is also affected with markedly restricted movement of the septal and posterior leaflets and preserved motion of the anterior leaflet. The posterior leaflet is very small and identified by its posterior location away from the left ventricular outflow tract (LVOT) in the short-axis view. Marked systolic noncoaptation of the leaflet resulted in severe tricuspid regurgitation. (d) *En face* view from the ventricular aspect showing systolic noncoaptation (arrow) of the tricuspid valve in a different patient with rheumatic heart disease. A, anterior leaflet; AO, aorta; LA, left atrium; LV, left ventricle (also shown in Movie clip 6.2 D); P, posterior leaflet; S, septal leaflet; RV, right ventricle. (Reproduced from Pothineni *et al.* [3], with permission.)

Carcinoid heart disease, usually in patients with hepatic metastases [5], also results in significant leaflet restriction, and this can be imaged with 3DTTE (Figure 6.3).

Tricuspid valve prolapse is a more common condition in which 3DTTE offers significant incremental value over 2DTTE techniques. By cropping from the atrial aspect in a plane that is parallel to the orifice to a level just above the tricuspid annulus, prolapsing segments of the tricuspid valve can be identified in systole (Figure 6.4)[4]. Prolapsing segments appear brighter or more echogenic, and can be easily identified from this *en face* image (Figures 6.4a and 6.4b). Each leaflet is arbitrarily divided into three equal segments numbered 1, 2, and 3, as demonstrated in Figure 6.4c, and tricuspid prolapse should be denoted by segment.

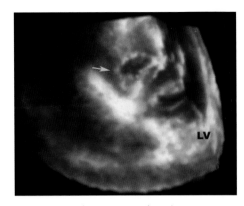

Figure 6.3 Live/real time 3D transthoracic echocardiography. Carcinoid heart disease. The arrow points to the restricted tricuspid valve orifice viewed in short axis. LV, left ventricle. Movie clip 6.3. (Reproduced from Pothineni *et al.* [3], with permission.)

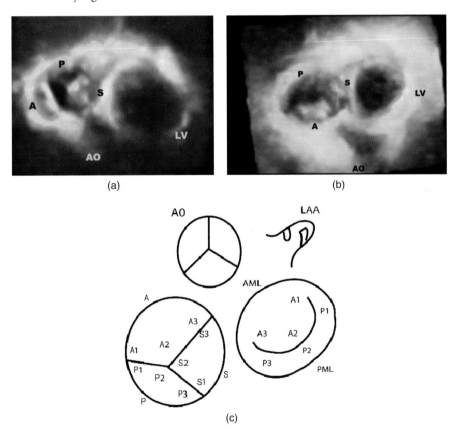

(a)

(b)

(c)

Figure 6.4 Live/real time 3D transthoracic echocardiography. Tricuspid valve prolapse. (a) *En face* view from atrial aspect showing systolic prolapse of S1, S2, A2, A3, P1, and P2 tricuspid valve segments. (b) *En face* view in another patient showing prominent systolic prolapse of A1, A2, A3, S2, and S3 tricuspid valve segments. Mild prolapse of P2 segment of tricuspid valve is also noted. (c) Schematic shows proposed division of all three tricuspid valve leaflets into three equal segments numbered 1, 2, and 3. A, anterior leaflet; AML, anterior mitral leaflet; AO, aorta; LAA, left atrial appendage; LV, left ventricle; P, posterior leaflet; PML, posterior mitral leaflet; S, septal leaflet. Movie clip 6.4A. (Reproduced from Pothineni *et al.* [3], with permission.)

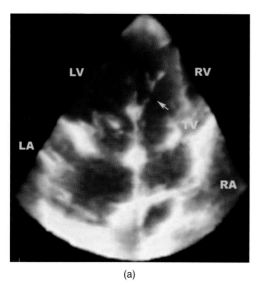

(a)

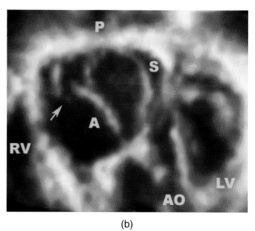

(b)

Figure 6.5 Live/real time 3D transthoracic echocardiography. Flail tricuspid valve. (a, b) The arrow points to site of chordae rupture to the anterior tricuspid valve leaflet visualized in four-chamber (a) and short-axis (b) views. In Movie clip 6.5 A Part 1, no prolapse of the anterior tricuspid leaflet is initially noted in the apical four-chamber view. Subsequent postero-anterior cropping demonstrates marked prolapse and a small dot-like hypermobile echo density in the distal right ventricle consistent with chordae rupture. Movie clip 6.5 A Part 2 shows, in addition, mobile chordal components in the right ventricle adjacent to the tricuspid valve. In Movie clip 6.5 A Part 3, the arrow points to one of the sites of chordae rupture. A, anterior leaflet; AO, aorta; LA, left atrium; LV, left ventricle; P, posterior leaflet; S, septal leaflet; RA, right atrium; RV, right ventricle. (Reproduced from Pothineni et al. [3], with permission.)

Flail tricuspid valve is an increasingly more common finding in tertiary care centers with cardiac transplant programs as an acquired defect from right ventricular biopsies, but may also be due to blunt chest trauma and myxomatous degeneration. TR from flail leaflets is a serious medical condition associated with significant excess mortality (39% at 10 years in one series) [6]. In order to accurately localize sites of individual chordae rupture in patients with flail tricuspid valves, we have found that a combination of short-axis planes and longitudinal planes with side-to-side cropping are useful (Figure 6.5) [4]. By localizing the site of rupture in a long-axis view (Figure 6.5a), quick conversion to a short axis view at that level can help to localize the site of rupture (Figure 6.5b). Similarly, 3DTTE has been found helpful in the comprehensive assessment of tricuspid papillary muscle rupture (Figures 6.6–6.8) [3,7,8].

Severe TR can also result from endocarditis of the tricuspid valve (Figure 6.9) [4,9]. Our initial report of this important tricuspid valve pathol-

ogy was from cropping of a dataset acquired from the right parasternal window (Figure 6.9a) [9]. Affected leaflets containing echogenic material and associated abscess can be accurately identified with 3DTTE (Figures 6.9b and 6.9c and Figure 6.10), often obviating the need for a TEE in this condition.

Besides delineating the etiology of TR, the addition of color Doppler to 3DTTE imaging offers the ability to quantify TR through measurements of vena contracta area (VCA) [10]. From an apically acquired dataset, the optimal TR jet is visualized in its long axis by postero-anterior cropping (Figure 6.11a). Next, the dataset is cropped from the top to the level of the vena contracta, or its narrowest portion, using a cropping plane that is exactly perpendicular to the regurgitant jet (Figure 6.11b). The image is then tilted en face (Figure 6.11c), and the previously cropped postero-anterior data are added back to visualize the vena contracta (Figure 6.11d). Using video planimetry, QLAB, or TomTec software packages (TomTec, Inc., Munich, Germany), the vena contracta can be quantified and essentially

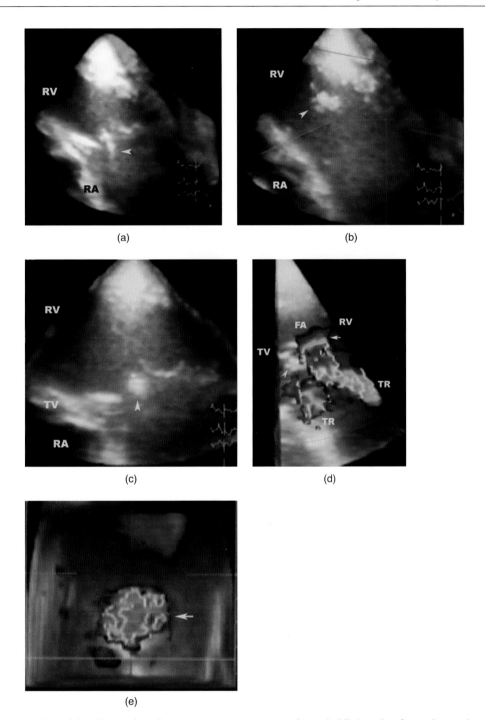

(a)

(b)

(c)

(d)

(e)

Figure 6.6 Live/real time 3D transthoracic echocardiography. Right ventricular papillary muscle rupture. (a–c) The arrowhead points to the ruptured muscle which prolapses into the right atrium (RA) in diastole. (d, e) Color Doppler examination shows a large flow acceleration (FA, arrow in (d)) as well as a large vena contracta (arrow in (e)) viewed *en face* and measuring 1.0 cm^2 in area indicative of very severe tricuspid regurgitation (TR) [8] . The arrowhead in (d) points to the prolapsing papillary muscle. RV, right ventricle; TV, tricuspid valve. Movie clip 6.6. (Reproduced from Pothineni *et al.* [3], with permission.)

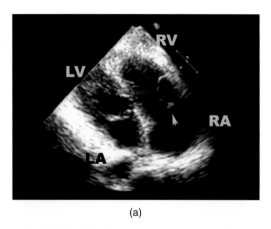

(a)

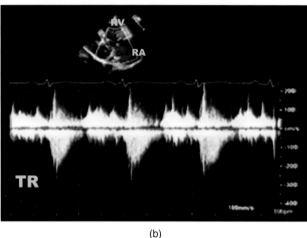

(b)

Figure 6.7 Traumatic tricuspid papillary muscle and chordae rupture. 2D transthoracic echocardiography. (a) The arrow points to the ruptured anterior papillary muscle which has prolapsed into the right atrium. (b) Continuous wave Doppler interrogation of the tricuspid regurgitation jet showing a "V"-shaped slightly concave spectral waveform consistent with severe tricuspid regurgitation. The peak velocity is only 2.2 m/s indicative of absence of pulmonary hypertension. LA, left atrium; LV, left ventricle; RA, right atrium; RV, right ventricle; TR, tricuspid regurgitation. Movie clip 6.7. (Reproduced from Reddy et al. [7], with permission.)

represents the "hole" in the valve. It is important to note that this "hole" takes a form that represents the complex geometry of the trileaflet valve, as was demonstrated by us (Figures 6.11e and 6.11f). This is particularly notable since many of the 2D measures of TR severity rely upon geometric assumptions of a circular or elliptical shape. Evaluation of the 3D architecture of the TR jet has led to the realization that many of these assumptions are fraught with error.

Despite the shortcomings of the 2D measures of TR, 3D measurements of TR VCA do correlate well with the time-honored indices of TR severity [10]. 3D VCA agrees with 2D measurements of maximum tricuspid regurgitant jet area (RJA) to right atrial area (RAA) (Figure 6.12) and to measurements of RJA alone (Figure 6.13). Using the time-honored criteria of RJA to RAA of greater than

35% and RJA >10 cm^2, we demonstrated ability to discern severity of TR in the 93 patients studied by us (Figures 6.14 and 6.15). As further evidence suggests that 2D evaluation may inadequately appreciate the complex geometry of the TR vena contracta, calculations of VCA from 2D measures of vena contracta width correlated poorly with the actual 3D VCA measurements (Figure 6.16). Our experience suggested the following criteria for VCA assessment of TR: <0.5 cm^2 for grade I, 0.5–0.75 cm^2 for grade II, and >0.75 cm^2 for grade III. In addition, a TR VCA that was greater than >1.0 cm^2 marked torrential TR.

Pulmonary regurgitation

The evaluation of pulmonary regurgitation (PR) is limited by the lack of a gold standard for

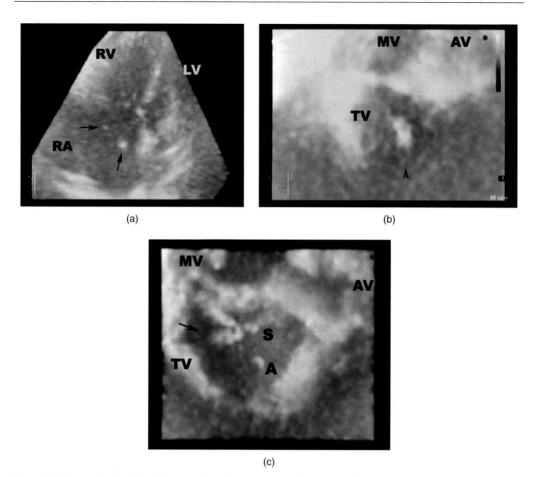

(a)

(b)

(c)

Figure 6.8 Traumatic tricuspid papillary muscle and chordae rupture. Live/real time 3D transthoracic echocardiography. (a) The vertical arrow points to the ruptured anterior papillary muscle in the right atrium. The horizontal arrow points to a ruptured chord imaged in the right atrium. In Movie clip 6.8 A , the lower arrowhead points to the ruptured papillary muscle and the upper arrowhead to a ruptured chord. (b) *En face* view of the ruptured anterior papillary muscle (arrowhead). In Movie clip 6.8 B, the vertical arrowhead shows a site of papillary muscle rupture in the right ventricle and the horizontal arrow points to a ruptured head in the right atrium. The horizontal arrowhead identifies a ruptured chord in the right atrium. (c) *En face* view of the tricuspid valve showing a flail posterior tricuspid valve leaflet (arrow in the figure and arrowhead in Movie clip 6.8 C). A, anterior tricuspid leaflet; AV, aortic valve; LV, left ventricle; MV, mitral valve; RA, right atrium; RV, right ventricle; S, septal tricuspid leaflet; TV, tricuspid valve. (Reproduced from Reddy *et al.* [7], with permission.)

assessing its severity [11]. Invasive angiography has been used for the quantification of PR, but since the catheter lies across the valve, the severity of PR is not accurate [11,12]. With this limitation in mind, the assessment of PR severity using color Doppler 2DTTE has been shown to correlate well with the severity of PR on angiography [13]. The most common assessment of PR severity using 2DTTE has utilized similar criteria to those used for aortic regurgitation (discussed at length in Chapter 5) ac-

knowledging the difference in pressures between the two situations [14–16]. Essentially, severe PR is diagnosed when the proximal PR jet width (which corresponds to the vena contracta of the aortic regurgitation jet) is more than 65% of the right ventricular outflow tract. The corresponding ratios for mild, moderate, moderately severe and severe PR are <25%, 25–46%, and 47–64% and greater than 65% [14–16]. However, since the geometry of the vena contracta is complex and not circular or

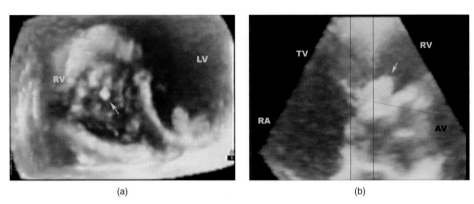

(a)   (b)

Figure 6.9 Live/real time 3D transthoracic echocardiography. Tricuspid valve endocarditis. (a) The arrow points to a vegetation on the tricuspid valve viewed in short axis. No echolucencies were noted on sectioning the vegetation. (b) The arrow shows a large abscess at the junction of the tricuspid valve and aorta in another patient. AV, aortic valve; LV, left ventricle; RA, right atrium; RV, right ventricle; TV, tricuspid valve. Other abbreviations as in Figures 6.1–6.6. (Reproduced from Pothineni *et al.* [3], with permission.)

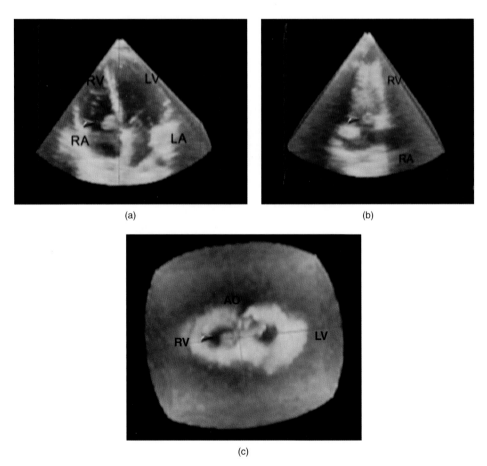

(a)   (b)

(c)

Figure 6.10 Live/real time 3D echocardiography. Tricuspid valve endocarditis. (a–c) The arrowhead shows a large vegetation attached to the septal tricuspid leaflet. Echolucent areas within the vegetation are consistent with abscess formation. AO, aorta; LA, left atrium; LV, left ventricle; RA, right atrium; RV, right ventricle. (Reproduced from Panwar *et al.*, *Echocardiography* 2007;24:272–3, with permission.)

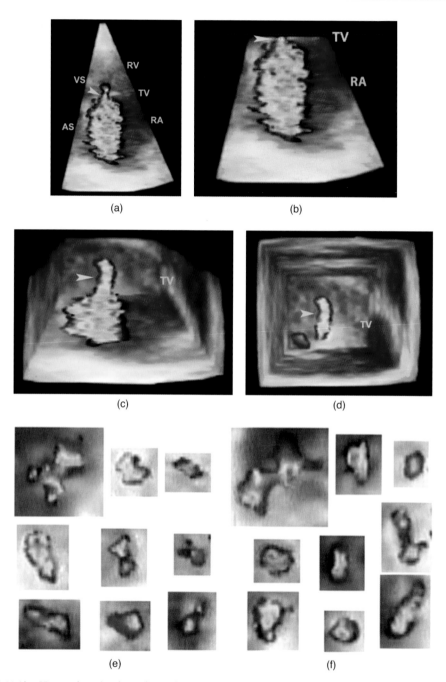

(a)

(b)

(c)

(d)

(e)

(f)

Figure 6.11 Live 3D transthoracic echocardiographic assessment of tricuspid valve (TV) regurgitation. (a) Shows optimal visualization of the TV regurgitation jet and the vena contracta (arrowhead) acquired using the apical four-chamber view. This was done by postero-anterior cropping of 3D dataset. (b) Next, the dataset was cropped from top to the level of the vena contracta. (c, d) It was then tilted *en face* and the previously cropped postero-anterior tissue data added back. Subsequently, the maximum size of the banana-shaped TV regurgitation vena contracta was planimetered. (e, f) Depict complex geometric shapes of the vena contracta in different patients with TV regurgitation. Right lower corner picture in (e) shows two individual vena contractas in same patient. AS, atrial septum; RA, right atrium; RV, right ventricle; VS, ventricular septum. Movie clips 6.11 A Part 1, 6.11 A Part 2, 6.11 B, 6.11 C. D, 6.11 D. (Reproduced from Velayudhan *et al.* [10], with permission.)

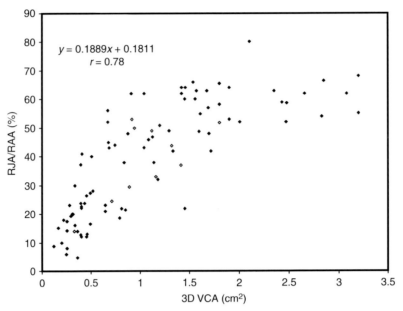

Figure 6.12 Shows correlation between percent ratio of 2D transthoracic echocardiography-derived maximum tricuspid regurgitant jet area (RJA) to right atrial area (RAA) and 3D transthoracic echocardiography-derived vena contracta area (3D VCA). Open diamonds represent patients with eccentric tricuspid regurgitant jets. (Reproduced from Velayudhan et al. [10], with permission.)

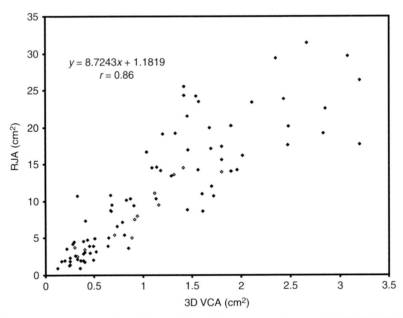

Figure 6.13 Correlation between regurgitant jet area (RJA) and 3D vena contracta area (3D VCA). (Reproduced from Velayudhan et al. [10], with permission.)

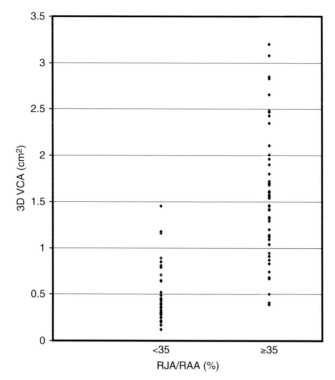

Figure 6.14 Shows percent ratio of regurgitant jet area (RJA) to right atrial area (RAA) of <35% and ≥35% plotted against 3D vena contracta area (3D VCA). (Reproduced from Velayudhan *et al*. [10], with permission.)

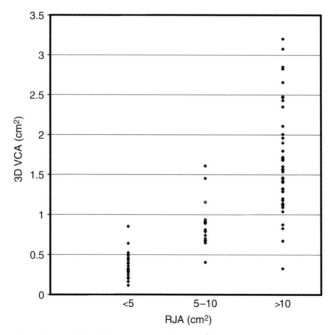

Figure 6.15 Shows regurgitant jet area (RJA) of <5, 5–10, and >10 cm² plotted against 3D vena contracta area (3D VCA). (Reproduced from Velayudhan *et al*. [10], with permission.)

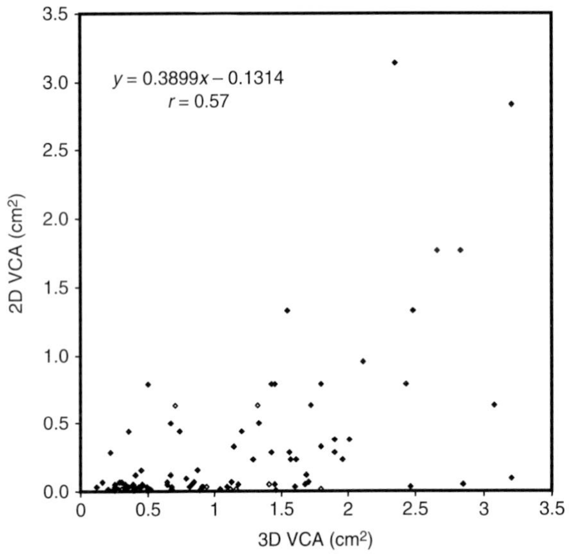

y = 0.3899x – 0.1314
r = 0.57
2D VCA (cm²)
3D VCA (cm²)
0.0
0.5
1.0
1.5
2.0
2.5
3.0
3.5
0
0.5
1
1.5
2
2.5
3
3.5

Figure 6.16 Correlation between 2D vena contracta area (2D VCA) and 3D VCA. (Reproduced from Velayudhan *et al.* [10], with permission.)

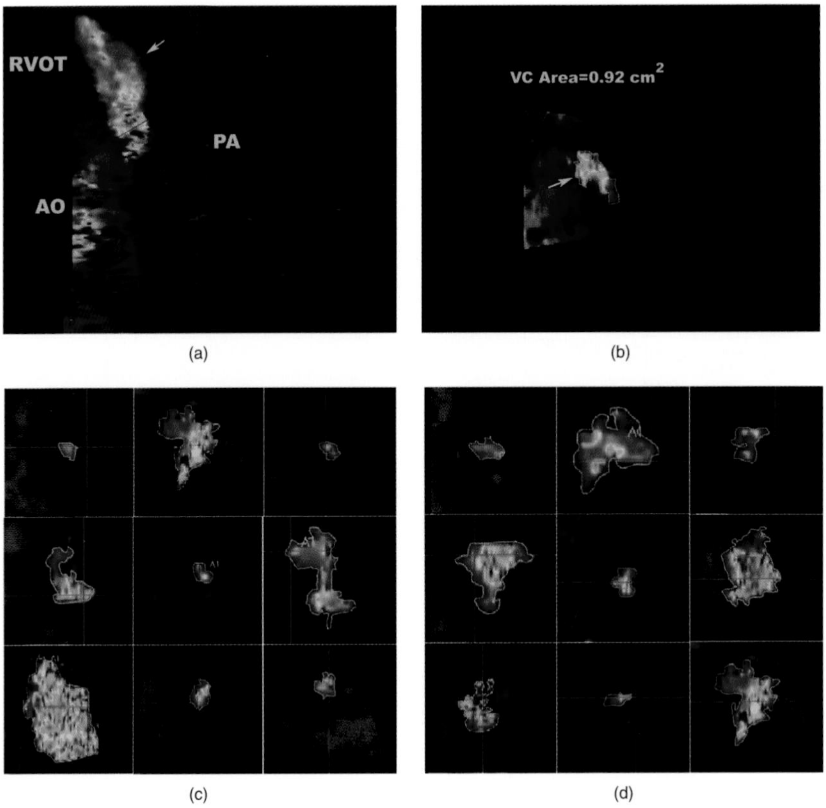

RVOT
PA
AO
(a)
VC Area=0.92 cm²
(b)
(c)
(d)

Figure 6.17 Live/real time 3D transthoracic echocardiography. (a) Shows pulmonary regurgitation (PR) jet (arrow) with the cropping plane (blue line) at the level of the vena contracta (VC) and aligned parallel to it. (b) *En face* view of the VC (arrow), which measures 0.92 cm^2 by planimetry. This is consistent with grade 3/4 PR. Movie clip 6.17 A–B Part 1 shows PR VC assessment by QLAB. Movie clip 6.17 A–B Part 2 shows the same with regular cropping. (c, d) Randomly selected VC in 18 of our patients with PR. Note the complex geometric shapes. AO, aorta; PA, main pulmonary artery; RVOT, right ventricular outflow tract. (Reproduced from Pothineni *et al.* [17], with permission.)

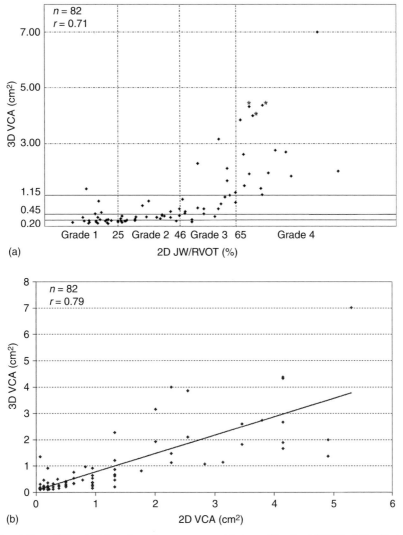

Figure 6.18 Correlation of 3D and 2D transthoracic echocardiographic findings in our patients. (a) 3D-derived vena contracta area (VCA) versus maximum proximal pulmonary regurgitation (PR) jet width (JW) to right ventricular outflow tract (RVOT) width ratio by 2D. Asterisks represent three patients who underwent pulmonary valve replacement for severe PR. (b) 3D VCA versus 2D VCA. (*Continued on next page*)

elliptical, the measurement of its area in 2D space is problematic. Furthermore, the identification of the plane at which the VCA is supposed to be measured is not straightforward, especially with cardiac motion. These limitations can be averted with 3DTTE since the dataset used for assessment can include the pulmonary valve itself as well as the full extent of the proximal portion of the PR jet area. Using cropping planes, the echocardiographer can then identify with certainty a plane parallel to the vena contracta, and with back and forth cropping position, the plane at the narrowest diameter of the regurgitant jet, and then with planimetry, the VCA (Figure 6.17) [17]. Using this feature, we studied 82 patients with at least mild PR reported on 2DTTE using a Philips iE33 (Philips Medical Systems, Inc., Andover, MA) ultrasound system and a 4-MHz matrix transducer that provides both B-mode and color Doppler 3D images. The area of the vena contracta was then palnimetered using

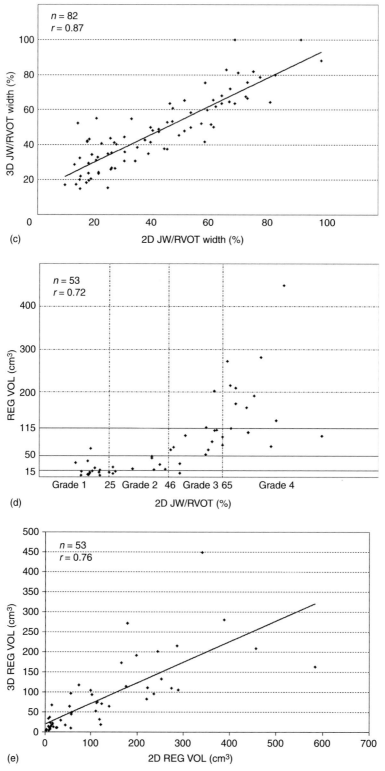

Figure 6.18 (*Continued*) (c) 3D JW to RVOT width ratio versus 2D JW to RVOT width ratio. (d) 3D regurgitant volumes (REG VOL) versus 2D JW to RVOT width ratio. (e) 3D REG VOL versus 2D REG VOL. (Reproduced from Pothineni *et al*. [17], with permission.)

QLAB version 5.0 with a B-mode gain of 5, brightness of 5, and color gain of 50 [17]. The area of the vena contracta, as measured by 3DTTE, and the calculated regurgitant volume correlated closely with 2DTTE standard measures for PR (Figure 6.18). A vena contracta area of >1.15 cm^2 corresponded to severe PR, and regurgitant volumes of <15, 15–50, 51–115, and >115 mL were effective as cutoffs for grades 1, 2, 3, and 4 PR, respectively [17]. As expected, the vena contracta had complex geometries from almost all patients (Figure 6.17). Therefore, although 3DTTE measurements of PR correlated well with 2DTTE measures, the 3DTTE are more quantitative and are theoretically more accurate than their 2DTTE counterparts [17].

References

1. Raman SV, Sparks EA, Boudoulas H, Wooley CF. Tricuspid valve disease: tricuspid valve complex perspective. *Curr Probl Cardiol* 2002;27(3):103–42.

2. Faletra F, La Marchesina U, Bragato R, De Chiara F. Three dimensional transthoracic echocardiography images of tricuspid stenosis. *Heart* 2005;91(4):499.

3. Pothineni KR, Duncan K, Yelamanchili P, *et al.* Live/real time three-dimensional transthoracic echocardiographic assessment of tricuspid valve pathology: incremental value over the two-dimensional technique. *Echocardiography* May 2007;24(5):541–52.

4. Connolly HM, Oh JK. Echocardiography. In: Libby P, Bonow RO, Mann DL, Zipes DP, eds. *Braunwald's Heart Disease: A Text Book of Cardiovascular Medicine.* 8th edn. Philadelphia: Saunders; 2007:267–79.

5. Bernheim AM, Connolly HM, Pellikka PA. Carcinoid heart disease in patients without hepatic metastases. *Am J Cardiol* 2007;99(2):292–4.

6. Messika-Zeitoun D, Thomson H, Bellamy M, *et al.* Medical and surgical outcome of tricuspid regurgitation caused by flail leaflets. *J Thorac Cardiovasc Surg* 2004;128(2):296–302.

7. Reddy VK, Nanda S, Bandarupalli N, Pothineni KR, Nanda NC. Traumatic tricuspid papillary muscle and chordae rupture: emerging role of three-dimensional echocardiography. *Echocardiography* 2008;25(6):653–7.

8. Trocino G, Salustri A, Roelandt JR, Ansink T, van Herwerden L. Three-dimensional echocardiography of a flail tricuspid valve. *J Am Soc Echocardiogr* 1996;9(1):91–3.

9. Patel V, Nanda NC, Upendram S, *et al.* Live three-dimensional right parasternal and supraclavicular transthoracic echocardiographic examination. *Echocardiography* 2005;22(4):349–60.

10. Velayudhan DE, Brown TM, Nanda NC, *et al.* Quantification of tricuspid regurgitation by live three-dimensional transthoracic echocardiographic measurements of vena contracta area. *Echocardiography* 2006;23(9):793–800.

11. Zoghbi WA, Enriquez-Sarano M, Foster E, *et al.* Recommendations for evaluation of the severity of native valvular regurgitation with two-dimensional and Doppler echocardiography. *J Am Soc Echocardiogr* 2003;16(7):777–802.

12. Bouzas B, Kilner PJ, Gatzoulis MA. Pulmonary regurgitation: not a benign lesion. *Eur Heart J* 2005;26(5):433–9.

13. Williams RV, Minich LL, Shaddy RE, Pagotto LT, Tani LY. Comparison of Doppler echocardiography with angiography for determining the severity of pulmonary regurgitation. *Am J Cardiol* 2002;89(12):1438–41.

14. Nanda NC. *Atlas of Color Doppler Echocardiography.* Philadelphia: Lea & Febiger; 1989:229–30.

15. Nanda NC. *Textbook of Color Doppler Echocardiography.* Philadelphia: Lea & Febiger; 1989:160–167.

16. Perry GJ, Helmcke F, Nanda NC, Byard C, Soto B. Evaluation of aortic insufficiency by Doppler color flow mapping. *J Am Coll Cardiol* 1987;9(4):952–9.

17. Pothineni KR, Wells BJ, Hsiung MC, *et al.* Live/real time three-dimensional transthoracic echocardiographic assessment of pulmonary regurgitation. *Echocardiography* 2008;25:911–17.

CHAPTER 7

Prosthetic Valves

Introduction

Evaluation of prosthetic valves with echocardiography has been traditionally accomplished through Doppler and 2D transthoracic echocardiographic (2DTTE) studies to characterize valve gradients, regurgitation, and leaflet movement [1]. However, mechanical prosthetic valve gradients do not consistently correlate with valve function. When we looked at valve gradients of mechanical prostheses shortly after implantation in one study, we found no significant correlation for implanted valve sizes and actual orifice areas with Doppler-measured peak and mean pressure gradients and effective orifice area due to locally high velocities found in prostheses of some patients [2]. For this reason, the most important assessment is a qualitative description of leaflet movement [3]. However, this is also often very difficult when visualized from a thin 2D plane incapable of capturing multiple leaflets and often subject to artifacts created by the valve's metallic components. Because all of the components of a mechanical prosthesis can be captured in a 3D dataset, 3D echocardiography offers incremental value in evaluating prosthetic valve function.

3D assessment of prosthetic valve function

Early investigation of 3D echocardiography demonstrated value in differentiating transvalvular from paravalvular regurgitant jets [4,5]. These studies were limited by reconstructive techniques with-

out live imaging. Using contemporary live/real time 3DTTE, a complete assessment of prosthetic valve function is possible.

In a recent series reported by us, we evaluated with 3DTTE 31 patients who had a mechanical, bioprosthetic, or homograft prosthetic valve and correlated the findings with 2DTTE, TEE, and surgery [6]. These valvular prostheses included 14 St. Jude mechanical prostheses and 4 bioprostheses in the mitral position; 4 St. Jude mechanical prostheses, 4 bioprostheses, and 6 homografts in the aortic position; and 1 St. Jude mechanical prosthesis and 2 bioprostheses in the tricuspid position. In almost all patients, 3DTTE added incremental information to that obtained by the 2DTTE examination. While 2DTTE was able to visualize both leaflets of mechanical prosthetic valves in only a small minority of patients, with 3DTTE it was possible to crop the dataset in such a way as to observe both leaflets simultaneously. This greatly increased the confidence level of the echocardiographer that indeed both leaflets were seen in normally functioning valves, and also detected abnormal motion in prosthetic valves missed by 2DTTE [6]. With the systemic cropping of the 3D dataset, a more comprehensive examination could be performed, which led to a more robust identification and localization of thrombi in addition to the visualization of clot lysis when the thrombi were cropped open, as detailed elsewhere in this book. In prosthetic valves affected by endocarditis, 3DTTE proved to be very useful, not only in identifying vegetations missed by 2DTTE, but also in detailing the extent of the

Live/Real Time 3D Echocardiography, 1st edition.
By Navin C. Nanda, Ming Chon Hsiung, Andrew P. Miller, and Fadi G. Hage. Published 2010 by Blackwell Publishing Ltd.

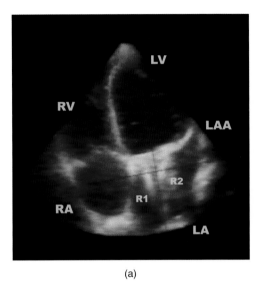

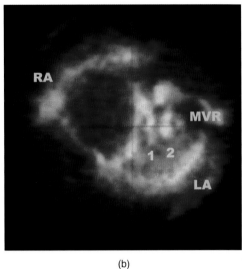

(a)   (b)

Figure 7.1 Live/real time 3D transthoracic echocardiographic assessment of St. Jude mitral prosthesis. QLAB analysis. (a) Apical four-chamber view. R1 and R2 represent reverberations from the two leaflets of mitral valve replacement (MVR) in the open position. (b) Short-axis view showing the two leaflets numbered 1 and 2. Movie clips 7.1 Parts 1–4 demonstrate normal opening and closing movement of MVR. The arrowhead in Part 2 points to the prosthetic valve imaged in short axis. Parts 3 and 4 show cropping of the 3D dataset to comprehensively examine the prosthetic valve and its reverberations which serve as surrogates of prosthetic leaflet motion. Cropping of the left atrial appendage reveals no clots. LA, left atrium; LAA, left atrial appendage; LV, left ventricle; RA, right atrium; RV, right ventricle. (Reproduced from Singh *et al.* [6], with permission.)

vegetative process and quantifying the volume of vegetations. 3DTTE was also superior to 2DTTE in revealing complications of endocarditis, such as abscess formations, fistulas, and paravalvular regurgitation. In patients with regurgitation, 3DTTE provided essential information related to the severity of the regurgitant jet as well as identifying the cause of regurgitation such as a flail leaflet or perforations (Figures 7.1–7.12).

In summary, 3D echocardiography provides incremental value in assessing prosthetic valve function and associated pathology since it offers: (1) superior differentiation of transvalvular versus paravalvular regurgitation and quantification of regurgitation severity [7–9], (2) simultaneous visualization of multiple leaflets, which is especially useful in the case of mechanical prostheses, and (3) complete visualization of the valve apparatus through systematic cropping [6]. The ability to view the live motion of each valve leaflet overcomes past difficulties created by locally created high velocities in prostheses that may lead to inaccurate characterization of normally functioning valves [2]. Further, 3D echocardiography provides live images that can be tilted and cropped to detect pathologic lesions, such as thrombus and vegetations on valve leaflets/apparatus, and localize their exact attachment points and size. Taken together, 3D echocardiography provides a comprehensive view of prosthetic valves that greatly enhances our ability to characterize their function and diagnose pathologic changes.

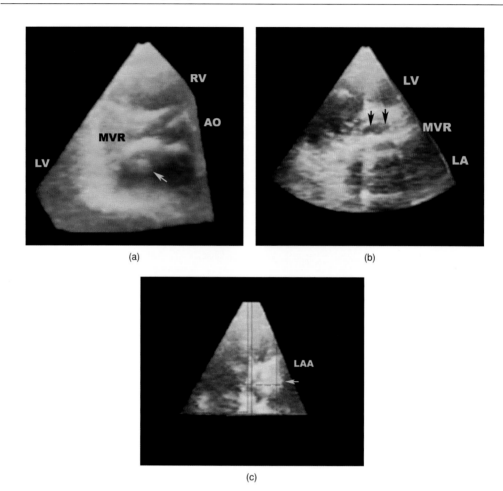

(a)

(b)

(c)

Figure 7.2 Live/real time 3D transthoracic echocardiographic assessment of St. Jude mitral prosthesis. (a) The arrow points to a large thrombus on the atrial aspect of mitral valve replacement (MVR). (b) The arrows point to two thrombi on the ventricular aspect. (c) The arrow points to a thrombus in the left atrial appendage (LAA). Movie clips 7.2 Part 1–3. The arrowheads in Movie clip 7.2 Part 1 show thrombi on the atrial aspect of the prosthesis. The arrowhead in Movie clip 7.2 Part 2 denotes an irregular thrombus with some mobility in the left atrial appendage. Movie clip 7.2 Part 3 shows virtually no motion of the prosthetic valve, only ring motion. AO, aorta; LA, left atrium; LAA, left atrial appendage; LV, left ventricle; RV, right ventricle; R,reverberations from MVR. (Reproduced from Singh *et al.* [6], with permission.)

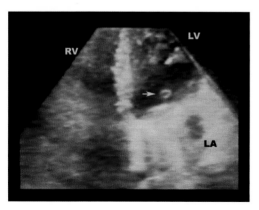

Figure 7.3 Live/real time 3D transthoracic echocardiographic assessment of St. Jude mitral prosthesis. The arrow (arrowhead in Movie clip 7.3) points to a thrombus on the ventricular aspect of mitral valve replacement (MVR) showing prominent central lysis. LA, left atrium; LV, left ventricle; RV, right ventricle (Reproduced from Singh *et al.* [6], with permission.)

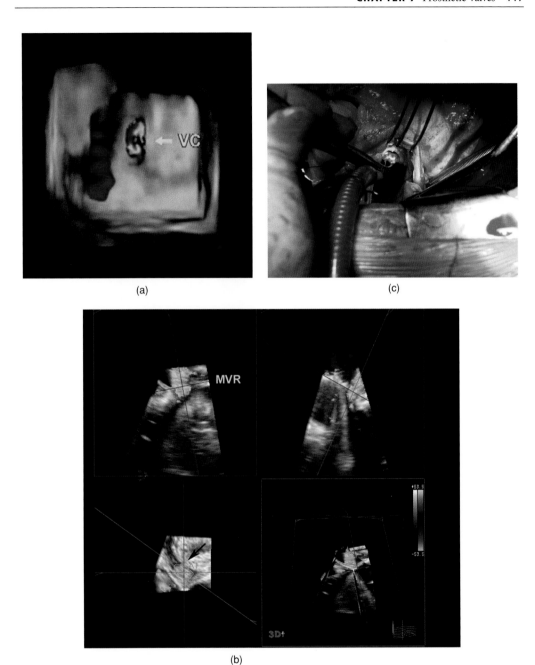

(a)

(c)

(b)

Figure 7.4 Live/real time 3D transthoracic echocardiographic assessment of St. Jude mitral prosthesis. (a, b) The arrow points to the vena contracta (VC) of paravalvular mitral regurgitation (MR) viewed *en face* using regular cropping (a) and QLAB analysis package (b). (c) Paravalvular defect seen at surgery. The arrows in the movie clips point to paravalvular MR. Movie clips 7.4 Part 1–3 show cropping for VC. Movie clips 7.4 Part 4 and 7.4 Part 5 show localization of MR (arrow) just below the aortic valve (AV) at 12 o'clock position. MVR, mitral valve replacement. (Reproduced from Singh *et al.* [6], with permission.)

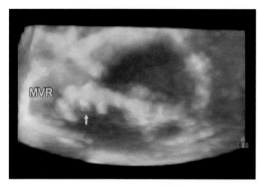

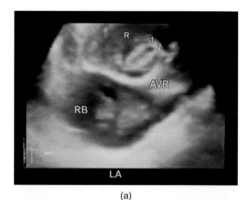

(a)

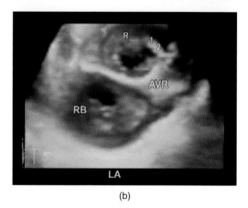

(b)

Figure 7.5 Live/real time 3D transthoracic echocardiographic assessment of tissue mitral prosthesis. The arrow points to a tear in one of the leaflets of mitral valve replacement (MVR), which is prolapsing into left atrium (LA). Movie clips 7.5 Part 1–3. AV, aortic valve. (Reproduced from Singh *et al.* [6], with permission.)

Figure 7.7 Live/real time 3D transthoracic echocardiographic assessment of St. Jude aortic prosthesis. (a, b) 1 and 2 represent two leaflets of aortic valve replacement (AVR) shown in the open (a) and closed (b) positions viewed from the aortic aspect. LA, left atrium; R, prosthetic ring; RB, reverberations from AVR. Movie clip 7.7.

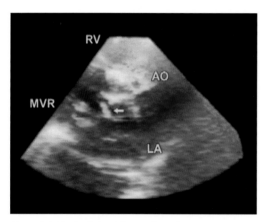

Figure 7.6 Live/real time 3D transthoracic echocardiographic assessment of tissue mitral prosthesis. The arrow points to a portion of mitral valve replacement (MVR) which shows rocking motion (see Movie clip 7.6 Part 1). Movie clips 7.6 Part 2 and 7.6 Part 3 show dehiscence and prominent rocking motion (arrow) of MVR viewed *en face*. Movie clip 7.6 Part 4 shows 2D transthoracic rocking motion of the medial portion of MVR and mitral regurgitation (MR). AO, aorta; LA, left atrium; RV, right ventricle. (Reproduced from Singh *et al.* [6], with permission.)

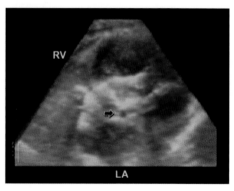

Figure 7.8 Live/real time 3D transthoracic echocardiographic assessment of St. Jude aortic prosthesis. The arrow points to severe aortic valve replacement (AVR) stenosis. The dataset was cropped to view the prosthesis *en face*. LA, left atrium; RV, right ventricle. (Reproduced from Singh *et al.* [6], with permission.)

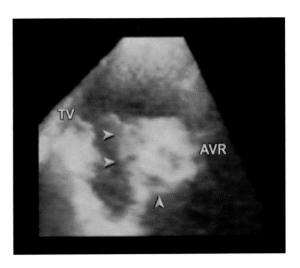

Figure 7.9 Live/real time 3D transthoracic echocardiographic assessment of St. Jude aortic prosthesis. The arrowheads point to multiple abscess cavities involving aortic valve replacement (AVR). The arrowhead in Movie clip 7.9 Part 1 points to AVR vegetation prolapsing into left ventricular outflow tract in the same patient. The arrowhead in Movie clip 7.9 Part 2 shows an abscess cavity communicating with right atrium. The arrowhead in Movie clip 7.9 Part 3 points to a fistulous communication between AVR and right atrium just beneath the tricuspid valve and above the one shown in Part 2. TV, tricuspid valve. (Reproduced from Singh *et al.* [6], with permission.)

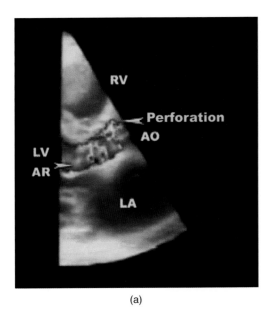

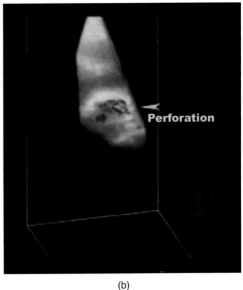

(a)

(b)

Figure 7.10 Live/real time 3D transthoracic echocardiographic assessment of homograft aortic prosthesis. (a) The upper arrowhead points to a perforation in the aortic valve. The lower arrowhead denotes severe aortic regurgitation (AR). Color Doppler signals fill the whole extent of proximal left ventricular outflow tract in diastole. (b) *En face* view of the large perforation. AO, aorta; LA, left atrium; LV, left ventricle; RV, right ventricle.. Movie clips 7.10 Part 1 and 7.10 Part 2. (Reproduced from Singh *et al.* [6], with permission.)

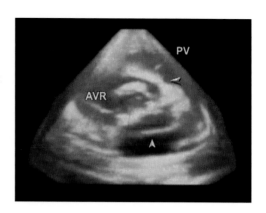

Figure 7.11 Live/real time 3D transthoracic echocardiographic assessment of homograft aortic prosthesis. The arrowheads point to a large echo-free space around aortic valve replacement (AVR). Movie clips show a large communication (arrow) from the prosthesis into the echo-free space posteriorly consistent with pseudoaneurysm found at surgery. Note rocking motion of the posterior aspect of the prosthesis. PV, pulmonary valve. Other abbreviations as in previous figures. Movie clips 7.11 Part 1 and 7.11 Part 2. (Reproduced from Singh *et al.* [6], with permission.)

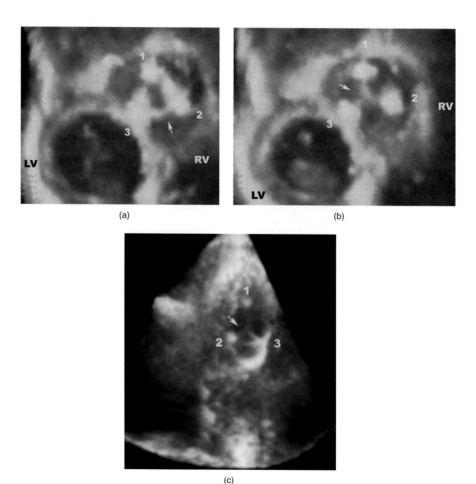

(a)

(b)

(c)

Figure 7.12 Live/real time 3D transthoracic echocardiography. Tricuspid valve prosthesis. (a, b) Normal bioprosthetic tricuspid valve leaflets (arrow) seen in open (a) and closed (b) positions. Numbers 1, 2, and 3 represent the three struts of the prosthetic valve. (c) The arrow shows systolic noncoaptation of the leaflets in another patient with a bioprosthesis. LV, left ventricle; RV, right ventricle. Movie clip 7.12. (Reproduced from Singh *et al.* [6], with permission.)

References

1. Seiler C. Management and follow up of prosthetic heart valves. *Heart* 2004;90(7):818–24.
2. Keser N, Nanda NC, Miller AP, *et al.* Hemodynamic evaluation of normally functioning Sulzer Carbomedics prosthetic valves. *Ultrasound Med Biol* 2003;29(5):649–57.
3. Muratori M, Montorsi P, Teruzzi G, *et al.* Feasibility and diagnostic accuracy of quantitative assessment of mechanical prostheses leaflet motion by transthoracic and transesophageal echocardiography in suspected prosthetic valve dysfunction. *Am J Cardiol* 2006;97(1):94–100.
4. Li Z, Wang X, Xie M, Nanda NC, Hsiung MC. Dynamic three-dimensional reconstruction of abnormal intracardiac blood flow. *Echocardiography* 1997;14(4):375–82.
5. Ansingkar K, Nanda NC, Aaluri SR, *et al.* Transesophageal three-dimensional color Doppler echocardiographic assessment of valvular and paravalvular mitral prosthetic regurgitation. *Echocardiography* 2000;17(6 Pt 1):579–83.
6. Singh P, Inamdar V, Hage FG, Karakus G, Suwanjutah T, Hsiung MC, Nanda NC. Usefulness of live/real time three-dimensional transthoracic echocardiography in evaluation of prosthetic valve function. *Echocardiography* 2009;26:1236–49.
7. Khanna D, Vengala S, Miller AP, *et al.* Quantification of mitral regurgitation by live three-dimensional transthoracic echocardiographic measurements of vena contracta area. *Echocardiography* 2004;21(8):737–43.
8. Fang L, Hsiung MC, Miller AP, *et al.* Assessment of aortic regurgitation by live three-dimensional transthoracic echocardiographic measurements of vena contracta area: usefulness and validation. *Echocardiography* 2005;22(9):775–81.
9. Velayudhan DE, Brown TM, Nanda NC, *et al.* Quantification of tricuspid regurgitation by live three-dimensional transthoracic echocardiographic measurements of vena contracta area. *Echocardiography* 2006;23(9):793–800.

CHAPTER 8

Left Ventricular and Right Ventricular Function Assessment

Introduction

The most commonly requested information from transthoracic echocardiography (TTE) is an assessment of left ventricular (LV) function. An accurate and unbiased measurement of LV ejection fraction (LVEF) is a vital component for decision-making in the practice of clinical cardiology. Traditionally, 2D and M-mode TTE (2DTTE) has been the primary noninvasive imaging modality, but it is limited by observer variability, reliance on geometric modeling, and foreshortening [1,2]. Since the early reports using rotational reconstruction methods, 3DTTE has shown potential for overcoming these limitations [3–5]. These pioneering studies bloomed into wider applications of 3DTTE with the advent of live/real time imaging coupled to online image analysis software. Numerous contemporary series have now been published that demonstrate the added value of live/real time 3DTTE in assessing LV function, volumes, and mass [1,6–17]. In addition, 3DTTE has been applied to right ventricular (RV) function and volumes with success [7,18,19]. While many of the tools to assess function and volume are now built into the online software packages, some attention to pitfalls and spatial techniques is still needed.

Left ventricular function

Since 3DTTE permits quick acquisition of a dynamic pyramidal dataset that encompasses the en-

tire left ventricle, it offers direct assessment of LV function, volume, and mass without the need for plane selection or geometric modeling. Online software packages, such as QLAB, as well as offline processing with the TomTec Echoview (TomTec, Inc., Munich, Germany) permit rapid determination of LV function, volumes, and mass. Numerous investigators have compared results of 3DTTE with 2DTTE demonstrating superior performance of 3DTTE when compared with 2DTTE and similar accuracy when compared with other 3D noninvasive imaging modalities such as computed tomography (CT) or magnetic resonance imaging (MRI).

Using real time 3DTTE datasets acquired on a Philips 7500 system (Philips Medical Systems, Inc., Andover, MA) and offline processing with the 4D-LV Analysis software (TomTec Imaging systems GmbH, Unterschleissheim, Germany), Sugeng *et al.* demonstrated correlation for 3DTTE measurements of LVEF that were superior to cardiac CT measurements, when compared with cardiac MRI measurements as a reference standard [12]. In 31 patients, 3DTTE measures of LVEF showed no significant bias (+0.3%; $p = 0.68$) when compared with cardiac MRI measures, while cardiac CT significantly underestimated LVEF (by −2.8%). Likewise, 3DTTE demonstrated superior volume measurements, underestimating end-diastolic and end-systolic volumes only slightly (by 5 and 6 mL, respectively), while cardiac CT significantly overestimated end-diastolic and end-systolic volumes (by 26 and 19 mL, respectively). Observer input is yet required with 3DTTE, and it did demonstrate its observer bias, however, with roughly twofold variability in interobserver measurements when compared with cardiac CT.

Live/Real Time 3D Echocardiography, 1st edition.
By Navin C. Nanda, Ming Chon Hsiung, Andrew P. Miller, and Fadi G. Hage. Published 2010 by Blackwell Publishing Ltd.

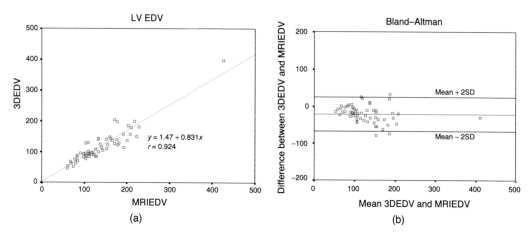

Figure 8.1 (a, b) Comparison of 3D echocardiographic and magnetic resonance imaging (MRI)-derived measures of left ventricular end-diastolic volumes (LV EDV). (Reproduced from Qi *et al*. [16], with permission.)

We reported our experience in a series of 58 patients with diverse cardiac disorders and clinical characteristics, who underwent both cardiac MRI and 3DTTE evaluations [16]. A full-volume apical scan using the Philips iE33 echocardiographic system (Philips Medical Systems, Inc., Andover, MA) was evaluated offline with the TomTec Echoview version 5.2 (TomTec, Inc., Munich, Germany), and LV volumes, EF, and mass were calculated with comparison to cardiac MRI measurements as the reference standard. In a population that included subjects with severe forms of dilated cardiomyopathy (LV end-diastolic volumes above 400 mL), correlations of LV volumes, EF, and mass between 3DTTE and MRI were very good ($r > 0.9$), with an overall

small negative bias for the 3DTTE measurements of volumes (e.g., +15 mL for LV end-systolic volume) and small positive bias for mass (+8 g). Inter- and intraobserver variability was very low in our study ($r \sim 0.95$ for all parameters assessed) (Figures 8.1–8.5). Together, these studies, and others like them, suggest that real time 3DTTE offers rapid and accurate assessment of LV volumes, EF, and mass, which overcome 2D pitfalls and closely compare to other noninvasive imaging modalities.

Right ventricular function

In addition to assessment of LV volumes and function, 3DTTE has been applied to right

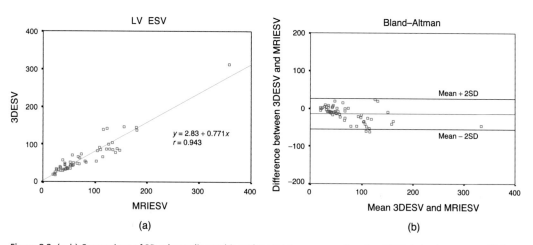

Figure 8.2 (a, b) Comparison of 3D echocardiographic and magnetic resonance imaging (MRI)-derived measures of left ventricular end-systolic volumes (LV ESV). (Reproduced from Qi *et al*. [16], with permission.)

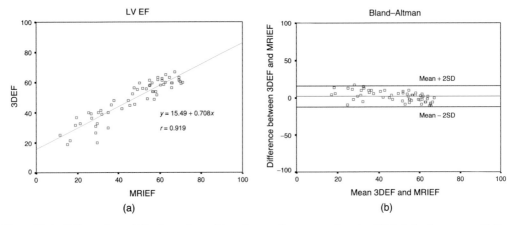

Figure 8.3 (a, b) Comparison of 3D echocardiographic and magnetic resonance imaging (MRI)-derived measures of left ventricular ejection fraction (LVEF). (Reproduced from Qi *et al.* [16], with permission.)

ventricular (RV) volumes and function [7,18,19]. Prakasa *et al.* studied 58 patients [23 with arrhythmogenic right ventricular dysplasia (ARVD), 20 first-degree relatives with no ARVD, 8 with idiopathic ventricular tachycardia, and 7 healthy volunteers] using the Philips 7500 or iE33 ultrasound system (Philips Medical Systems, Inc., Andover, MA) and an offline TomTec workstation (TomTec, Inc., Munich, Germany) to assess RV volumes and EFs [18]. Compared with cardiac MRI-derived measures as a reference standard, there were good correlations for real time 3DTTE-derived measures of RVEF ($r = 0.88$; $p < 0.001$), RV end-systolic volume ($r = 0.72$; $p < 0.0001$), and RV end-diastolic volume ($r = 0.50$; $p < 0.0001$), with intra- and interobserver differences for EF and end-diastolic

volume of less than 3% and 3 mL, respectively. While this evaluation is not currently integrated into the QLAB analysis software, the potential for online RV analysis is appealing in its application to disease processes such as ARVD, but also as a prognostic index or indicator for surgical interventions in patients with other cardiac disorders. Movie clips parts 6 and 7 in Figure 8.5 demonstrate the technique for estimation of RV volumes and EF using a recently developed offline method.

Techniques and applications

Online and offline processing permits quick and accurate assessment of ventricular volumes and function from a single apically acquired 3DTTE dataset

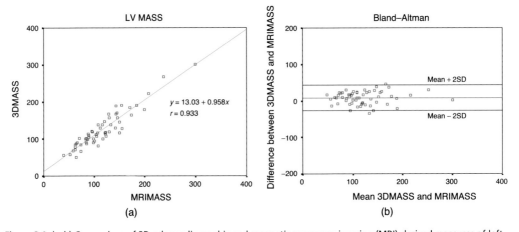

Figure 8.4 (a, b) Comparison of 3D echocardiographic and magnetic resonance imaging (MRI)-derived measures of left ventricular mass (LV MASS). (Reproduced from Qi *et al.* [16], with permission.)

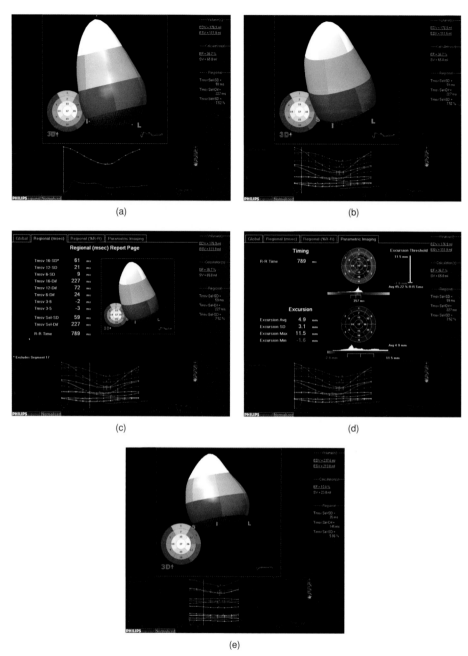

(a)

(b)

(c)

(d)

(e)

Figure 8.5 Live/real time 3D transthoracic echocardiographic assessment of left (LV) and right ventricular (RV) function. (a) Shows global function in this patient. The LV end-diastolic volume (EDV) was 176.9 mL, end-systolic volume (ESV) 111.9 mL, stroke volume (SV) 65.0 mL, and ejection fraction (EF) 36.7%. (b) Shows segmental volume curves in the same patient. (c) Standard deviations from different segment groups are given and help in the assessment of cardiac dyssynchrony. (d) Shows parametric imaging maps. (e) Demonstrates very poor left ventricular function in another patient. The SV is 23.8 mL and ejection fraction 10.0%. Movie clip 8.5 Part 1 shows steps in the assessment of LV function using QLAB. The EF is in the range of 37%. Movie clip 8.5 Part 2 from another patient shows EF of 27.5%. Movie clip 8.5 Part 3 shows normal left ventricular EF. Calculation of left ventricular mass is also demonstrated. Movie clip 8.5 Part 4 shows evaluation of LV function in a different patient using an offline TomTec software. Movie clip 8.5 Part 5 demonstrates assessment of RV volumes and EF using the same QLAB technique as LV. RV EDV was measured as 148.0 mL, ESV 119.4 mL, and EF 20%. Movie clips 8.5 Part 6 and 8.5 Part 7 demonstrate the technique for assessment of RV volumes and EF using a newly developed TomTec software. IN, right ventricular inflow; LV, left ventricle; OUT, right ventricular outflow tract; RV, right ventricle. (Courtesy of Bernhard Mumm, TomTec Imaging Systems GmbH, Unterschleissheim, Germany.)

(Figure 8.5). Sequential processing for the LV is performed as follows:

1 The apically acquired dataset is imported into an online or offline software package.

2 First, the apex is defined in order to assure no foreshortening. This is easily accomplished by playing the image and manipulating the longitudinal cropping planes until the largest ventricular dimensions are created. If the apex was not captured, which occurs not infrequently with ventricular dilatation, the dataset should be re-acquired using a standoff applied to the chest wall. End-diastolic and end-systolic frames should then be identified by playing the clip frame by frame.

3 Second, from the end-diastolic frame, the mitral annulus is defined in four planes and the apex is selected from either longitudinal view. Orientation to the septum may also need to be selected.

4 Next, the imaging software's border detection fills in an estimate of end-diastolic volume. This may require editing, but often is capable of accurately depicting segments with low echo signal or "dropout." In order to ensure that border detection was accurate, it is helpful to pan from apex to base in the short-axis plane, watching the endocardium. The end-diastolic volume can be edited after automatic acquisition, but care should be given toward creating segment deformation that will contaminate segmental analysis.

5 The process is then repeated for the end-systolic frame of selecting basal and apical borders, and then assessing accuracy and editing, as in steps 3 and 4.

6 Once the end-diastolic and end-systolic frames are properly defined, segmental analysis is accomplished automatically and accurate volumes, EF, and segmental contraction are obtained.

Since 3DTTE obviates use of geometric assumptions, ensures inclusion of the apex, and directly detects segmental motion, these processing techniques provide reliable assessment for clinical applications, including stress echocardiography, cardiac resynchronization therapy, and critical decisions for defibrillator therapy. 3DTTE can also be used to assess LV dyssynchrony in patients with heart failure in order to guide resynchronization therapy [20–23]. Moreover, newer applications have been generated to assess RV volume and function.

References

1. Jenkins C, Bricknell K, Hanekom L, Marwick TH. Reproducibility and accuracy of echocardiographic measurements of left ventricular parameters using real-time three-dimensional echocardiography. *J Am Coll Cardiol* 2004;44:878–86.

2. Lang RM, Mor-Avi V, Sugeng L, Nieman PS, Sahn DJ. Three-dimensional echocardiography: the benefits of the additional dimension. *J Am Coll Cardiol* 2006;48:2053–69.

3. Ghosh A, Nanda NC, Maurer G. Three-dimensional reconstruction of echo-cardiographic images using the rotation method. *Ultrasound Med Biol* 1982;8:655–61.

4. Gopal AS, Schnellbaecher MJ, Shen Z, Boxt LM, Katz J, King DL. Freehand three-dimensional echocardiography for determination of left ventricular volume and mass in patients with abnormal ventricles: comparison with magnetic resonance imaging. *J Am Soc Echocardiogr* 1997;10:853–61.

5. Mele D, Maehle J, Pedini I, Alboni P, Levine RA. Three-dimensional echocardiographic reconstruction: description and applications of a simplified technique for quantitative assessment of left ventricular size and function. *Am J Cardiol* 1998;81:107G–110G.

6. Kuhl HP, Schreckenberg M, Rulands D, et al. High-resolution transthoracic real-time three-dimensional echocardiography: quantitation of cardiac volumes and function using semi-automatic border detection and comparison with cardiac magnetic resonance imaging. *J Am Coll Cardiol* 2004;43:2083–90.

7. Yang Y, Wang XF, Xie MX, Wang J. Real-time three-dimensional echocardiography in assessment of left ventricular and right ventricular volumes. *Chin Med Sci J* 2004;19:236.

8. Caiani EG, Corsi C, Zamorano J, et al. Improved semi-automated quantification of left ventricular volumes and ejection fraction using 3-dimensional echocardiography with a full matrix-array transducer: comparison with magnetic resonance imaging. *J Am Soc Echocardiogr* 2005;18:779–88.

9. Corsi C, Coon P, Goonewardena S, et al. Quantification of regional left ventricular wall motion from real-time 3-dimensional echocardiography in patients with poor acoustic windows: effects of contrast enhancement tested against cardiac magnetic resonance. *J Am Soc Echocardiogr* 2006;19:886–93.

10. Smith SC, Jr., Feldman TE, Hirshfeld JW, Jr., et al. ACC/AHA/SCAI 2005 guideline update for percutaneous coronary intervention: a report of the American College of Cardiology/American Heart Association Task

Force on Practice Guidelines (ACC/AHA/SCAI Writing Committee to update 2001 Guidelines for Percutaneous Coronary Intervention). *Circulation* 2006;113:e166–286.

11. Jenkins C, Chan J, Hanekom L, Marwick TH. Accuracy and feasibility of online 3-dimensional echocardiography for measurement of left ventricular parameters. *J Am Soc Echocardiogr* 2006;19:1119–28.

12. Sugeng L, Mor-Avi V, Weinert L, *et al.* Quantitative assessment of left ventricular size and function: side-by-side comparison of real-time three-dimensional echocardiography and computed tomography with magnetic resonance reference. *Circulation* 2006;114:654–61.

13. Van Den Bosch AE, Robbers-Visser D, Krenning BJ, *et al.* Real-time transthoracic three-dimensional echocardiographic assessment of left ventricular volume and ejection fraction in congenital heart disease. *J Am Soc Echocardiogr* 2006;19:1–6.

14. Jenkins C, Bricknell K, Chan J, Hanekom L, Marwick TH. Comparison of two- and three-dimensional echocardiography with sequential magnetic resonance imaging for evaluating left ventricular volume and ejection fraction over time in patients with healed myocardial infarction. *Am J Cardiol* 2007;99:300–306.

15. Jenkins C, Leano R, Chan J, Marwick TH. Reconstructed versus real-time 3-dimensional echocardiography: comparison with magnetic resonance imaging. *J Am Soc Echocardiogr* 2007;20:862–8.

16. Qi X, Cogar B, Hsiung MC, *et al.* Live/real time three-dimensional transthoracic echocardiographic assessment of left ventricular volumes, ejection fraction, and mass compared with magnetic resonance imaging. *Echocardiography* 2007;24:166–73.

17. Mor-Avi V, Jenkins C, Kuhl HP, *et al.* Real-time 3-dimensional echocardiographic quantification of left ventricular volumes. *J Am Coll Cardiol Cardiol Img* 2008;1:413–23.

18. Prakasa KR, Dalal D, Wang J, *et al.* Feasibility and variability of three dimensional echocardiography in arrhythmogenic right ventricular dysplasia/cardiomyopathy. *Am J Cardiol* 2006;97:703–9.

19. Chen G, Sun K, Huang G. In vitro validation of right ventricular volume and mass measurement by real-time three-dimensional echocardiography. *Echocardiography* 2006;23:395–9.

20. Baker GH, Hlavacek AM, Chessa KS, Fleming DM, Shirali GS. Left ventricular dysfunction is associated with intraventricular dyssynchrony by 3-dimensional echocardiography in children. *J Am Soc Echocardiogr* 2008;21:230–233.

21. Kapetanakis S, Kearney MT, Siva A, Gall N, Cooklin M, Monaghan MJ. Real-time three-dimensional echocardiography: a novel technique to quantify global left ventricular mechanical dyssynchrony. *Circulation* 2005;112:992–1000.

22. Liodakis E, Al Sharef O, Dawson D, Nihoyannopoulos P. The use of real time three dimensional echocardiography for assessing mechanical synchronicity. *Heart* 2009;95:1865–71.

23. Soliman OI, Geleijnse ML, Theuns DA, *et al.* Usefulness of left ventricular systolic dyssynchrony by real-time three-dimensional echocardiography to predict long-term response to cardiac resynchronization therapy. *Am J Cardiol* 2009;103:1586–91.

9 CHAPTER 9

Ischemic Heart Disease

Introduction

2D transthoracic echocardiography (2DTTE) is widely used for the study of ischemic heart disease. On resting 2DTTE, myocardial infarction can be detected as wall motion abnormality, and more importantly global left ventricular function can be measured [1]. These functions serve diagnostic and prognostic roles. The sensitivity of 2DTTE for the detection of coronary artery disease has been greatly augmented with the introduction of exercise and Dobutamine stress 2DTTE [1]. Furthermore, the direct visualization of the coronary arteries with 2DTTE is possible, at least for the ostium and proximal portions of these vessels [2]. Perhaps an equally important role of echocardiography in ischemic heart disease is the detection of complications of myocardial infarction, including the development of cardiogenic shock [3,4], left ventricular aneurysm formation [5], mural left ventricular thrombus [6], cardiac rupture [7,8], ventricular septal rupture [7], ischemic mitral regurgitation (papillary muscle dysfunction or rupture or mitral annular dilatation) [4,7,9], and pericardial effusion and pericarditis [10,11]. The introduction of 3DTTE has greatly expanded the field and facilitated the detection of ischemic heart disease and its complications.

Coronary stenosis

Even prior to the development of live/real time 3DTTE, 3DTTE reconstruction was used for the

examination of coronary artery anatomy [12]. However, using live/real time 3DTTE, a full-volume 3D image of the proximal and mid-coronary arteries can be visualized in real time, and the 3D color flow velocity signal can also be obtained using Doppler imaging [13]. Using this technology, coronary artery narrowing by plaques can be clearly seen, even with hints to the composition of the plaque which can have clinical implications. It is also possible to visualize smaller coronary arteries using color Doppler imaging (Figures 9.1–9.3) [13]. After the pyramidal dataset is obtained, it is always possible to crop the coronary arteries from any angulation and even to view the cross-section of the vessel *en face* which is not possible with 2DTTE. This technique can, therefore, be a safer substitute to the more invasive coronary angiography, especially in cases that involve proximal coronary artery narrowing or congenital coronary artery anomalies. However, visualization of the distal vessels is still suboptimal, and coronary angiography is still a must in those circumstances.

Wall motion abnormalities, left ventricular aneurysm, and pseudo-aneurysm

Since the entire left ventricle can be acquired in a single 3D dataset, wall motion abnormalities can be comprehensively evaluated by meticulous systematic cropping of the full-volume pyramidal dataset. This also allows full assessment of left ventricular clots, which can then be sectioned to look for the presence and extent of clot lysis. Left ventricular aneurysms are also well visualized by 3DTTE and easily differentiated from pseudo-aneurysms by their broad neck (Figures 9.4 and 9.5) [14].

Live/Real Time 3D Echocardiography, 1st edition.
By Navin C. Nanda, Ming Chon Hsiung, Andrew P. Miller, and Fadi G. Hage. Published 2010 by Blackwell Publishing Ltd.

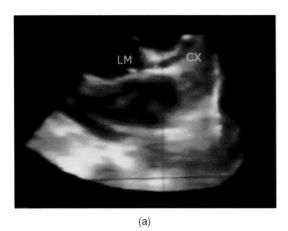

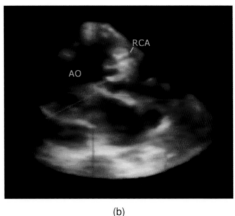

(a)   (b)

Figure 9.1 Live/real time 3D transthoracic echocardiography of coronary arteries. Sixty-nine-year-old female. (a) The pyramidal section has been cropped to show normal left main (LM) and proximal circumflex (CX) coronary arteries. The left anterior descending coronary artery is located in a different plane. (b) Another section in the same patient demonstrates a normal proximal right coronary artery (RCA). AO, aorta. (Reproduced from Vengala *et al.* [13], with permission.)

The patch used surgically for left ventricular size reduction can be viewed *en face* by 3DTTE and the sutures securing it to the ventricular walls detected.

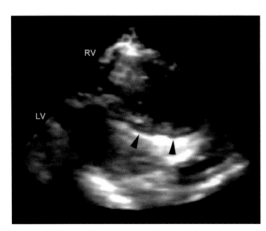

Figure 9.2 Live/real time 3D transthoracic echocardiography of coronary arteries. Twenty-six-year-old male. The arrowheads demonstrate the mid-portion of the left anterior descending (LAD) coronary artery located in the anterior interventricular groove. LV, left ventricle; RV, right ventricle. (Reproduced from Vengala *et al.* [13], with permission.)

Other complications of myocardial infarction

3DTTE has been used to diagnose serious complications that occur after acute myocardial infarction. Ventricular rupture occurs after almost 5% of all myocardial infarctions and account for more than one-third of all deaths following infarction [7]. Ventricular rupture encompasses three conditions that occur after myocardial infarction, namely, free wall rupture, ventricular septal rupture, and papillary muscle rupture. Presentation of all three conditions is dramatic, and mortality is very high; therefore, prompt diagnosis and surgical treatment are essential [7,15]. Septal rupture from inferior infarctions are usually located in the basal inferior septum, while those secondary to anterior infarctions are in the apical septum. The location, shape, and size of the septal defect may influence prognosis as well as management and, therefore, are important to determine preoperatively. Although these can ideally be visualized by 2DTTE, this may prove difficult on occasion for any 2D imaging modality [16]. 3D imaging, on the other hand, allows for full description of the defect and its visualization *en face* from either chamber which may help surgical planning. Originally, such imaging was carried out with

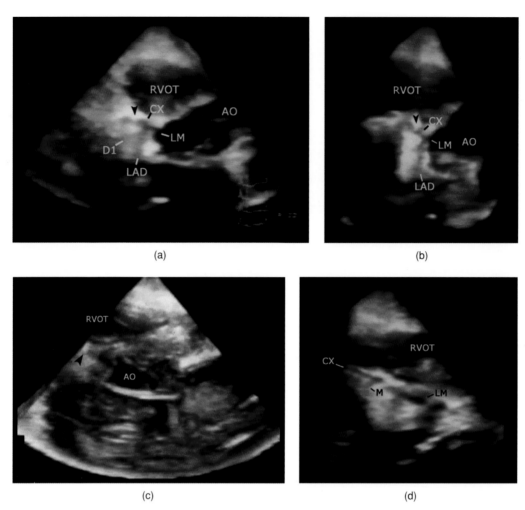

Figure 9.3 Live/real time 3D transthoracic echocardiography of coronary arteries. Thirty-year-old male, status postorthotopic cardiac transplantation. (a) The arrowhead points to severe stenosis at the origin of the first obtuse marginal branch of circumflex (CX). Movie clip 9.3 shows the plaque producing the stenosis to be somewhat mobile indicating its soft consistency and probable propensity to rupture. (b) The image in (a) has been cropped and rotated to provide an *en face* view of the stenosis (arrowhead). (c) The arrowhead shows almost total stenosis of the proximal right coronary artery (RCA). (d) The pyramidal section has been cropped to delineate a longer segment of CX, which shows no significant stenosis. M represents another marginal branch of CX with a normal lumen. (e) 3D color Doppler flow imaging shows flow signals in the visualized coronary arteries. Note that the baseline on the color Doppler bar has been shifted to provide an estimate of coronary flow velocities. (f) 3D color Doppler flow imaging demonstrates a segment of left anterior descending (LAD) adjacent to ventricular septum (VS). This segment was not visualized by B-mode 3D imaging. (g, h) The arrowheads point to multiple septal perforators imaged in short axis within the VS. Note also the presence of an intramural coronary artery branch (arrow) in the left ventricular posterior wall (PW) in (g). AO, aorta; D1, first diagonal branch of LAD; D2, second diagonal branch of LAD; LM, left main; RV, right ventricle; RVOT, right ventricular outflow tract. (Reproduced from Vengala *et al.* [13], with permission.)

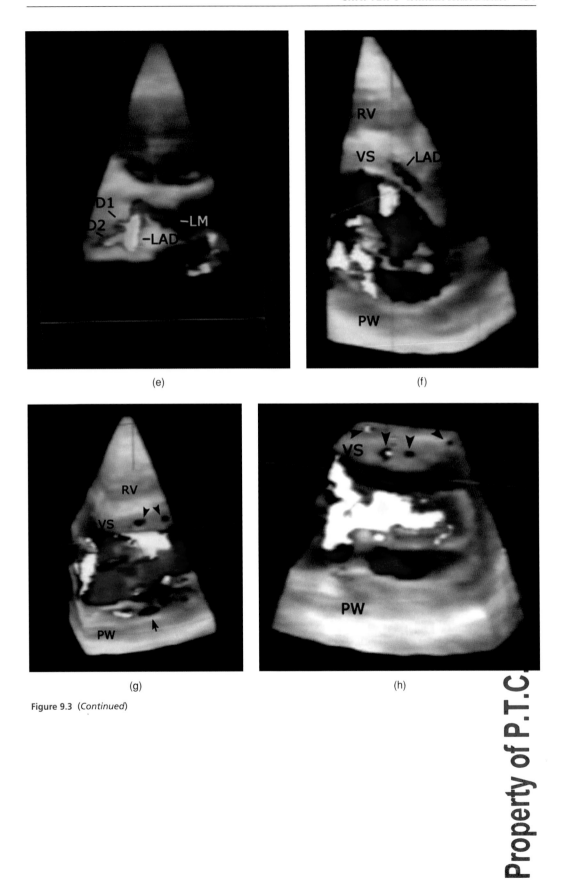

(e)

(f)

(g)

(h)

Figure 9.3 (*Continued*)

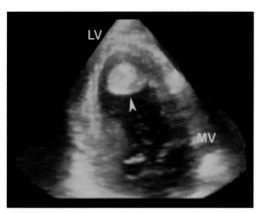

Figure 9.4 Live/real time 3D transthoracic echocardiographic assessment of left ventricular wall motion abnormalities and clot. The arrowhead points to a large clot in the left ventricular apex. Movie clip 9.4 Part 1 shows thinning out of the distal portion of the ventricular septum which is markedly hypokinetic. Sectioning of the clot shows areas of lysis. Movie clip 9.4 Part 2 from another patient shows no evidence of aneurysm in the apical four-chamber view. However, cropping of the dataset reveals a large posterior wall aneurysm (arrow) with a broad base indicative of a true aneurysm. Some sections show a narrow base mimicking a pseudo-aneurysm. No clot is seen but a small loculated pericardial effusion is present behind the aneurysm. Color Doppler study shows flow signals in the aneurysm. Movie clip 9.4 Part 3 from a different patient shows a surgically placed patch (arrowhead) to close off the aneurysm and reduce the size of the left ventricle in an attempt to improve its function. The patch is visualized *en face* from both the aneurysm and ventricular aspects. Small arrows point to individual sutures used to secure the patch to ventricular walls. LV, left ventricle; MV, mitral valve.

multiplane 3DTEE [12,17,18], but with the advent of real time 3DTTE, this became a less invasive, more convenient, and accessible approach (Figure 9.6 and 9.7) [19,20]. In a similar fashion, 3DTTE can also be used to assess left ventricular free wall rupture [21].

Finally, 3DTTE might enhance risk stratification after myocardial infarction when compared with traditional 2DTTE [22].

3DTTE for stress testing

Since with 3DTTE the acquisition of a full pyramidal dataset allows for the visualization of all the left ventricular walls, performing stress tests with 3DTTE is posed to have an advantage over 2DTTE imaging. The feasibility of 3DTTE stress testing has been verified for vasodilator as well as for Dobutamine stress [23–25]. Since with 3DTTE all the left ventricular walls are imaged in a single acquisition, the reduction of imaging time may enhance ischemia detection [25]. Furthermore, the visualization of the true apex by 3DTTE (which is often difficult by 2DTTE) may enhance the detection of left anterior descending artery disease [24,25]. Further studies in this field will no doubt further define the role of 3DTTE in the diagnosis of ischemic heart disease as well as in predicting prognosis.

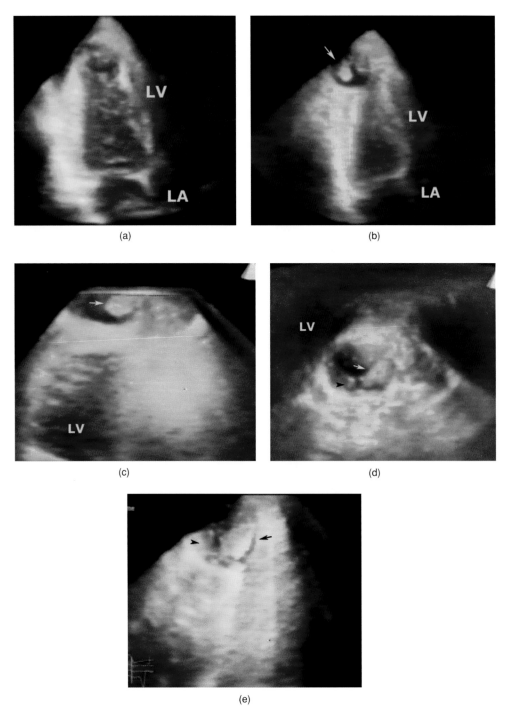

(a)

(b)

(c)

(d)

(e)

Figure 9.5 Live/real time 3D transthoracic echocardiogram in a patient with left ventricular pseudo-aneurysm. (a) Apical view showing no aneurysm or thrombus in the left ventricle (LV). (b) Posterior–anterior cropping demonstrates the pseudo-aneurysm containing thrombus (arrow; arrowhead in Movie clip 9.5). (c, d) Sectioning of thrombus (c) and viewing it *en face* (d) shows no evidence of clot lysis or liquefaction. In addition, a highly mobile component (arrowhead) is visualized. (e) Sagittal section also shows no lysis in thrombus; the arrowhead shows mobile component. LA, left atrium. (Reproduced from Duncan, *Echocardiography* 2006;23:68–72, with permission.)

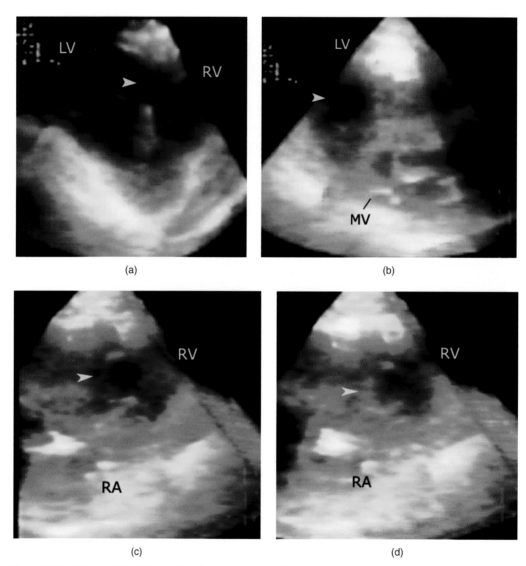

(a)

(b)

(c)

(d)

Figure 9.6 (a–d) Live/real time 3D transthoracic echocardiography. (a) Septal defect (arrowhead) viewed in modified four-chamber view. (b) Septal defect (arrowhead) viewed *en face* from LV aspect. (c, d) Septal defect (arrowhead) viewed from RV side. LA, left atrium; MV, mitral valve; RA, right atrium. (Reproduced from Vengala *et al.* [19], with permission.)

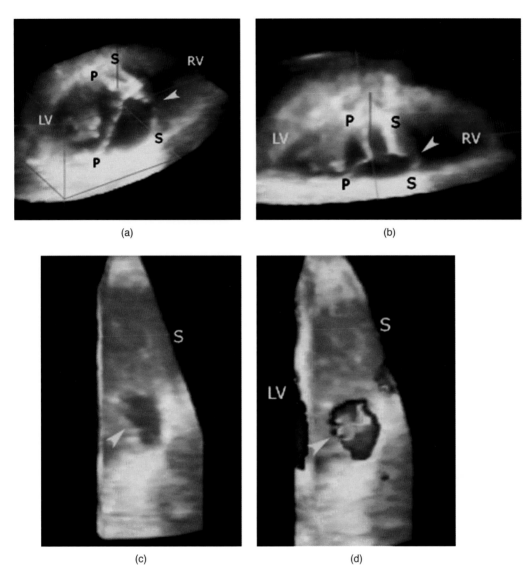

(a)

(b)

(c)

(d)

Figure 9.7 (a, b) Live/real time three-dimensional echocardiography in a 58 year old male with ventricular septal rupture following myocardial infarction and closure patch dehiscence. The arrowhead shows a defect in the ventricular septum (S). P represents the dehisced patch. (c, d) *En face* view of the defect (arrowhead) without (c) and with (d) color Doppler flow signals. LV, left ventricle; RV, right ventricle. Movie clips 9.7 Parts 1–7. (Reproduced from Mehmood *et al.* [22], with permission.)

References

1. Armstrong WF, Ryan T. Stress echocardiography from 1979 to present. *J Am Soc Echocardiogr* 2008;21:22–8.

2. Rigo F, Murer B, Ossena G, Favaretto E. Transthoracic echocardiographic imaging of coronary arteries: tips, traps, and pitfalls. *Cardiovasc Ultrasound* 2008;6:7.

3. Hameed AK, Gosal T, Fang T, *et al*. Clinical utility of tissue Doppler imaging in patients with acute myocardial infarction complicated by cardiogenic shock. *Cardiovasc Ultrasound* 2008;6:11.

4. Hutyra M, Skala T, Marek D, *et al*. Acute severe mitral regurgitation with cardiogenic shock caused by two-step complete anterior papillary muscle rupture during acute myocardial infarction. *Biomed Pap Med Fac Univ Palacky Olomouc Czech Repub* 2006;150:293–7.

5. Friedman BM, Dunn MI. Postinfarction ventricular aneurysms. *Clin Cardiol* 1995;18:505–11.

6. Keeley EC, Hillis LD. Left ventricular mural thrombus after acute myocardial infarction. *Clin Cardiol* 1996; 19:83–6.

7. Davis N, Sistino JJ. Review of ventricular rupture: key concepts and diagnostic tools for success. *Perfusion* 2002;17:63–7.

8. Raposo L, Andrade MJ, Ferreira J, *et al*. Subacute left ventricle free wall rupture after acute myocardial infarction: awareness of the clinical signs and early use of echocardiography may be life-saving. *Cardiovasc Ultrasound* 2006;4:46.

9. Birnbaum Y, Chamoun AJ, Conti VR, Uretsky BF. Mitral regurgitation following acute myocardial infarction. *Coron Artery Dis* 2002;13:337–44.

10. Gregor P, Widimsky P. Pericardial effusion as a consequence of acute myocardial infarction. *Echocardiography* 1999;16:317–20.

11. Wilansky S, Moreno CA, Lester SJ. Complications of myocardial infarction. *Crit Care Med* 2007;35:S348–54.

12. Nanda NC, Sorrell VL. *Atlas of Three-Dimensional Echocardiography*. Armonk, NY: Futura Publishing Company, 2002.

13. Vengala S, Nanda NC, Agrawal G, *et al*. Live three-dimensional transthoracic echocardiographic assessment of coronary arteries. *Echocardiography* 2003;20: 751–4.

14. Gatewood RP, Jr., Nanda NC. Differentiation of left ventricular pseudoaneurysm from true aneurysm with two

dimensional echocardiography. *Am J Cardiol* 1980;46: 869–78.

15. Deja MA, Szostek J, Widenka K, *et al*. Post infarction ventricular septal defect—can we do better? *Eur J Cardiothorac Surg* 2000;18:194–201.

16. Helmcke F, Mahan EF, III, Nanda NC, *et al*. Two-dimensional echocardiography and Doppler color flow mapping in the diagnosis and prognosis of ventricular septal rupture. *Circulation* 1990;81:1775–83.

17. Gabriel H, Binder T, Globits S, Zangeneh M, Rothy W, Glogar D. Three-dimensional echocardiography in the diagnosis of postinfarction ventricular septal defect. *Am Heart J* 1995;129:1038–40.

18. Nekkanti R, Nanda NC, Zoghbi GJ, Mukhtar O, McGiffin DC. Transesophageal two- and three-dimensional echocardiographic diagnosis of combined left ventricular pseudoaneurysm and ventricular septal rupture. *Echocardiography* 2002;19:345–9.

19. Vengala S, Nanda NC, Mehmood F, *et al*. Live three-dimensional transthoracic echocardiographic delineation of ventricular septal rupture following myocardial infarction. *Echocardiography* 2004;21: 745–7.

20. Mehmood F, Miller AP, Nanda NC, *et al*. Usefulness of live/real time three-dimensional transthoracic echocardiography in the characterization of ventricular septal defects in adults. *Echocardiography* 2006;23:421–7.

21. Little SH, Ramasubbu K, Zoghbi WA. Real-time 3-dimensional echocardiography demonstrates size and extent of acute left ventricular free wall rupture. *J Am Soc Echocardiogr* 2007;20:538 e1–3.

22. Gopal AS, Chukwu EO, Mihalatos DG, *et al*. Left ventricular structure and function for postmyocardial infarction and heart failure risk stratification by three-dimensional echocardiography. *J Am Soc Echocardiogr* 2007;20:949–58.

23. Varnero S, Santagata P, Pratali L, Basso M, Gandolfo A, Bellotti P. Head to head comparison of 2D vs real time 3D dipyridamole stress echocardiography. *Cardiovasc Ultrasound* 2008;6:31.

24. Aggeli C, Giannopoulos G, Misovoulos P, *et al*. Real-time three-dimensional dobutamine stress echocardiography for coronary artery disease diagnosis: validation with coronary angiography. *Heart* 2007;93:672–5.

25. Takeuchi M, Lang RM. Three-dimensional stress testing: volumetric acquisitions. *Cardiol Clin* 2007;25:267–72.

CHAPTER 10

Cardiomyopathies

Introduction

Cardiomyopathy is a general term that refers to diseases of the myocardium that result in cardiac dysfunction. Broadly, the cardiomyopathies can be divided into ischemic and nonischemic cardiomyopathy. Echocardiography is well established in managing these disorders, from diagnosis and identifying the etiology to prognostication and monitoring therapy [1]. Since Chapter 9 has addressed the role of 3D transthoracic echocardiography (3DTTE) in coronary artery disease and ischemic cardiomyopathy, we will concentrate here on the nonischemic cardiomyopathies. After coronary artery disease has been excluded as the etiology of cardiomyopathy, the most common variety has been termed dilated cardiomyopathy and is mostly idiopathic, familial, or caused by viral infections (Figure 10.1; see also Figure 12.1). However, other well-characterized forms of cardiomyopathy include hypertrophic cardiomyopathy (HCM) and isolated left ventricular noncompaction among others. 3DTTE has proven its value on top of traditional 2DTTE in some of these disorders, and its role is being investigated in others.

Hypertrophic cardiomyopathy

HCM is a common genetic cardiac disease that is characterized by hypertrophy of the left ventricle, most commonly asymmetric, in the absence of other causes that are capable of generating similar degrees of hypertrophy such as systemic hypertension or aortic valve stenosis [2]. 2DTTE is the most

commonly used diagnostic test for HCM, but more recent studies suggest that there could be an additional value to 3DTTE in differentiating HCM from other forms of left ventricular hypertrophy that occur in patients with systemic hypertension or in trained athletes and can more accurately determine left ventricular mass and volume [3,4]. Although the most common form of HCM involves asymmetric septal hypertrophy, other forms are well characterized, and variants such as apical HCM are more difficult to diagnose by 2DTTE. Apical HCM is most common in Japan but does occur in other parts of the world and in the United States, and since it does have prognostic implications, this condition should be recognized by noninvasive imaging. 2DTTE is usually the test of choice for most forms of HCM, but in the case of apical HCM, it is well known to miss the diagnosis due to the inability to visualize or recognize the markedly narrowed left ventricular apical cavity. In order to circumvent this, some sonographers advocate the use of echo contrast agent to facilitate the visualization of the apex [5–7]. However, even with the use of echo contrast, 2DTTE might still miss the diagnosis, and in this case 3DTTE might be helpful to visualize the apical hypertrophy [8]. Intravenous contrast infusion could be utilized with 3DTTE to help delineate the endocardium near the apex to demonstrate the hypertrophy, where in severe cases a slit-like cavity is visualized (Figures 10.2–10.4) [8].

Almost one-fourth of HCM patients exhibit dynamic left ventricular outflow tract (LVOT) obstruction secondary to systolic anterior motion (SAM) of the mitral valve in a narrow left ventricular outflow [9]. Due to its ability for better and more realistic geometrical visualization of cardiac structures, 3DTTE has been utilized for the study of SAM in HCM, and it has been determined that

Live/Real Time 3D Echocardiography, 1st edition.
By Navin C. Nanda, Ming Chon Hsiung, Andrew P. Miller, and Fadi G. Hage. Published 2010 by Blackwell Publishing Ltd.

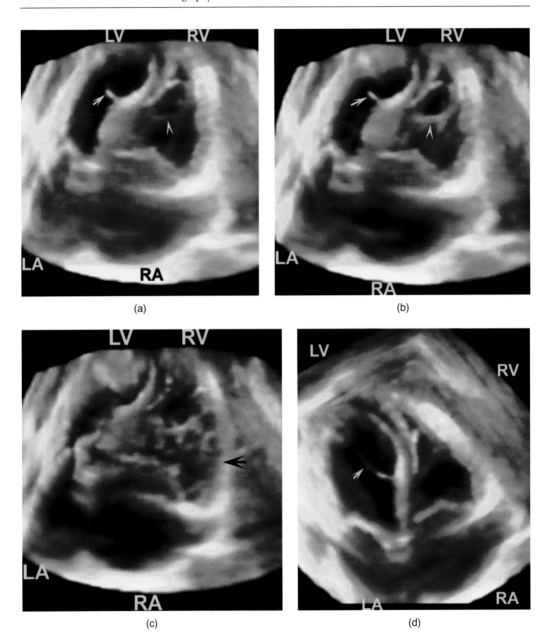

(a)

(b)

(c)

(d)

Figure 10.1 Live/real time 3D transthoracic echocardiography (3DTEE) in dilated cardiomyopathy. (a–c) Systematic and sequential anteroposterior cropping of right ventricle (RV) demonstrates the moderator band (arrowhead) as well as other trabeculations and papillary muscles (black arrow) in the RV. (d, e) Further cropping shows only a few trabeculations in the RV apex. There is no evidence of noncompaction. Also, there is no evidence of a mass or clot in the RV apex which was suspected on the 2D study. A prominent trabeculation in the RV apex very clearly delineated by 3DTTE (arrows in Movie clip 10.1 Part 1) was most likely the culprit for the mass-like lesion suspected on the 2D echocardiogram. Both ventricles are dilated and show globally poor motion typical of dilated cardiomyopathy. Yellow arrow in (a), (b), (d), and (e) points to a false tendon in left ventricle (LV). Movie clip 10.1 Part 2 shows another patient with dilated cardiomyopathy and globally poor biventricular function. The arrowhead shows a large clot in the left ventricle which, when further cropped, demonstrates a central echolucency consistent with clot lysis. A few trabeculations are also seen. LA, left atrium; RA, right atrium. (Reproduced from Bodiwala *et al.* [18], with permission.)

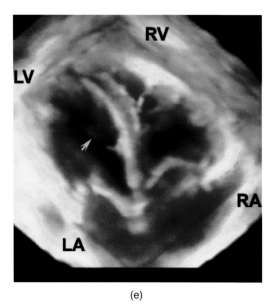

(e)

Figure 10.1 *(Continued)*

the anterior segment of the anterior mitral leaflet is essential in the development of the gradient, and that SAM occurs predominantly on the medial side, resulting in a laterally located LVOT opening [10,11]. However, LVOT obstruction in HCM is not solely due to SAM of the mitral valve but could happen in the mid-ventricular cavity secondary to myocardial hypertrophy that has also been studied by 3DTTE which can visualize the mid-cavity obliteration during systole as well as identify other

causes for LVOT obstruction [12,13]. Furthermore, Fukuda *et al.* [14] used 3DTTE to measure the area of the LVOT in patients with HCM and showed that it inversely correlated with the pressure gradient and, therefore, can quantitate the severity of LVOT obstruction.

In HCM patients who do exhibit an LVOT gradient and have symptoms that are refractory to medical therapy, management options include surgical septal myomectomy versus percutaneous alcohol septal ablation [9]. We have reported on the benefit of 3DTTE in studying the complications of surgical myomectomy. One of the complications is a septal perforator coronary artery—LV fistula. When a comprehensive examination of the LV septum is performed with systemic cropping of the pyramidal dataset and viewing the images *en face*, a better assessment of septal perforator coronary artery—LV fistulas—can be performed than 2DTTE. Further, with *en face* viewing, the area of the fistula can be accurately determined (Figures 10.5 and 10.6) [15]. We have also used 3DTTE to follow the effect of alcohol septal ablation in patients with HCM [16]. Since left atrial volume and ejection fraction are well-known indexes of diastolic function, we used 3DTTE to assess the effect of alcohol septal ablation on these variables. We showed that after alcohol septal ablation, the left atrial end systolic volume decreases and its ejection fraction increases, signifying an improvement in diastolic function (Figure 10.7). More importantly, these changes were

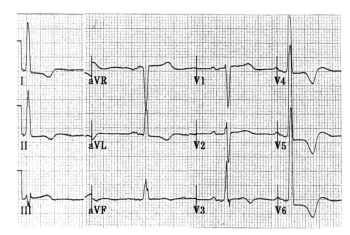

Figure 10.2 Electrocardiogram in apical hypertrophic cardiomyopathy. Shows left ventricular hypertrophy with ST depression and T-wave inversion in leads I, II, aVL, and V_4–V_6. (Reproduced from Frans *et al.* [8], with permission.)

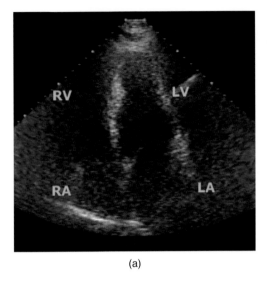

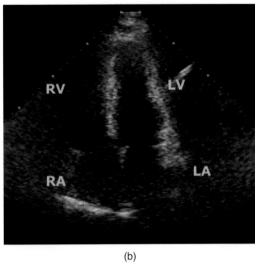

(a)   (b)

Figure 10.3 Real time 2D transthoracic echocardiography in apical hypertrophic cardiomyopathy. Apical four-chamber view. End-diastolic (a) and end-systolic (b) images show apparent left ventricular apical hypokinesis with no evidence of apical hypertrophy. LA, left atrium; LV, left ventricle; RA, right atrium; RV, right ventricle. Movie clip 10.3. (Reproduced from Frans et al. [8], with permission.)

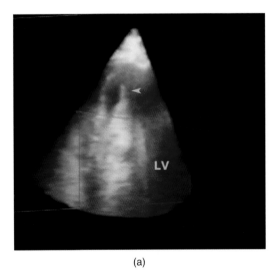

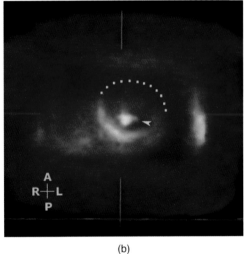

(a)   (b)

Figure 10.4 Live/real time 3D transthoracic contrast echocardiography in apical hypertrophic cardiomyopathy. (a) The arrowhead points to a slit-like left ventricular (LV) apical cavity with marked hypertrophy well demonstrated by echo contrast injection. (b) En face transverse section of LV apex shows the asymmetric nature of hypertrophy which is more marked anteriorly than posteriorly. The arrowhead points to the contrast-filled apical cavity. (c) En face transverse section through the body of LV showing a much larger contrast-filled cavity (arrow) at this level. Orientation symbols: A, anterior; P, posterior; L, left; R, right. Movie clips 10.4 A–10.4 C. (Reproduced from Frans et al. [8], with permission.)

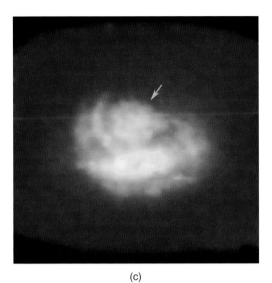

(c)

Figure 10.4 (*Continued*)

accompanied by clinical improvement and a decrease in the LVOT gradient. Significantly, the rise in left atrial ejection fraction correlated with the decrease in the resting left ventricular outflow gradient [16].

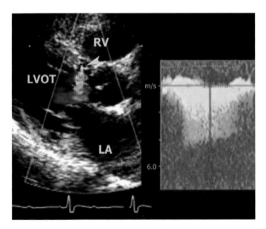

Figure 10.5 2D transthoracic echocardiographic demonstration of septal perforator coronary artery-left ventricle fistula following septal myectomy. The arrowhead points to turbulent flow signals moving into the left ventricular outflow tract (LVOT) from ventricular septum. In some patients, they mimic aortic regurgitation. Color Doppler-guided continuous wave Doppler interrogation shows a peak velocity of approximately 4.3 m/s in diastole consistent with a coronary artery fistula (inset). LA, left atrium; RV, right ventricle. (Reproduced from Patel *et al.* [15], with permission.)

Isolated left ventricular noncompaction

Isolated left ventricular noncompaction (ILVNC), labeled under the unclassified cardiomyopathies, is a rare form of cardiomyopathy in adults that has been discovered more than 20 years ago [17]. This condition is assumed to occur secondary to the arrest of the compaction process during normal ventricular morphogenesis [17]. The clinical presentation involves to various extents a combination of heart failure, thromboembolic events, and arrhythmias. The diagnostic method that has been used most to diagnose ILVNC is 2DTTE which usually reveals multiple prominent trabeculations, most commonly in the apical portion of the LV but also in the inferior and lateral walls, and deep intertrabecular recesses that communicate with the LV cavity, as seen on color Doppler imaging [17]. This results in a myocardial wall that has two layers, a thin compacted myocardium on the epicardial side and a thicker noncompacted myocardium on the endocardial side (with a typical ratio of noncompacted to compacted layer of ≥ 2). We examined eight patients with ILVNC using a 4-MHz, 4 matrix probe with approximately 5–7 seconds of breath holding to obtain 3DTTE images [18]. We then cropped the 3D pyramidal dataset systematically to create an *en face* view of the ventricular septum and apex. The extent of noncompaction was then determined using a segmental approach that divided the LV into basal, mid, and apical regions of the septal, inferior, posterolateral, and anterior walls. In this report, 3DTTE was able to visualize the honeycomb appearance in the apical area in all patients while 2DTTE was nondiagnostic in five of these eight patients. In addition, 3DTTE was able to show the involvement of the right ventricle in some patients. Significantly, in one patient, both 2DTTE and MRI suggested the presence of a tumor extending across the septum into the right and left ventricles, while 3DTTE revealed the presence of combined right and left ventricular noncompaction. We have diagnosed right ventricular noncompaction, either isolated or combined with ILVNC, if trabeculations occupy more than 80% of right ventricular cavity or if they completely fill at least one-third of the right ventricle. Stringent criteria are necessary for diagnosing right ventricular noncompaction since normally several

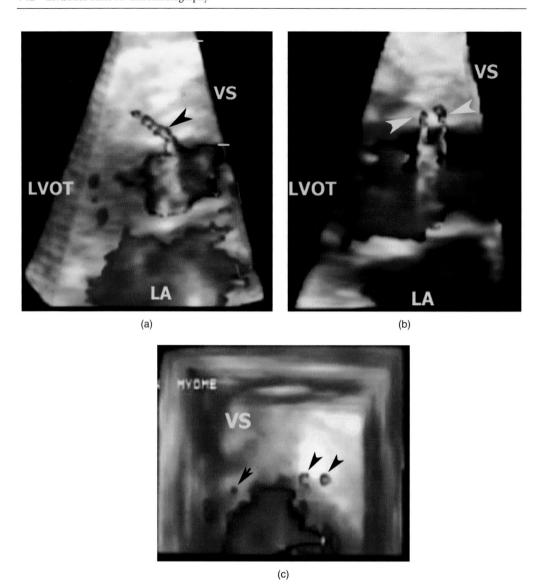

Figure 10.6 Live/real time 3D transthoracic echocardiographic (3DTEE) demonstration of septal perforator coronary artery—left ventricular (LV) fistulas—following septal myectomy. (a) The arrowhead points to intramyocardial course of a fistulous septal perforator coronary artery. (b) The arrowheads point to two adjacent but separate septal perforator coronary arteries—LVOT fistulas. (c) *En face* viewing of ventricular septum. The arrowheads point to the two fistulous coronary arteries which demonstrate turbulent flow signals and are larger as compared to a normal septal perforator coronary artery (arrow) that shows laminar flow signals. Movie clip 10.6 Part 1 demonstrates septal perforator—LV fistula—using both 2DTTE and 3DTTE. Note the superiority of 3DTTE in finding a second fistula not visualized by 2DTTE. Movie clip 10.6 Part 2 shows a patient with classical hypertrophic cardiomyopathy cropped using QLAB. Medial site of obstruction of the left ventricular outflow tract (LVOT) (arrowhead) by the systolic anterior motion of the mitral valve is clearly demonstrated in the short-axis view. Movie clip 10.6 Part 3 shows another patient with typical hypertrophic cardiomyopathy. Regular cropping demonstrates very severe obstruction, and the LVOT in short axis does not appear much larger than a pin hole (arrowhead) in late systole. LA, left atrium; VS, ventricular septum. (Reproduced from Patel *et al.* [15], with permission.)

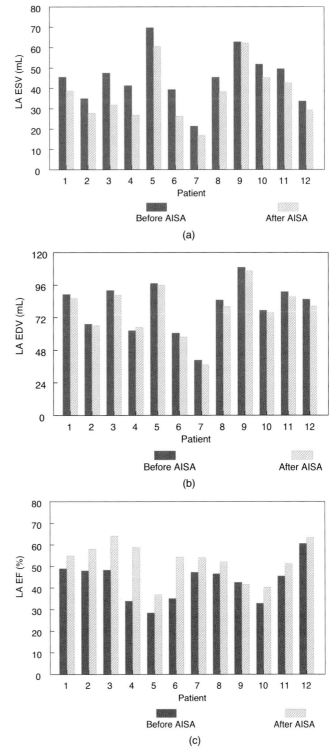

Figure 10.7 (a) Left atrial end-systolic volumes, (b) end-diastolic volumes, and (c) ejection fraction, as measured by live/real time 3D transthoracic echocardiography in 12 individual patients with hypertrophic cardiomyopathy before and after alcohol-induced septal ablation. AISA, alcohol-induced septal ablation; LA EDV, left atrial end-diastolic volume; LA ESV, left atrial end-systolic volume; LA EF, left atrial ejection fraction. (Reproduced from Hage *et al.* [16], with permission.)

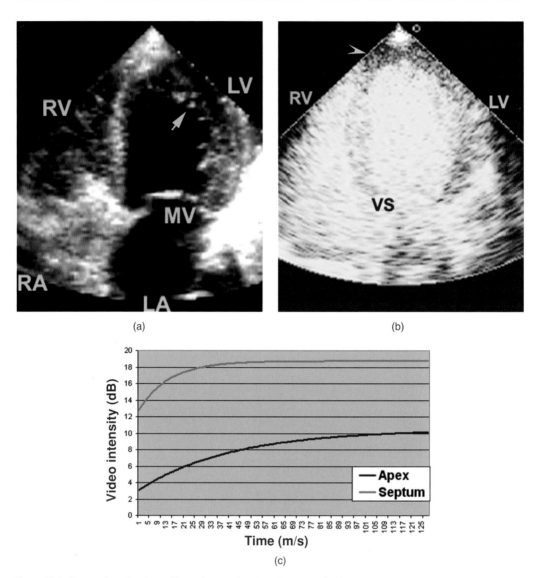

(a)   (b)

(c)

Figure 10.8 2D transthoracic echocardiography in isolated left ventricular (LV) noncompaction. (a) The arrow points to prominent trabeculations involving the whole extent of LV posterolateral wall consistent with noncompaction. (b) Myocardial perfusion study using perflutren lipid microspheres demonstrated apical hypoperfusion (arrowhead). (c) Echo contrast time intensity curves show diminished rate of filling as well as peak filling in the LV apex as compared to the ventricular septum (VS). LA, left atrium; MV, mitral valve; RA, right atrium; RV, right ventricle. (Reproduced from Bodiwala *et al.* [18], with permission.)

trabeculations and muscle bands are present in the right ventricle, more so when it is hypertrophied. It is unusual to find more than four trabeculations in the normal left ventricle, and hence noncompaction should be suspected if five or more trabeculations are noted. 3DTTE in these patients shows the characteristic "honeycomb-like" appearance of ILVNC when viewed *en face* in short axis. This is differentiated from dilated cardiomyopathy, which could include trabeculations, but they are less extensive, usually spare the apex, and lack the presence of truly noncompacted tissue [18]. The 3DTTE exam could, therefore, add significant value on top of 2DTTE for the identification of ILVNC and differentiating it from other entities. In some cases, intravenous echo contrast can be used to augment 3D imaging by enhancing the endocardial border definition just as in 2D imaging (Figures 10.8–10.12).

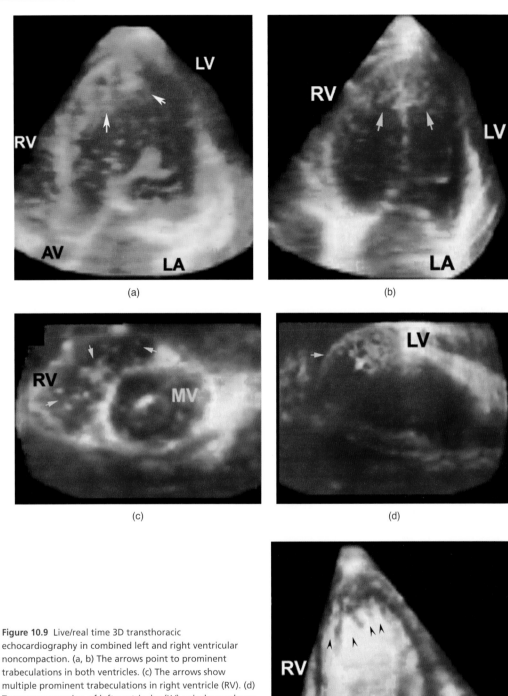

(a)

(b)

(c)

(d)

Figure 10.9 Live/real time 3D transthoracic echocardiography in combined left and right ventricular noncompaction. (a, b) The arrows point to prominent trabeculations in both ventricles. (c) The arrows show multiple prominent trabeculations in right ventricle (RV). (d) Transverse cropping of left ventricular (LV) apical area shows a honeycomb-like appearance (arrow) typical of noncompaction. (e) Echo contrast study using perflutren lipid microspheres shows filling of intertrabecular recesses with the contrast agent (arrows). See Movie clip 10.9 Part 1. Movie clips 10.9 Part 2–5 are from another patient with isolated left ventricular noncompaction. Systemic cropping of the 3D dataset demonstrates extensive trabecular involvement of the left ventricle (arrowheads). AV, aortic valve; LA, left atrium; MV, mitral valve. (Reproduced from Bodiwala *et al.* [18], with permission.)

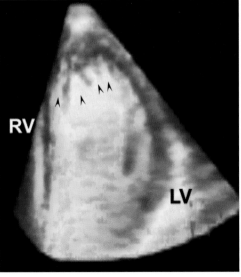

(e)

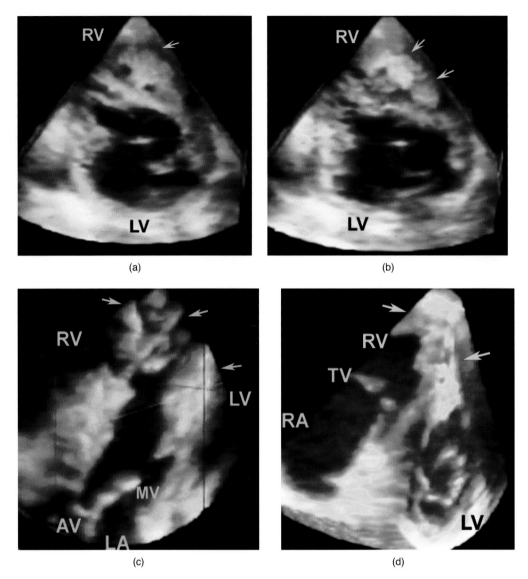

(a)

(b)

(c)

(d)

Figure 10.10 Live/real time 3D transthoracic echocardiography in combined left (LV) and right ventricular (RV) noncompaction in another patient. (a, b) The arrows point to a cauliflower-like mass in RV mimicking a tumor. Magnetic resonance imaging in this patient erroneously suggested a ventricular septal tumor. (c–e) The arrows point to massive trabeculations in both LV and RV consistent with noncompaction. (f, g) Transverse (f) and anteroposterior (g) cropping of LV apical area shows a honeycomb-like appearance (arrow) typical of noncompaction. (h) The arrowheads point to multiple trabeculations occupying over 80% of RV cavity. (i, j) The arrow points to massive trabeculations in the ventricular septal area. (k) The arrows point to multiple trabeculations crossing the RV cavity transversely. AO, ascending aorta; AV; aortic valve; MV, mitral valve; RA, right atrium; RCA, right coronary artery; TV, tricuspid valve; #1, anterior leaflet of tricuspid valve; #2, septal leaflet of tricuspid valve. Movie clip 10.10. (Reproduced from Bodiwala et al. [18], with permission.)

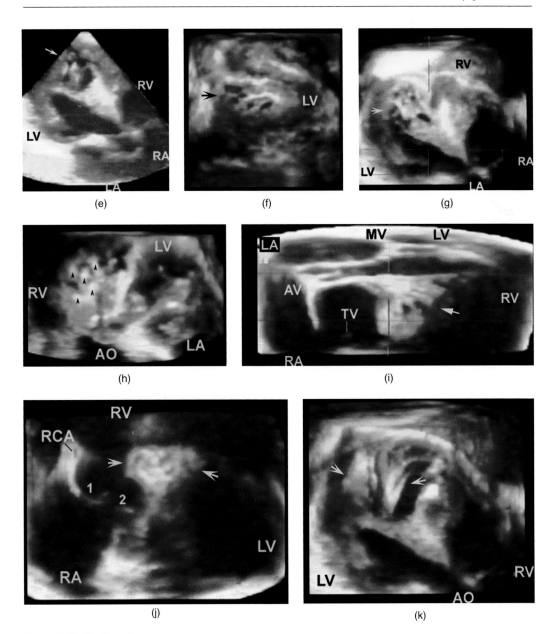

Figure 10.10 (*Continued*)

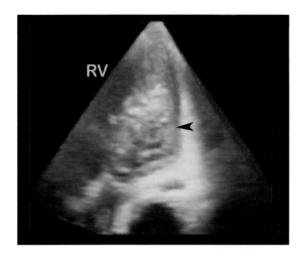

Figure 10.11 Live/real time 3D echocardiography in isolated right ventricular (RV) noncompaction. In this patient, prominent trabeculations (arrowhead) occupy over 80% of the RV cavity.

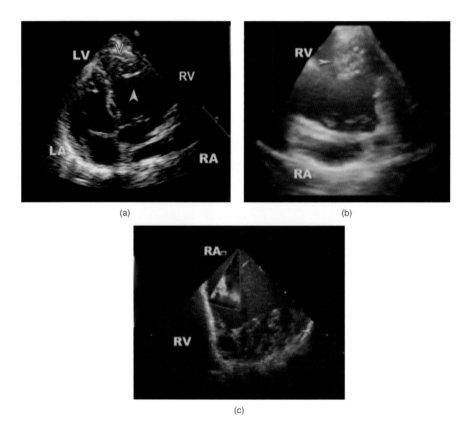

(a)

(b)

(c)

Figure 10.12 Live/real time 2D and 3D transthoracic echocardiography in isolated right ventricular noncompaction. (a) 2D study. The arrowheads point to a few muscle bands in the right ventricular apex but there is no clear-cut evidence for noncompaction. (b) 3D study. Cropping of the image reveals a honeycombed appearance typical of right ventricular noncompaction. Trabeculations (arrowhead) fill the distal 40% of right ventricle (RV) almost completely. (c) Intracardiac echocardiography. Shows right ventricular noncompaction (arrowhead). LA, left atrium; LV, left ventricle; RA, right atrium. Movie clips 10.12 A–10.12 C. (Reproduced from Reddy *et al.*, *Echocardiography* 2009;26:598–609, with permission.)

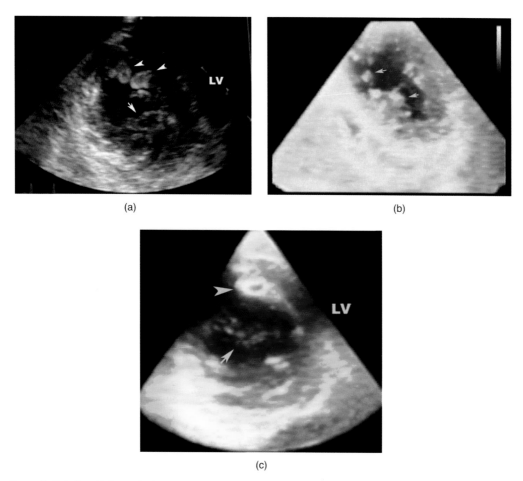

(a)

(b)

(c)

Figure 10.13 Isolated left ventricular noncompaction and thrombi in an adult patient. (a) 2D transthoracic echocardiography. The arrowheads show echodensities in the left ventricle (LV) suggestive of thrombi with areas of echolucency consistent with clot lysis. The arrow points to adjacent trabeculations which are relatively less echogenic. (b, c) Live/real time 3D transthoracic echocardiography. The arrows point to multiple trabeculations in LV. In (c), one of the echodensities (arrowhead) was cropped revealing a prominent echolucency, typical of clot lysis. Movie clips 10.13 A–10.13 C. (Reproduced from Yelamanchili *et al.* [19], with permission.)

Another benefit of 3DTTE over 2DTTE in ILVNC is its ability to identify thrombi within the trabeculations at the apex. Patients with ILVNC are known to have a high incidence of thromboembolic events which could be due to LV clot formations that result from poor LV function, or in patients with preserved ejection fraction, due to sluggish flow in the deep recesses between trabeculations. Therefore, the identifications of clots in these patients could have prognostic and therapeutic implications. Although 2DTTE can sometimes, but not always, suspect the presence of a clot in these patients, the diagnosis can be made with more certainty using 3DTTE [19,20]. Furthermore, by systemic cropping and with a comprehensive assessment from multiple perspectives, clots can be easily differentiated from adjacent trabeculations on 3DTTE, and by viewing the cropped sections of the clot *en face*, areas of clot lysis can be visualized as echolucencies while trabeculations appear solid on serial sectioning [19]. Clots appear more echogenic as compared to trabeculations on 3DTTE, and this feature, in addition to their hypermobility and "gel-like" appearance, is most useful in their identification (Figures 10.13 and 10.14).

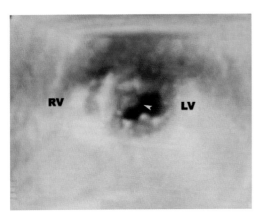

Figure 10.14 Isolated left ventricular noncompaction and thrombus in another patient. Live/real time 3D transthoracic echocardiography. The arrowhead points to a clot in the left ventricle (LV). RV, right ventricle. Clot hypermobility (arrowhead) is demonstrated in Movie clip 10.14 Part 1. Movie clip 10.14 Part 2 is from another patient with isolated left ventricular noncompaction with thrombi in the left ventricular cavity. Thrombi are easily differentiated from trabeculations (arrowheads) by their much higher echogenicity. Thrombi are denoted by arrowheads in sections of the movie containing no trabeculations. (Reproduced from Yelamanchili et al. [19], with permission.)

More recently, Rajdev et al. [21] studied 21 patients with ILVNC using 2DTTE and 3DTTE using the Philips iE33 ultrasound imaging system (Philips Medical Systems, Inc., Andover, MA) and a 3.5-MHz transducer for 2DTTE and a 4-MHz, 4 matrix array transducer for 3DTTE. The LV mass was calculated using 3DTTE by tracing the endocardial and epicardial borders in the apical four-chamber and two-chamber views and in planes 45° orthogonal to these views. The LV mass was then recalculated with the exclusion of the trabeculations allowing for the calculation of the trabecular mass as the difference of the two values. The same was done using 2DTTE from the apical four-chamber view. Interestingly, the number of trabeculations, and the calculated trabecular mass were both significantly larger using 3DTTE than 2DTTE (Figures 10.15–10.18) [21]. This suggested that 2DTTE can underestimate the extent and severity of noncompaction. 2DTTE examination in these patients is complicated by the altered geometry of the LV and the fact that 2DTTE allows for the visualization of a single plane at any particular time. With

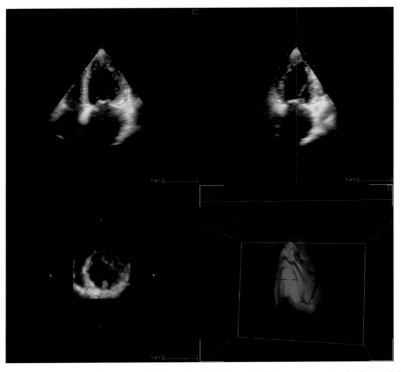

Figure 10.15 Shows the technique of estimating left ventricular (LV) mass in LV noncompaction by live/real time 3D transthoracic echocardiography. (Reproduced from Rajdev et al. [21], with permission.)

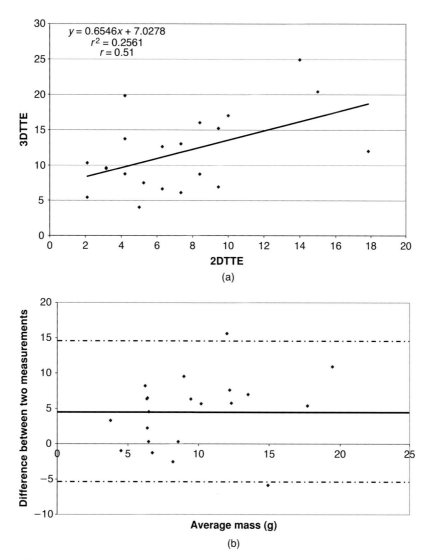

Figure 10.16 (a) Shows left ventricular trabecular mass assessed by 2D transthoracic echocardiography (2DTTE) and live/real time 3D transthoracic echocardiography (3DTTE) in 21 patients. (b) Bland–Altman plot of left ventricular trabecular mass assessed by 2DTTE and live/real 3DTTE. The 95% confidence intervals are indicated by the dashed lines. (Reproduced from Rajdev *et al.* [21], with permission.)

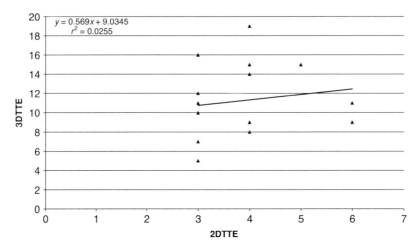

Figure 10.17 Shows number of left ventricular trabeculations assessed by 2D transthoracic echocardiography (2DTTE) and live/real time 3D transthoracic echocardiography (3DTTE) in 17 patients. (Reproduced from Rajdev *et al.* [21], with permission.)

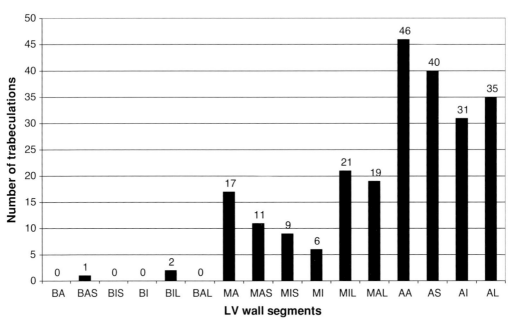

Figure 10.18 Shows segmental distribution of left ventricular (LV) trabeculations using live/real time 3D transthoracic echocardiography (3DTTE). AA, apical anterior; AI, apical inferior; AL, apical lateral; AS, apical septal; BA, basal anterior; BAL, basal anterolateral; BAS, basal anteroseptal; BI, basal inferior; BIL, basal inferolateral; BIS, basal inferoseptal; MA, mid anterior; MAL, mid anterolateral; MAS, mid anteroseptal; MI, mid inferior; MIL, mid inferolateral; MIS, mid inferoseptal. (Reproduced from Rajdev *et al.* [21], with permission.)

3DTTE, after the generation of the full 3D pyramidal dataset, systemic comprehensive cropping allows for a more accurate assessment of the extent of noncompaction.

Other cardiomyopathies

3DTTE has also shown promise in the study of other cardiomyopathies. For example, Kjaergaard et al. [22] showed that 3DTTE can demonstrate decreased right ventricular ejection fraction in patients with arrhythmogenic right ventricular dysplasia. Other groups have used the technology to evaluate LV regional wall motion in patients with takotsubo cardiomyopathy [23,24].

References

1. Wood MJ, Picard MH. Utility of echocardiography in the evaluation of individuals with cardiomyopathy. *Heart* 2004;90:707–12.

2. Maron BJ, McKenna WJ, Danielson GK, *et al.* American College of Cardiology/European Society of Cardiology clinical expert consensus document on hypertrophic cardiomyopathy. A report of the American College of Cardiology Foundation Task Force on Clinical Expert Consensus Documents and the European Society of Cardiology Committee for Practice Guidelines. *J Am Coll Cardiol* 2003;42:1687–713.

3. Caselli S, Pelliccia A, Maron M, *et al.* Differentiation of hypertrophic cardiomyopathy from other forms of left ventricular hypertrophy by means of three-dimensional echocardiography. *Am J Cardiol* 2008;102:616–20.

4. Bicudo LS, Tsutsui JM, Shiozaki A, *et al.* Value of real time three-dimensional echocardiography in patients with hypertrophic cardiomyopathy: comparison with two-dimensional echocardiography and magnetic resonance imaging. *Echocardiography* 2008;25:717–26.

5. Acarturk E, Bozkurt A, Donmez Y. Apical hypertrophic cardiomyopathy: diagnosis with contrast-enhanced echocardiography—a case report. *Angiology* 2003;54:373–6.

6. D'Andrea A, Liccardo B, Scarafile R, Esposito N, Calabro R. Apical hypertrophic cardiomyopathy: quickly noninvasive diagnosis by intravenous contrast echocardiography. *Minerva Cardioangiol* 2008;56:578–9.

7. Ward RP, Weinert L, Spencer KT, *et al.* Quantitative diagnosis of apical cardiomyopathy using contrast echocardiography. *J Am Soc Echocardiogr* 2002;15:316–22.

8. Frans EE, Nanda NC, Patel V, *et al.* Live three-dimensional transthoracic contrast echocardiographic assessment of apical hypertrophic cardiomyopathy. *Echocardiography* 2005;22:686–9.

9. Elliott P, McKenna WJ. Hypertrophic cardiomyopathy. *Lancet* 2004;363:1881–91.

10. Song JM, Fukuda S, Lever HM, *et al.* Asymmetry of systolic anterior motion of the mitral valve in patients with hypertrophic obstructive cardiomyopathy: a real-time three-dimensional echocardiographic study. *J Am Soc Echocardiogr* 2006;19:1129–35.

11. Perez De Isla L, Zamorano J, Malangatana G, *et al.* Morphological determinants of subaortic stenosis in hypertrophic cardiomyopathy: insights from real-time 3-dimensional echocardiography. *J Am Soc Echocardiogr* 2005;18:802–4.

12. de Gregorio C, Recupero A, Grimaldi P, Coglitore S. Can transthoracic live 3-dimensional echocardiography improve the recognition of midventricular obliteration in hypertrophic obstructive cardiomyopathy? *J Am Soc Echocardiogr* 2006;19:1190 e1–4.

13. Yang HS, Lee KS, Chaliki HP, *et al.* Anomalous insertion of the papillary muscle causing left ventricular outflow obstruction: visualization by real-time three-dimensional echocardiography. *Eur J Echocardiogr* 2008;9:855–60.

14. Fukuda S, Lever HM, Stewart WJ, *et al.* Diagnostic value of left ventricular outflow area in patients with hypertrophic cardiomyopathy: a real-time three-dimensional echocardiographic study. *J Am Soc Echocardiogr* 2008;21:789–95.

15. Patel V, Nanda NC, Vengala S, *et al.* Live three-dimensional transthoracic echocardiographic demonstration of septal perforator coronary artery-left ventricle fistulas following myectomy. *Echocardiography* 2005;22:273–5.

16. Hage FG, Karakus G, Luke WD, Jr, Suwanjutah T, Nanda NC, Aqel RA. Effect of alcohol-induced septal ablation on left atrial volume and ejection fraction assessed by real time three-dimensional transthoracic echocardiography in patients with hypertrophic cardiomyopathy. *Echocardiography* 2008;25:784–9.

17. Engberding R, Yelbuz TM, Breithardt G. Isolated noncompaction of the left ventricular myocardium—a review of the literature two decades after the initial case description. *Clin Res Cardiol* 2007;96:481–8.

18. Bodiwala K, Miller AP, Nanda NC, *et al.* Live three-dimensional transthoracic echocardiographic assessment of ventricular noncompaction. *Echocardiography* 2005;22:611–20.

19. Yelamanchili P, Nanda NC, Patel V, *et al.* Live/real time three-dimensional echocardiographic demonstration of

left ventricular noncompaction and thrombi. *Echocardiography* 2006;23:704–6.

20. Duncan K, Nanda NC, Foster WA, Mehmood F, Patel V, Singh A. Incremental value of live/real time three-dimensional transthoracic echocardiography in the assessment of left ventricular thrombi. *Echocardiography* 2006;23:68–72.

21. Rajdev S, Singh A, Nanda NC, Baysan O, Hsiung MC. Comparison of two- and three-dimensional transthoracic echocardiography in the assessment of trabeculations and trabecular mass in left ventricular noncompaction. *Echocardiography* 2007;24:760–67.

22. Kjaergaard J, Hastrup Svendsen J, Sogaard P, *et al.* Advanced quantitative echocardiography in arrhythmogenic right ventricular cardiomyopathy. *J Am Soc Echocardiogr* 2007;20:27–35.

23. Fujikawa M, Iwasaka J, Oishi C, *et al.* Three-dimensional echocardiographic assessment of left ventricular function in takotsubo cardiomyopathy. *Heart Vessels* 2008;23:214–16.

24. Breithardt OA, Becker M, Kalsch T, Haghi D. Follow-up in Tako-tsubo cardiomyopathy by real-time three-dimensional echocardiography. *Heart* 2008;94:210.

CHAPTER 11

Congenital Heart Disease

Introduction

Congenital heart disease (CHD) is arguably the most complex discipline in cardiology. This has been attributed to the intricacy of the multiple CHD conditions that a cardiologist might have to address and the difficulty to make a diagnosis, and ultimately plan of management based on the physical exam alone. In response, CHD has depended heavily on imaging modalities to guide its progress [1–4]. 2D transthoracic echocardiography (2DTTE) has been the most widely used imaging modality for the study of CHD, particularly in the pediatric population [4]. 2DTTE is particularly attractive and has advantages over computed tomography (CT) and magnetic resonance imaging (MRI) since it is entirely noninvasive, does not depend on potentially harmful radiation, and requires minimal cooperation from the patient. Nevertheless, despite its multiple advantages and widespread use, 2DTTE is limited in comparison to the other imaging modalities in the 3D visualization of these complex entities. It is, therefore, not surprising that with the development of 3DTTE and its application to clinical practice, it has enjoyed particular success in the assessment of multiple CHD conditions. With the increasing survival of CHD patients who undergo surgical correction during childhood, an exponentially higher number of adults with CHD will be under the care of clinical cardiologists in the coming years and this field will likely benefit from current improvements in imaging technology [5].

Live/Real Time 3D Echocardiography, 1st edition.
By Navin C. Nanda, Ming Chon Hsiung, Andrew P. Miller, and Fadi G. Hage. Published 2010 by Blackwell Publishing Ltd.

Shunt lesions

Atrial septal defects (Figures 11.1–11.14)

Patients with atrial septal defects (ASD) account for almost 10% of all patients with CHD [6]. The presence of an ASD allows blood to shunt from the left to the right side of the heart, therefore producing a state of volume overload [6]. There are four main types of ASDs: the most common is ostium secundum ASD, which occurs in the area of the fossa ovalis. Ostium primum ASDs are actually part of the spectrum of atrioventricular canals and are usually associated with a cleft mitral valve. Sinus venosus ASDs occur at the junction of the superior or inferior vena cava and the right atrium and are frequently accompanied by anomalous drainage of the pulmonary veins. The least common variety of ASDs is of the coronary sinus type which is located in the roof of the coronary sinus and basically represents an unroofed coronary sinus [6].

ASDs have traditionally been corrected surgically, but the recent evolution of percutaneous closure devices has made it a viable alternative [6]. Although the indications to undergo percutaneous or surgical repair are similar, there are specific attributes of ASDs that make them amenable to percutaneous closure which include the location of the defect, its shape and size, and the adequacy of its margins for the placement of such devices [6,7]. Although the diagnosis of ASD can be challenging with 2DTTE, 2D transesophageal echocardiography (2DTEE) has enjoyed widespread applicability in this field. Furthermore, 2DTTE can be used for the assessment of ASDs prior to treatment [7]. Nevertheless, since the defect cannot be visualized *en face* by either 2DTTE or 2DTEE, its maximum dimension cannot be ascertained and its geometrical shape cannot be defined. Since ASDs can have complex geometry that includes a Swiss cheese pattern

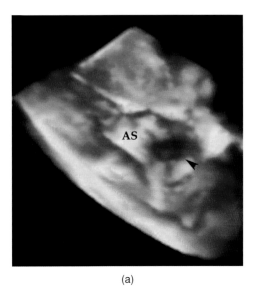

(a)   (b)

Figure 11.1 Live 3D transthoracic echocardiographic (3DTTE) assessment of atrial septal defect. The arrowhead points to a large secundum atrial septal defect visualized from both right (RA; a) and left atrial (LA; b) aspects. Note the large rim of tissue surrounding the defect. AS, atrial septum. Movie clip 11.1 Part 1 shows *en face* viewing of a small atrial septal defect from both the left and right atrial aspects. There is an ample rim of tissue surrounding the defect. Movie clip 11.1 Part 2 from another adult patient with a secundum atrial septal defect. Regular and QLAB (Philips Medical Systems, Andover, MA) cropping of the 3D dataset views the large defect *en face* (two arrowheads). Reasonable amount of atrial septal tissue surrounds the defect. The defect measures 3.2   3.1 cm, area 9.2 cm^2. Movie clip 11.1 Part 3 from another patient with a secundum atrial septal defect. The 2D study shows a large defect (arrowhead) in the apical four-chamber and subcostal views. Regular and QLAB croppings view the large defect *en face* (two arrowheads/arrows). Although the defect is similar in size to the previous patient, there is hardly any rim of the tissue adjacent to the aorta making it hazardous to close it in the catheterization laboratory. Movie clips 11.1 Part 4 and 11.1 Part 5. In this large patient, a secundum defect in the atrial septum (AS) was suspected during subcostal examination but a definitive diagnosis could not be made. When the images were acquired using a 3D transducer and cropped, the defect (arrow) was clearly visualized with left and right shunting. (Reproduced from Mehmood *et al.* [8], with permission.)

(multiple-hole types of defects) and friable borders, a direct *en face* view of the defect is very desirable, thus placing 3DTTE at a theoretical advantage over its 2D predecessor [8]. We have shown the usefulness, accuracy, and feasibility of the assessment of ASD with 3DTTE, particularly prior to percutaneous closure where it allowed for the assessment of the tissue surrounding the defect [8]. In this respect, we have found that an *en face* view of the ASD provides the most pertinent information regarding the rim of tissue surrounding the defect, and that the size of the inferior rim is more important than the superior rim [8]. When an ASD occluder device is placed in a patient with small rims, the risk of migration or embolization of the device is much higher [9]. In rare cases, the occluder device can embolize into the pulmonary artery and require surgical extraction [9]. 3DTTE measurements of the defect size agree closely with those obtained by 3DTEE in patients undergoing surgical repair and with those obtained by balloon sizing in patients undergoing percutaneous closure [8]. With the addition of saline contrast enhancement, one can characterize even a very small patent foramen ovale (<5 mm) and visualize the valve of the patent foramen ovale [8,10,11]. Furthermore, 3DTTE (with and without color Doppler) can be used for the accurate assessment of the morphology and efficacy

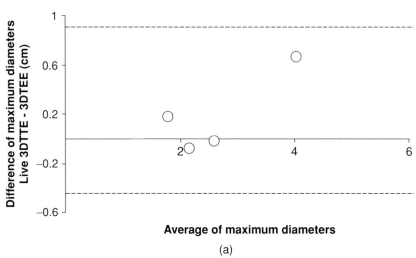

Maximum diameter by live 3DTTE vs 3DTEE

(a)

Circumferences live 3D TTE vs 3DTEE

(b)

Figure 11.2 Bland–Altman plots of maximum dimension, maximum circumference, and maximum area measurements of atrial septal defect (ASD) by live 3DTTE and 3D transesophageal echocardiographic reconstruction (3DTEE; a–c) and live 3DTTE and sizing balloon (d–h). The 95% confidence intervals are indicated by the dashed lines. (Reproduced from Mehmood et al. [8], with permission.)

Areas by live 3DTTE vs 3DTEE

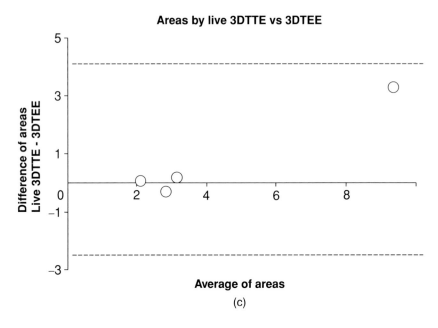

Average of areas

(c)

Maximum diameters by live 3DTTE vs sizing balloon

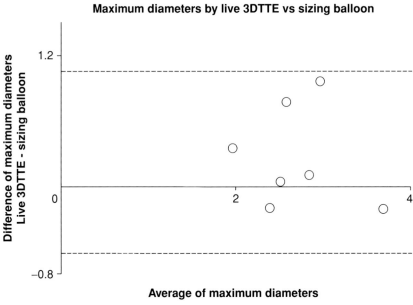

Average of maximum diameters

(d)

Figure 11.2 (*Continued*)

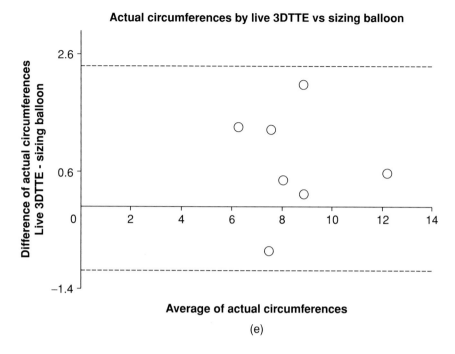

Actual circumferences by live 3DTTE vs sizing balloon

Average of actual circumferences

(e)

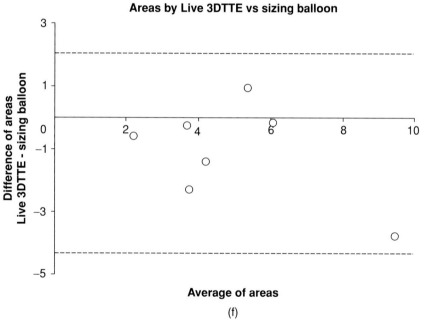

Areas by Live 3DTTE vs sizing balloon

Average of areas

(f)

Figure 11.2 (*Continued*)

Diameter derived from live 3DTTE circumference, assuming a circular ASD/sizing balloon

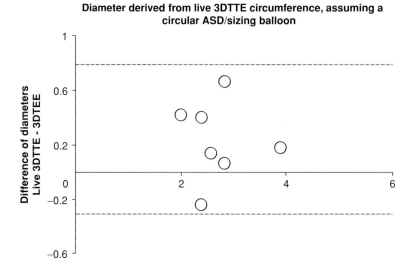

Average of diameters

(g)

Areas derived from diameter calculated from live 3DTTE circumference, assuming a circular ASD/sizing balloon

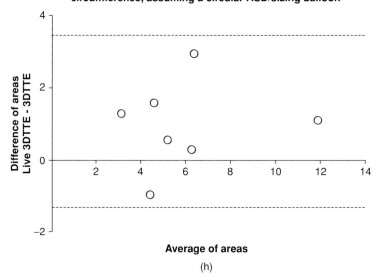

Average of areas

(h)

Figure 11.2 (*Continued*)

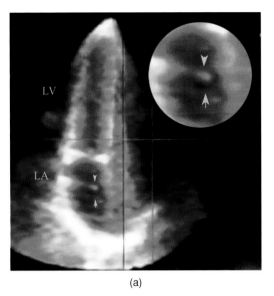

(a)

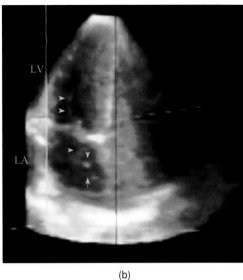

(b)

Figure 11.3 Live 3DTTE assessment of the patent foramen ovale (PFO). (a, b) The arrow shows the PFO, while the arrowheads point to contrast signals moving through the defect into the left atrium (LA) following an intravenous agitated saline injection. LV, left ventricle. (Reproduced from Mehmood *et al.* [8], with permission.)

of percutaneous closure devices used for the closure of ASD and even patent foramen ovale [10]. The visualization in 3D space of these closure devices may even help in the detection of the most serious postplacement complications such as residual shunts and device malposition, migration, embolization, and fracture [12]. In fact, with 3DTTE the right atrial and left atrial discs of the transcatheter closure device, the portion of the device that connects the two discs together, as well as the stainless steel screw thread located in the center of the device which is very echogenic, have been clearly visualized in in vitro settings and both discs are well seen in patients [10]. Interestingly, color Doppler 3DTTE showed a small residual shunt in some patients with an ASD occluder device which is considered a relatively normal finding seen early after device implantation and tends to disappear with time [10]. In vitro examination of an occluder device with 3DTTE has provided device measurements that correlated quite well with those from the manufacturer and revealed, in a manner that parallel in vivo studies, that the peripheral portions of both discs are more echogenic than the central mesh-like area [10]. Using 3DTTE patent foramen ovale can also be well visualized and the defect size measured, and on occasions the valve of the foramen ovale can be seen [11]. It is essential to have an adequate echocardiographic window to allow for a full 3DTTE assessment of ASDs. In our experience, this can be obtained in most patients from the right parasternal and the subcostal views. The right parasternal view is particularly helpful since patients with significant ASDs often have right ventricular enlargement which pushes the right lung away when the patient is placed in the right lateral decubitus position, affording a perpendicular ultrasound path to the atrial septum with this approach [8].

3DTTE can also be useful for the study of the more complex ostium primum ASD. These congenital defects are a consequence of incomplete fusion

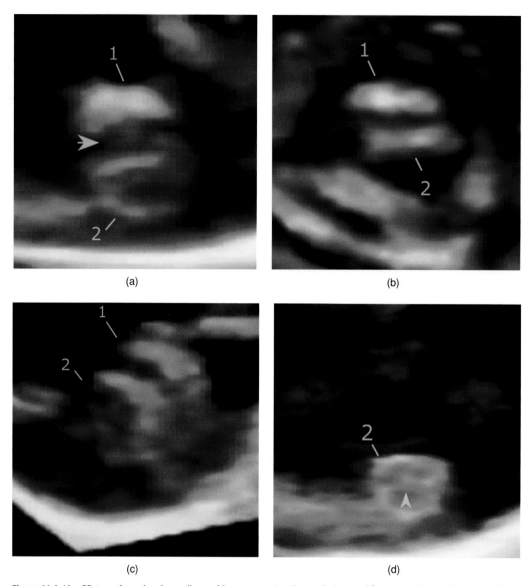

(a)

(b)

(c)

(d)

Figure 11.4 Live 3D transthoracic echocardiographic assessment of transcatheter closure of atrial septal defect. (a) The arrow points to the waist of the atrial septal defect (ASD) transcatheter closure device. (b, c) Show the device viewed from the top (b) and obliquely (c). Note that the left atrial disc (#1) is larger than the right atrial disc (#2). (d) The arrowhead points to the stainless steel screw thread located in the center of the right atrial disc viewed *en face*. (e) The arrow points to the small residual shunt seen one day after the device was positioned. (f)

Amplatzer device used for transcatheter closure of ASD. The arrowhead points to the metallic cap and the arrow points to the waist of the device. LA, left atrium; LV, left ventricle; MC, metallic cap; NW, nitinol winding; RA, right atrium; RV, right ventricle; ST, screw thread. Movie clip 11.4 shows 3DTTE examination of the atrial septal defect closure device 6 weeks after implantation. The device is well seated. (Reproduced from Sinha *et al.* [10], with permission.)

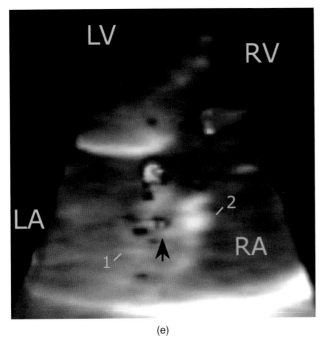

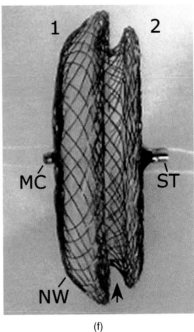

(e)

(f)

Figure 11.4 (*Continued*)

of the superior and inferior endocardial cushions resulting in complete or partial atrioventricular canal or septal defects with frequent abnormalities in the atrioventricular valves [6]. In complete atrioventricular canal, there is a large defect in the atrioventricular septum that includes both a primum ASD as well as an inlet ventricular septal defect (VSD). There is a single atrioventricular valve that consists of five leaflets, three lateral leaflets (mural lateral on the left, mural inferior, and anterosuperior on the right) and two bridging leaflets (superior and inferior). Complete atrioventricular defects are classified by Rastelli into types A, B, and C, based on the division and attachment of the superior bridging leaflet. In type A, the superior bridging leaflet is attached on the medial end to the crest of the interventricular septum by multiple chords and the leaflet itself may extend into the right ventricle attaching to the medial papillary muscle. In type B, the superior bridging leaflet extends further medially into the right ventricle and is attached to an anomalous papillary muscle arising from the

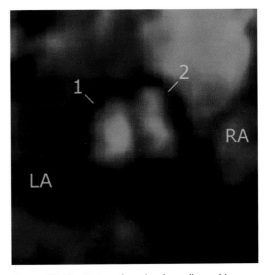

Figure 11.5 Live 3D transthoracic echocardiographic assessment of transcatheter closure of patent foramen ovale (PFO). 1 and 2 represent the left atrial and right atrial discs of the transcatheter device used to close the PFO. LA, left atrium; RA, right atrium. (Reproduced from Mehmood *et al.* [8], with permission.)

Figure 11.6 Live 3D transthoracic echocardiographic assessment of transcatheter closure of atrial septal defect. In vitro studies. (a, b) The arrowhead shows the stainless steel screw thread. #1 and #2 represent the left atrial and right atrial discs seen *en face* (a) and from the side (b). (c) The arrowhead points to the metallic cap seen in the middle of the left atrial disc. This is where the nitinol windings come together. (d–g) Real time 2D transthoracic echocardiography in embolization of atrial septal defect occlusion device. (d) The arrowhead points to the device located at the bifurcation of the main pulmonary artery. (e) Color Doppler-guided continuous wave Doppler interrogation demonstrates absence of significant obstruction. Peak velocity is only 1.47 m/s. (f–g) Live/real time 3D transthoracic echocardiography in embolization of atrial septal defect occlusion device. (f) The arrowhead points to the device located at the bifurcation of the main pulmonary artery. (g) Atrial septal defect viewed *en face* from the right atrial side (dotted line) after device embolization. Note the deficient inferior rim. AO, aorta; LPA, left pulmonary artery; PA, pulmonary artery; RPA, right pulmonary artery. Movie clip 11.6. ((a–c) Reproduced from Sinha *et al.* [10], with permission; (d–g) reproduced from Dod *et al.* [9], with permission.)

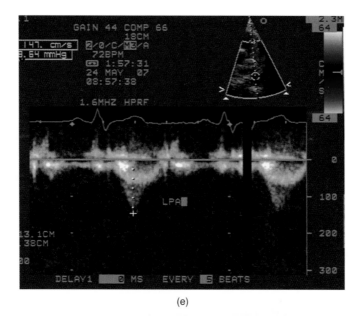

(e)

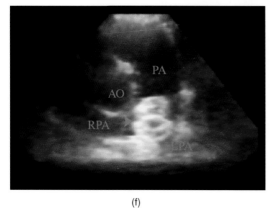

(f)

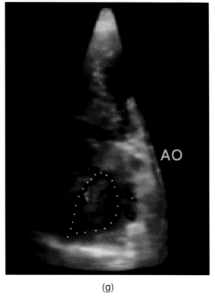

(g)

Figure 11.6 *(Continued)*

septomarginal trabeculation. In type C, there is a complete crossover of the superior bridging leaflet into the right ventricle where it attaches to the anterior papillary muscle [13]. The position of the great vessels is also dependent on the Raselli type where in type A, the aorta and the pulmonary artery tend to be positioned more to the left as compared to type C defects [14]. This classification system has important implications on surgical repair of this congeni-

tal entity [13]. In the partial form of atrioventricular septal defects, the extent of the defect is variable and can include the atrium septum (primum ASD), the ventricular septum, or both, and this form is characterized by separate right and left atrioventricular valve annuli [15]. It is important to recognize that in atrioventricular septal defects, there is anterior and superior displacement of the aorta and the left ventricular outflow tract which results in the elongation

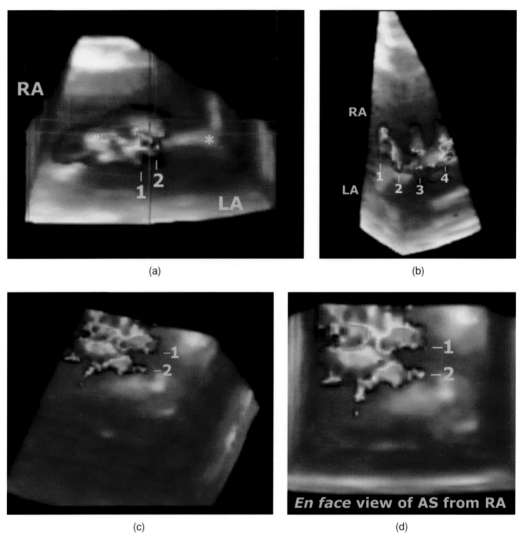

(a)   (b)

(c)   (d)

Figure 11.7 Live 3D right parasternal transthoracic echocardiographic examination of atrial septum and superior and inferior vena cavae. (a, b) Color Doppler examination in another patient showing four (numbered 1 through 4) separate secundum defects at different levels of the atrial septum (AS). (c, d) Two of these defects are viewed *en face*. In this 25-year-old female, four atrial septal defects at different levels of the atrial septum could be demonstrated by sequential cropping of the 3D dataset. Only two of these defects could be visualized by 2D transthoracic echocardiography. LA, left atrium; RA, right atrium. Movie clip 11.7. (Reproduced with permission from Patel *et al. Echocardiography* 2005;22:349–60.)

and narrowing of the left ventricular outflow tract and characteristic absence of wedging of the aorta between the mitral and tricuspid rings which is normally seen [16]. In addition, the papillary muscles can sometimes have abnormal arrangements that may result in subaortic obstruction of an already narrowed left ventricular outflow tract [17].

3DTTE provides a more comprehensive evaluation of this condition than 2DTTE [16]. Cropping the 3D dataset from multiple perspectives allows for the accurate assessment of the number and size of all five individual leaflets of the common atrioventricular valve and both the atrial and ventricular components of the septal defect, while this can

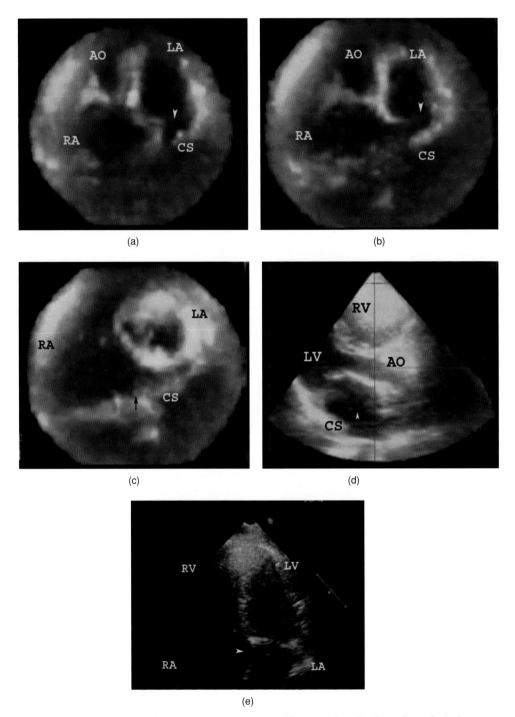

(a)

(b)

(c)

(d)

(e)

Figure 11.8 Real time/live 3D transthoracic echocardiographic findings in coronary sinus atrial septal defect. (a, b) The arrowhead points to unroofed coronary sinus (CS) which resulted in left atrial (LA) to right atrial (RA) shunting. (c) Shows opening (arrow) of CS into RA. (d) Parasternal long-axis view. The arrowhead points to a defect in the roof of CS resulting in communication with LA. (e) 2D transthoracic echocardiography in the same patient. The arrowhead points to a questionable defect in lower portion of atrial septum. AO, aorta; LA, left atrium; LV, left ventricle; RA, right atrium; RV, right ventricle. Movie clip 11.8. (Reproduced with permission from Singh et al. *Echocardiography* 2007;24:74–6.)

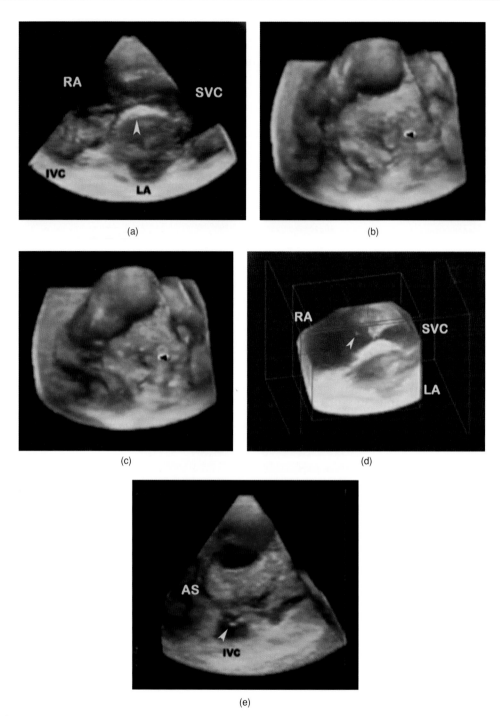

Figure 11.9 Real time/3D transthoracic echocardiographic visualization of the valve of foramen ovale. Right parasternal approach. (a) The arrowhead points to the atrial septum (AS). (b, c) *En face* view of the atrial septum from the left atrial (LA) side shows the valve of foramen of ovale in the closed (b) and open (c) positions. In the closed position, it completely covers the foramen ovale. (d) The arrowhead points to a mobile flap of tissue at the junction of superior vena cava (SVC) and right atrium (RA) representing a remnant of right-sided sinus venous valve. (e) The arrowhead shows the Eustachian valve. IVC, inferior vena cava. Movie clip 11.9 Part 1–8. (Reproduced from Panwar *et al.* [11], with permission.)

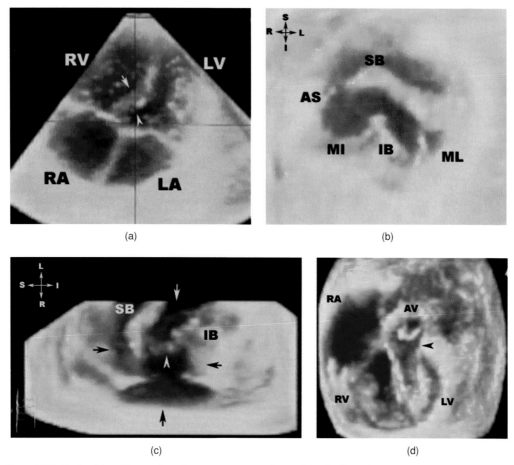

(a)

(b)

(c)

(d)

Figure 11.10 Live/real time 3D transthoracic echocardiography in complete atrioventricular septal defects. (a) The arrow shows attachment of common atrioventricular valve to a papillary muscle in the right ventricle (Rastelli type B). No attachments were seen to crest of ventricular septum (arrowhead). (b) *En face* view shows all five leaflets of common atrioventricular valve. (c) *En face* view of the defect viewed from top and sides (arrows). The arrowhead points to atrial septum. (d) The arrowhead points to elongated and narrowed left ventricular outflow tract. (*Continued on next page*)

be quite difficult if not impossible with 2DTTE. Furthermore, with 3DTTE subclassification of these defects, as described by Rastelli, is possible with more confidence than with 2DTTE [13,16]. The cleft in the atrioventricular valve can also be well appreciated in 3D with better assessment of its length, width, extent, and size of rim tissue from the valve margin than by 2DTTE. An isolated mitral valve cleft that is not associated with an ASD, a relatively rare anomaly, can also be well characterized by 3DTTE [18]. This cleft is directed toward the left ventricular outflow tract while the cleft asso-ciated with an atrioventricular canal defect points medially (toward the right ventricle). Also, in pa-tients with partial atrioventricular septal defects, 3DTTE showed only two scallops of the posterior leaflet of the left atrioventricular valve, compared to the usual three scallops, and the widened an-teroseptal commissure of the right atrioventricular valve ("cleft" tricuspid valve) which is hard to visu-alize with 2DTTE [16]. The 3D exam provides the advantage of better visualization of the relation-ship of the great vessels to each other and the atri-oventricular valve (unwedging of the aorta) and the

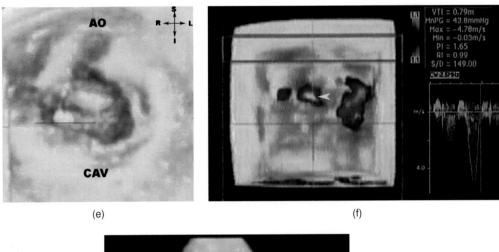

(e)   (f)

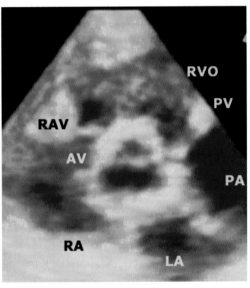

(g)

Figure 11.10 (*Continued*) (e) Shows absence of wedging of aorta (AO) in relation to common atrioventricular valve (CAV) annulus. (f) The arrowhead points to the vena contracta of CAV regurgitation jet. Its area measured 0.1 cm². Color Doppler-guided continuous wave Doppler interrogation of regurgitant jet showed a velocity time integral (VTI) of 79 cm. Regurgitant volume was calculated as 7.9 cm³. (g) Bicuspid aortic valve (AV). AS, anterosuperior leaflet; IB, inferior bridging leaflet; L, liver; LA, left atrium; LV, left ventricle; MI, mural inferior leaflet; ML, mural lateral leaflet; PA, pulmonary artery; PV, pulmonary valve; RA, right atrium; RV, right ventricle; RAV, right atrioventricular valve; RVO, right ventricular outflow tract; SB, superior bridging leaflet. Movie clips 11.10 A, 11.10 B, E, 11.10 C Part 1–3. (Reproduced from Singh *et al.* [16], with permission.)

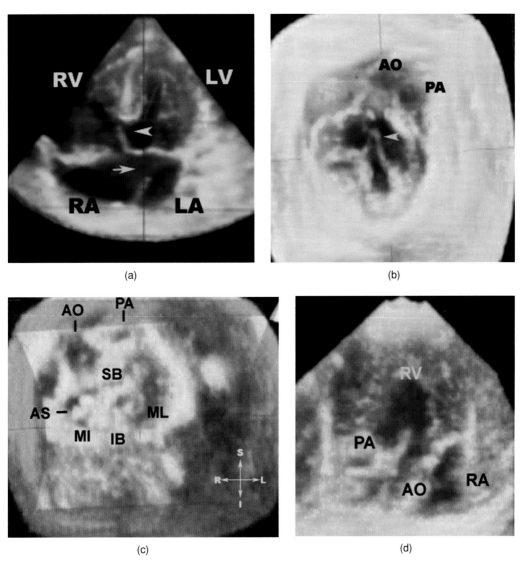

(a)

(b)

(c)

(d)

Figure 11.11 Live/real time 3D transthoracic echocardiography (3DTTE) in atrioventricular septal defects (AVSDs). (a) Complete AVSD. The arrowhead shows attachment of common atrioventricular valve (CAV) to crest of ventricular septum (Rastelli type A). The arrow points to atrial component of the defect. (b) Complete AVSD. The arrowhead points to an anomalous papillary muscle projecting into the left ventricular outflow tract causing subaortic obstruction. (c, d) Intermediate AVSD. (c) *En face* view of CAV shows superior bridging (SB) leaflet crossing over into the RV. (d) Both the aorta (AO) and the pulmonary artery (PA) are seen arising from the right ventricle (RV) consistent with double outlet RV. AS, anterosuperior leaflet; IB, inferior bridging leaflet; LA, left atrium; LV, left ventricle; MI, mural inferior leaflet; ML, mural lateral leaflet; RA, right atrium. Movie clips 11.11 B and 11.11 C. (Reproduced from Singh *et al.* [16], with permission.)

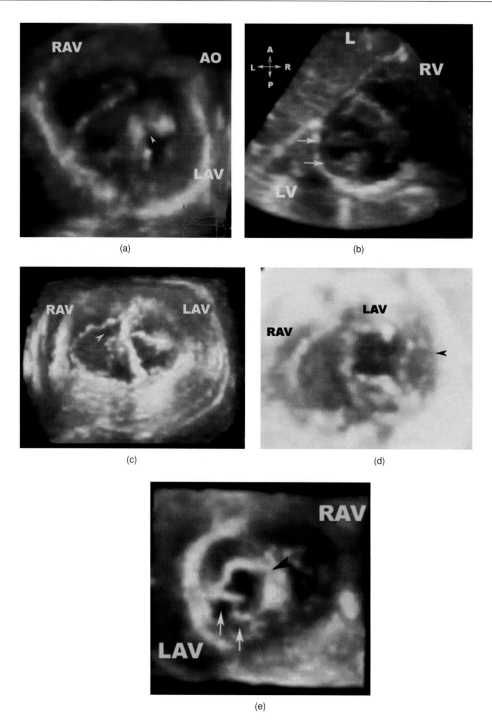

(a)

(b)

(c)

(d)

(e)

Figure 11.12 Live/real time 3D transthoracic echocardiography in partial atrioventricular septal defects. (a) The arrowhead points to a prominent cleft in the anterior leaflet of the left atrioventricular valve (LAV). (b) The arrows point to two left ventricular papillary muscles located close to each other. (c) The arrowhead points to a widened anteroseptal commissure ("cleft") of the right atrioventricular valve (RAV). (d) The arrowhead points to an accessory LAV orifice. (e) The arrows point to the presence of only two scallops in the posterior leaflet of LAV. The black arrowhead points to the anterior leaflet of LAV. AO, aorta; L, liver; LV, left ventricle; RV, right ventricle. Movie clip 11.12 C. (Reproduced from Singh *et al.* [16], with permission.)

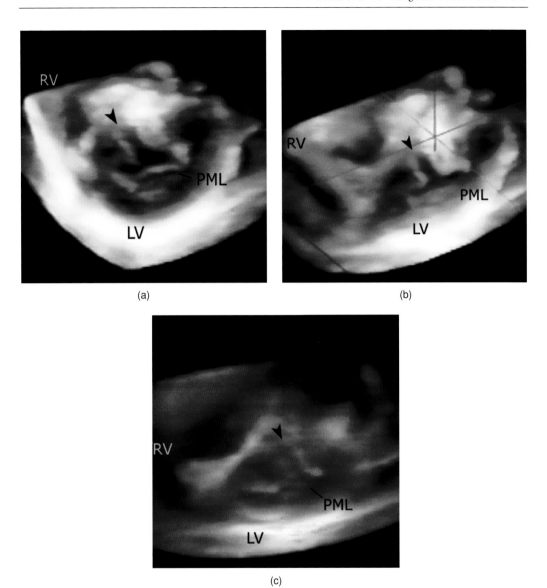

(a)

(b)

(c)

Figure 11.13 Live 3D transthoracic echocardiographic assessment of isolated cleft mitral valve. The arrowhead points to the cleft in the anterior mitral valve leaflet seen in the open (a, b) and closed (c) positions. LV, left ventricle; PML, posterior mitral leaflet; RV, right ventricle. The cleft is directed toward the left ventricular outflow tract unlike the atrioventricular septal defect where the cleft points medially. Movie clips 11.13 Part 1 and 11.13 Part 2 from another patient show an isolated cleft (arrow) in the anterior mitral leaflet in a 28-year-old female. Color Doppler examination shows prominent regurgitation (arrowhead) into the left atrium through the cleft. (Reproduced from Sinha *et al.* [18], with permission.)

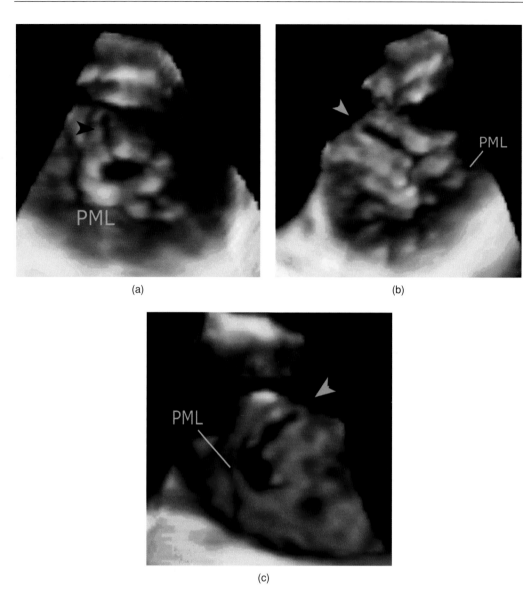

(a)

(b)

(c)

Figure 11.14 Live 3D transthoracic echocardiographic assessment of isolated cleft mitral valve. (a–c) The arrowhead points to the cleft in the anterior mitral valve leaflet. Note thickened mitral leaflets with a narrow orifice indicative of associated mitral stenosis. PML, posterior mitral leaflet. (Reproduced from Sinha *et al.* [18], with permission.)

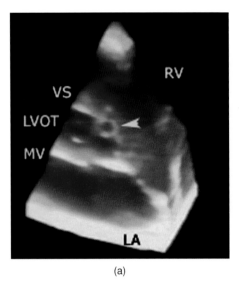

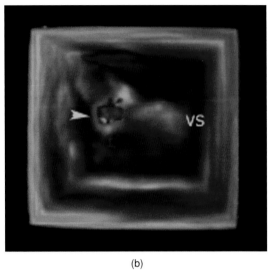

(a)

(b)

Figure 11.15 (a) The arrowhead points to a perimembranous ventricular septal (VS) defect viewed *en face*. (b) Shows color Doppler flow signals in the defect.

LA, left atrium; LVOT, left ventricular outflow tract; MV, mitral valve; RV, right ventricle. Movie clips 11.15 Part 1–4. (Reproduced from Mehmood *et al.* [22], with permission.)

identification of other related congenital conditions [16]. In particular, 3DTTE was very helpful in revealing abnormalities in the orientation or arrangement of the papillary muscles, such as an anomalous papillary muscle projecting into the narrowed and elongated left ventricular outflow tract causing subaortic obstruction or abnormally closely attached papillary muscles (paired papillary muscles), since both ventricles could be seen very well in 3D [16]. The severity of valvular regurgitation can be gauged as described in previous chapters. Therefore, 3DTTE can provide incremental value on top of 2DTTE in patients with both partial and complete forms of atrioventricular canal/septal defects.

Ventricular septal defects
(Figures 11.15–11.24)
VSDs account for the majority of patients with CHD (20% of all patients with CHD) [19,20]. When newborn infants are systematically screened with echocardiography, the incidence of these defects is as high as 5% [19]. Although the majority of these defects close spontaneously, some continue to be patent into adult life and require repair. Surgical closure of these defects has been the standard of care for decades, but over the last few years percutaneous closure has been advocated as a less invasive

alternative [20]. The success of such an approach depends on careful patient selection, and echocardiographic imaging of these defects plays a crucial role in presurgical planning [20]. Important considerations include the size, shape, and location of the defect in addition to the anatomy of the surrounding tissue [21]. 3DTTE, unlike 2DTTE, can show these defects *en face*, and therefore allow for the measurement of their circumference and area and for better characterization of the surrounding tissue, including the measurement of the distance from the margin of the VSD to the tricuspid valve [22]. These measurements show excellent intra- and interobserver variability by 3DTTE, and are closely correlated to those obtained by surgery and by 2DTEE, therefore allowing for better identification of patients that will be suitable for device closure and for preprocedural device sizing [22,23]. These measurements also allow for the exclusion of patients without adequate anatomical rim of the VSD, and therefore potentially decrease the complication rate [22]. The importance of the *en face* views, which can only be obtained with 3DTTE, for the proper assessment of the anatomy and facilitating surgical or percutaneous closure planning cannot be overstated. 3DTTE can also be quite useful in revealing failed VSD surgical repair (patch dehiscence) [22].

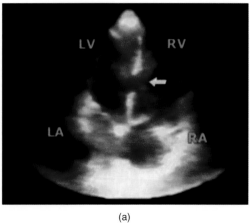

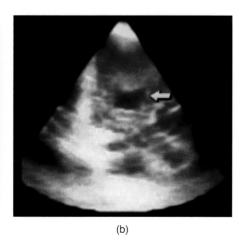

(a)   (b)

Figure 11.16 (a, b) Ventricular septal defect. The arrow in (a) points to a large defect in the trabecular ventricular system visualized in the apical 4-chamber view. The arrow in (b) shows the same defect viewed *en face* by cropping of the three-dimensional data set. Note the generous margins of the defect. Color Doppler examination shows flow signals moving through the defect. Movie clip 11.16.

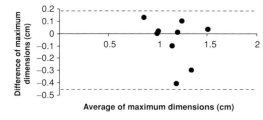

Figure 11.17 Bland–Altman plot of maximum dimensions of ventricular septal defect by live 3D transthoracic echocardiographic reconstruction (3DTTE) and surgery. The 95% confidence intervals are indicated by the dashed lines. (Reproduced from Mehmood et al. [22], with permission.)

Live 3DTTE vs 3DTEE maximum dimensions

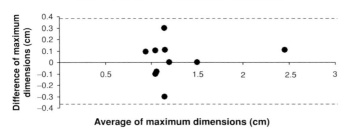

Figure **11.18** Bland–Altman plot of maximum dimension of ventricular septal defect by 3D transthoracic echocardiography (3DTTE) and 3D transesophageal echocardiographic reconstruction (3DTEE). The 95% confidence intervals are indicated by the dashed lines. (Reproduced from Mehmood *et al.* [22], with permission.)

Live 3DTTE vs 3DTEE circumferences

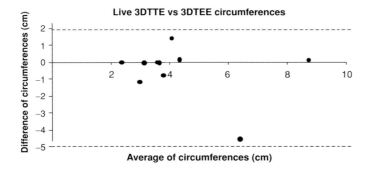

Figure **11.19** Bland–Altman plot of maximum circumferences of ventricular septal defect by 3D transthoracic echocardiography (3DTTE) and 3D transesophageal echocardiographic reconstruction (3DTEE). The 95% confidence intervals are indicated by the dashed lines. (Reproduced from Mehmood *et al.* [22], with permission.)

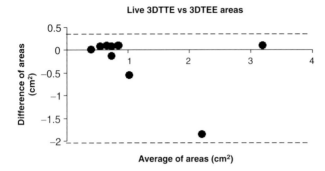

Figure 11.20 Bland–Altman plot of maximum areas of ventricular septal defect by 3D transthoracic echocardiography (3DTTE) and 3D transesophageal echocardiographic reconstruction (3DTEE). The 95% confidence intervals are indicated by the dashed lines. (Reproduced from Mehmood *et al.* [22], with permission.)

Aortopulmonary window (Figures 11.25 and 11.26)

An aortopulmonary window is an extremely rare congenital anomaly involving communication between the ascending aorta and the pulmonary artery. Although 2DTTE has been traditionally used for the diagnosis of this entity, it suffers from multiple limitations related to the characterization of associated congenital lesions and false positive results due to artifactual dropouts [24]. 3DTTE has been used successfully for the diagnosis of an aortopulmonary window and has resulted in an increased confidence in the diagnosis since the 3D datasets can be cropped and viewed from multiple angulations and varying degrees of tilt to comprehensively view the defect. *En face* views have allowed for the measurement of the defect size. Furthermore, 3DTTE allows for better characterization of associated anomalies like an interrupted aortic arch [24].

Patent ductus ateriosus
(Figures 11.27–11.30)

The ductus arteriosus, which connects the pulmonary artery to the descending thoracic aorta, is normally patent in the fetus but closes shortly after birth and remains patent into adult life in some individuals [25]. The diagnosis can be made by 2DTTE in the majority of patients, although the size and shape may not be reliably identified [26]. Other imaging modalities, such as MRI and CT, have also been used for the diagnosis and characterization of patent ductus arteriosus (PDA) [27]. Currently, almost all PDAs can be safely and effectively closed using percutaneous techniques [26]. Using 3DTTE, the shape, length, and width of the PDA can be well visualized as well as its connections

with the pulmonary artery and the descending thoracic aorta in a way that is not possible with 2DTTE [28]. The proximity of the opening of the PDA into the main pulmonary artery in relationship to the left pulmonary artery can also be well seen and measured by 3DTTE. Both the pulmonary and the aortic ends of the PDA can also be visualized in multiple projections and *en face* views. This comprehensive evaluation of the PDA allows for the better selection of patients for percutaneous correction, the selection of the best approach of percutaneous closure, and for the determination of the success of the procedure. 3DTTE can also identify complications from the placement of occluder devices used to treat PDAs [29].

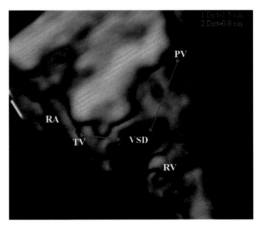

Figure 11.21 Shows the relationship and the distances of pulmonary valve (PV) and tricuspid valve (TV) from the ventricular septal defect (VSD). RA, right atrium; RV, right ventricle. (Reproduced from Chen *et al.* [23], with permission.)

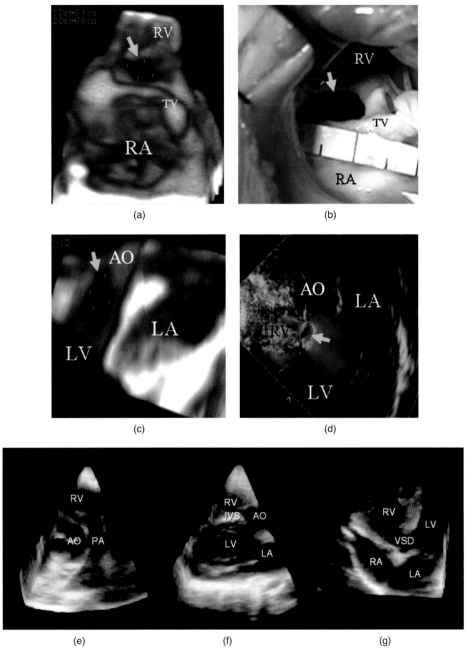

Figure 11.22 Perimembranous ventricular septal defect (VSD) (inlet) (arrow). (a) Real time 3D echocardiography (RT3DE) volume-rendered image of the right ventricle (RV) displaying the right aspect of the VSD. The location of the defect in relation to the tricuspid valve (TV) is shown. (b) Surgical view of VSD from the right aspect. (c) RT3DE volume-rendered image of the left ventricle (LV) displaying the left aspect of the VSD. The location of the defect in relation to left ventricular outflow tract is shown. (d) 2DE parasternal long-axis views showed the VSD in relation to aortic valve and RV. ((e–g) Live 3D transthoracic echocardiography in a patient with tetralogy of Fallot. (e) Note the wide aortic root (AO) and narrow pulmonary artery (PA). (f) The AO overrides the interventricular septum (IVS). (g) Four-chamber view. The VSD is located at the crux. LA, left atrium; RA, right atrium. ((a–d) Reproduced from Chen et al. [23], with permission; (e–g) reproduced from Wang et al. *Echocardiography* 2003;20:593–604, with permission.)

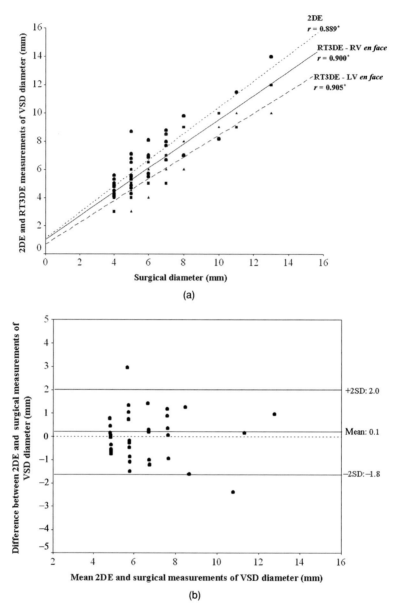

Figure 11.23 Population with ventricular septal defect (VSD) measured by 2D transthoracic echocardiography (2DTTE), real time 3D echocardiography (RT3DE), and surgical exploration. (a) Correlation between VSD diameter measured by 2DTTE and RT3DE from right ventricle (RV) *en face* and left ventricle (LV) *en face* projection. (b–d) Bland–Altman analysis showing excellent agreement between 2DE, RT3DE, and surgical diameter. *p value < 0.001 of statistical significance. (Reproduced from Chen *et al.* [23], with permission.)

Coronary artery anomalies (Figures 11.31–11.33)

Anomalies of the coronary artery occur in almost 1.3% of the population and could have serious complications, including myocardial infarction and sudden death [30]. A careful assessment of the anatomy of the anomalous coronaries can provide prognostic information and guide surgical repair

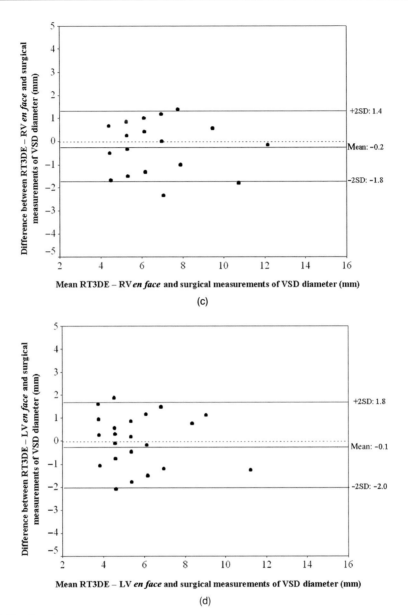

(c)

(d)

Figure 11.23 *(Continued)*

[30]. 3DTTE can be instrumental in the identification of the origin of such anomalies and the demonstration of coronary artery to pulmonary artery fistulas [31,32]. In patients with an anomalous origin of the left coronary artery from the pulmonary artery, the origin of the artery can be very well seen and the orifice can be measured *en face*. Postoperatively, the surgically created tunnel as well as the small defect in the tunnel that communicates with the pulmonary artery near the aortic end can be clearly visualized and 3D Doppler can show the tunnel-pulmonary artery shunting in 3D. By measuring the area of the defect in the tunnel and the time velocity integral, the shunt volume into the pulmonary artery can be calculated [31]. Coronary artery fistulas communicating with a cardiac chamber such as the left ventricle are also well delineated by 3DTTE.

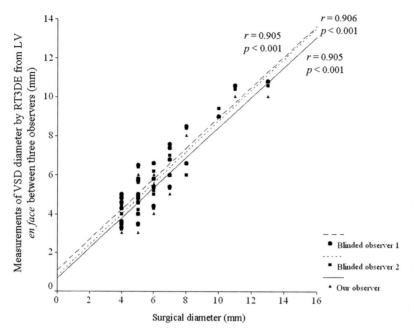

Figure 11.24 Interobserver variability between our observer and two blinded observers on measurement of ventricular septal defect (VSD) diameter by real time 3D echocardiography (RT3DE) from left ventricle (LV) *en face*. (Reproduced from Chen *et al.* [23], with permission.)

Obstructive lesions

Aortic stenosis (Figures 11.34–11.39)

Aortic stenosis has been described previously. Although the most common cause of aortic stenosis is acquired, namely calcific degeneration of the valve, congenital lesions (especially bicuspid aortic valve) are not uncommon [33]. With bicuspid aortic stenosis, symptom onset is, on average, in the fifth decade of life, while acquired aortic stenosis usually presents in the seventh to eighth decades. This lesion can be easily seen on 2DTTE and can result in aortic stenosis, regurgitation, or both. We recently observed a redundant aortic valve leaflet in a patient with bicuspid aortic valve and severe aortic regurgitation with no stenosis [34]. In order for equal-sized bicuspid valve leaflets to have midline closure without having leaflet redundancy, the length of the opposing surfaces of the valve cusps would be much smaller than the aortic circumference resulting in severe aortic stenosis. However, the presence of redundant folds in the leaflets increases the surface length of the leaflets so that when they open, they would reach the periphery of the aortic root resulting in no or minimal stenosis, but due to uneven closure of cusp margins, this may result in aortic regurgitation [34]. Another, rare cause, of congenital aortic stenosis is a quadricuspid aortic valve. This entity can be easily missed by 2DTTE but is amenable for a more comprehensive evaluation with 3DTTE [35]. Using this approach, not only the presence of a quadricuspid aortic valve can be made with more confidence than by 2DTTE, but also detailed assessment of aortic stenosis and regurgitation can be performed, as outlined previously.

Subaortic stenosis (Figures 11.40–11.45)

Obstruction to the left ventricular outflow tract may occur at the supravalvular, valvular, or subvalvular level [36]. Although obstruction at the subvalvular level can be dynamic due to systolic anterior motion of the mitral valve, as occurs in hypertrophic cardiomyopathy, fixed anatomic obstruction at the subaortic level also occurs. This obstruction can be secondary to a focal membranous structure or a diffuse tunnel-type lesion, with the focal form being more common [36,37]. The subaortic left ventricular outflow tract is a complex structure

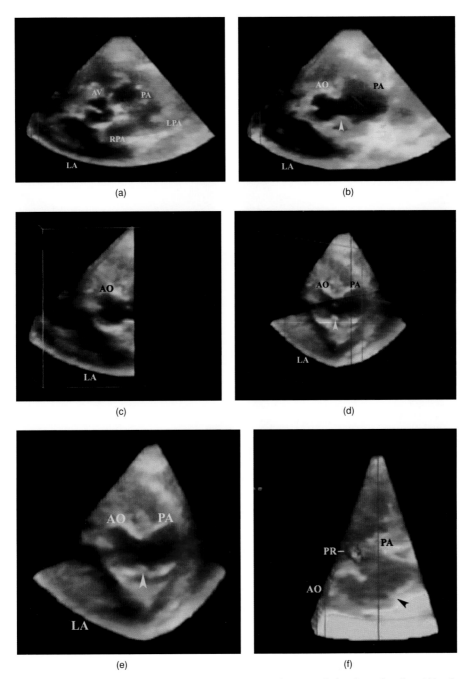

Figure 11.25 Live/real time 3D transthoracic echocardiographic assessment of aortopulmonary window. (a) Aortic short-axis view showing no evidence of an aortopulmonary window at this level. Movie clip 11.25 Part 2. The arrow points to the aortopulmonary window. (b) When the 3D dataset was cropped posteroanteriorly, a large communication between the aorta (AO) and pulmonary artery (PA) was revealed (arrowhead). (c–e) The aortopulmonary window (arrowhead) could be viewed *en face* by cropping the 3D dataset from the side (c) and rotating it (d, e). (f) Color Doppler exam shows mild pulmonic regurgitation (PR). The arrowhead points to the aortopulmonary window. AV, aortic valve; LA, left atrium; LPA, left pulmonary artery; RPA, right pulmonary artery. Movie clips 11.25 Part 1 and 11.25 Part 2. (Reproduced from Singh *et al.* [24], with permission.)

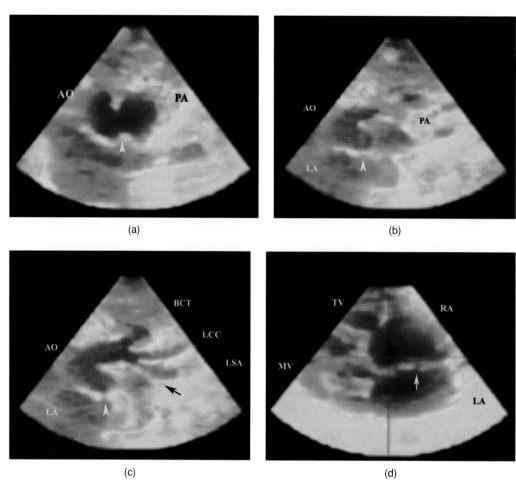

(a)

(b)

(c)

(d)

Figure 11.26 Live/real time 3D transthoracic echocardiographic assessment of aortopulmonary window. (a, b) The arrowhead points to the aortopulmonary window. Movie clips 11.26 Part 1 and 11.26 Part 2. The arrow points to the aortopulmonary window. The asterisk in Movie clip 11.26 Part 3 denotes the descending thoracic aorta. (c) The arrow points to the interrupted aortic arch. The arrowhead points to the aortopulmonary window. (d) The arrow points to a patent foramen ovale. AO, aorta; BCT, brachiocephalic trunk; LA, left atrium; LCC, left common carotid artery; LSA, left subclavian artery; MV, mitral valve; PA, pulmonary artery; RA, right atrium; TV, tricuspid valve. (Reproduced from Singh *et al.* [24], with permission.)

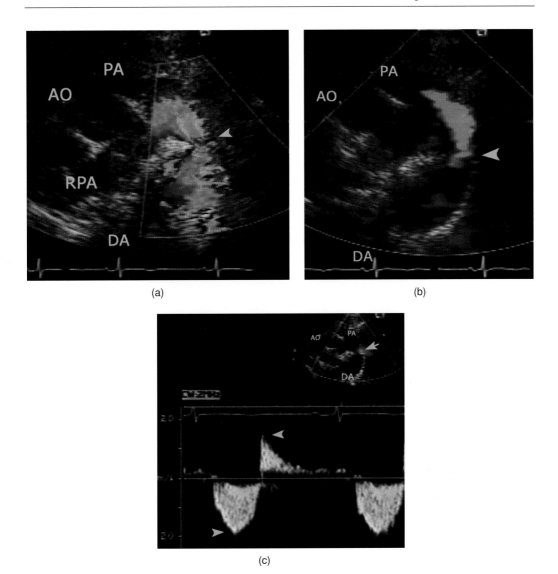

(a)

(b)

(c)

Figure 11.27 2D transthoracic echocardiography in an adult with patent ductus arteriosus. (a, b) Color Doppler examination demonstrates flow signals (arrowhead) moving between the main pulmonary artery (PA) and the descending thoracic aorta (DA) indicative of patent ductus arteriosus. (c) Color Doppler-guided continuous wave Doppler examination demonstrates flow signals moving from PA to DA in systole and back into PA in diastole (arrowheads). The arrow points to the continuous wave Doppler cursor line. AO, aorta; RPA, right pulmonary artery. (Reproduced from Sinha et al. [28], with permission.)

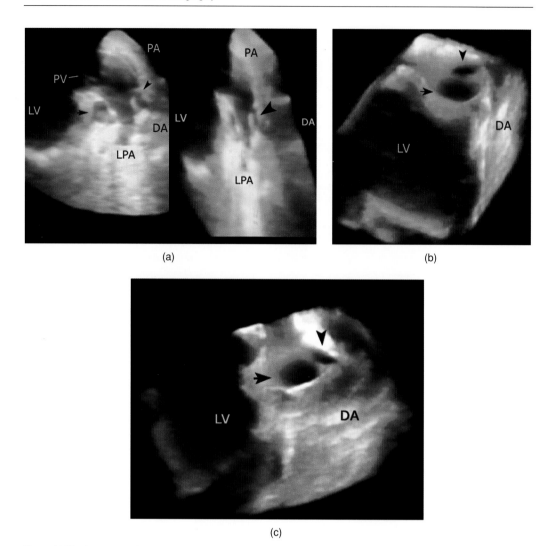

(a)

(b)

(c)

Figure 11.28 Live 3D transthoracic echocardiography in an adult with patent ductus arteriosus (PDA). B-mode images. (a) The pyramidal section has been cropped to show the full extent of the PDA (arrowhead) which connects the pulmonary artery (PA) to descending thoracic aorta (DA). The arrow points to the left atrial appendage. (b, c) The pyramidal section has been cropped from the top to show the opening of the PDA (arrowhead) into the pulmonary artery and its close location to the origin of the left pulmonary artery (arrow). LPA, left pulmonary artery; LV, left ventricle; PV, pulmonary valve. Movie clip 11.28. (Reproduced from Sinha *et al.* [28], with permission.)

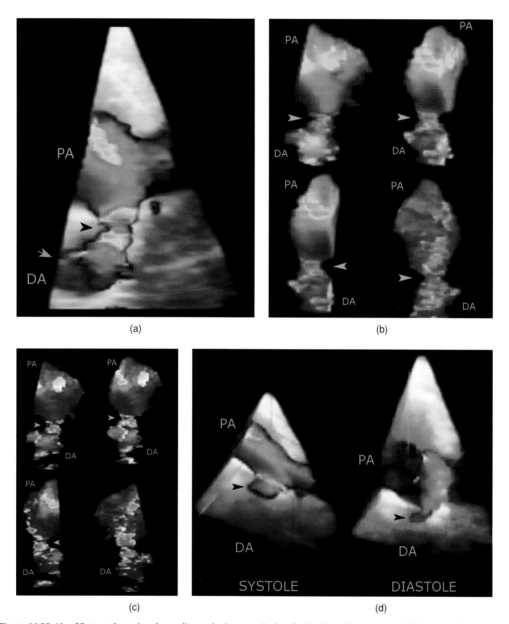

(a)   (b)

(c)   (d)

Figure 11.29 Live 3D transthoracic echocardiography in an adult with patent ductus arteriosus (PDA). Color Doppler images. The pyramidal section has been cropped to visualize flow signals in pulmonary artery (PA), PDA (arrowhead), and descending thoracic aorta (DA). (a) Shows the length of the PDA (arrowhead) connecting the PA and DA. The arrow points to an intercostal artery arising from DA. (b, c) Color Doppler images have been isolated by completely suppressing B-mode images. The isolated color Doppler images could be rotated from 0° to 176°, thus enabling comprehensive visualization of flows in PA, PDA (arrowhead), and DA in three dimensions. Images at 0° (top left), 45° (top right), 90° (lower left), and 176° (lower right) rotation are shown. (d) Frontal sections showing color Doppler signals moving from PA into DA in systole (left) and back into PA in diastole (right). (*Continued on next page*)

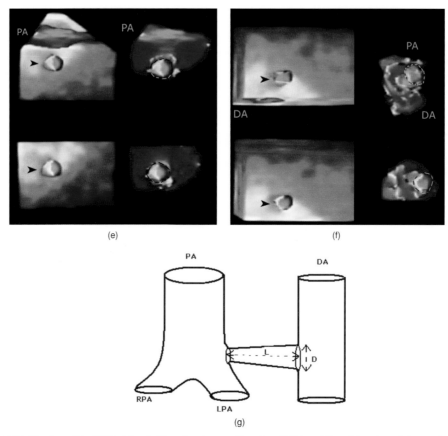

(e)   (f)

(g)

Figure 11.29 (*Continued*) (e, f) Tilted (top half) and *en face* (lower half) views of PDA (arrowheads) at aortic (e) and pulmonary (f) connections. On the right, B-mode signals have been suppressed resulting in only flow visualization. (g) Schematic. L, length of the ampulla, defined as the distance between the midportion of the narrowest diameter of PDA and the midportion of the aortic end. This measured 0.94 cm in our patient. D, PDA diameter at aortic insertion (ampulla diameter). This measured 1.31 cm in our patient. LPA, left pulmonary artery; RPA, right pulmonary artery. Movie clip 11.28, 11.29. (Reproduced from Sinha *et al.* [28], with permission.)

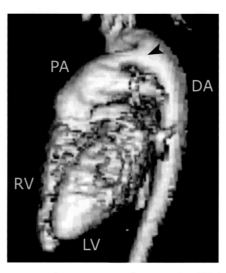

Figure 11.30 Thoracic magnetic resonance angiogram with gadolinium in the same patient. The arrowhead points to the patent ductus arteriosus (PDA) viewed in the left lateral position. DA, descending thoracic aorta; PA, pulmonary artery; RV, right ventricle. Other abbreviations as in Figure 11.29. (Reproduced from Sinha *et al.* [28], with permission.)

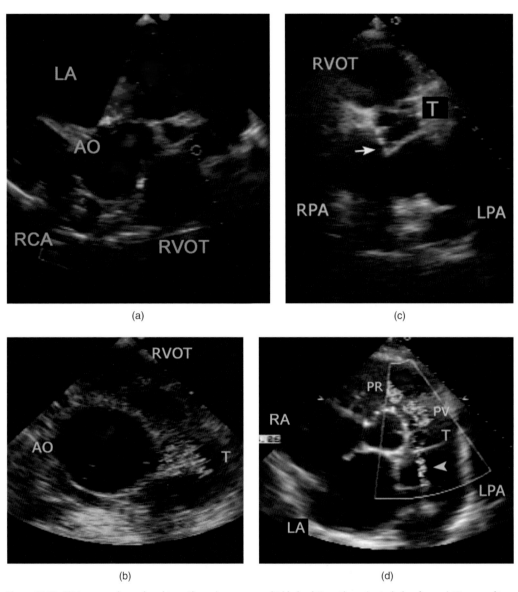

(a)

(c)

(b)

(d)

Figure 11.31 2D transesophageal and transthoracic echocardiography in an adult with anomalous origin of the left coronary artery from the pulmonary artery. (a, b) Intraoperative transesophageal study shows a dilated right coronary artery (RCA; a) and the surgically created tunnel (T; b). (c–e) Transthoracic study (performed 13 years after surgery). The arrow in (c) shows a small defect in the tunnel (T) near the aorta through which shunting occurs into the pulmonary artery (arrowhead in (d)). (*Continued on next page*)

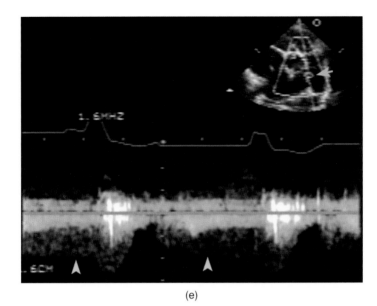

(e)

Figure 11.31 (*Continued*) Color Doppler-guided continuous wave Doppler examination (e) shows shunting occurring practically throughout the cardiac cycle (arrowheads). The arrow in (e) points to the Doppler cursor line. AO, aorta; LA, left atrium; LPA, left pulmonary artery; PR, pulmonary regurgitation; PV, pulmonary valve; RA, right atrium; RPA, right pulmonary artery; RVOT, right ventricular outflow tract. (Reproduced from Ilgenli *et al.* [31], with permission.)

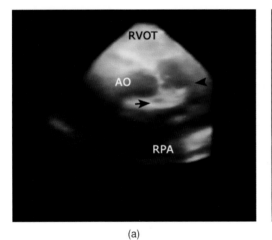

(a)

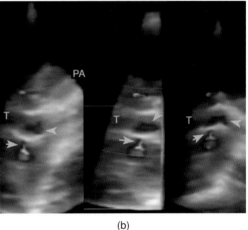

(b)

Figure 11.32 Live 3D transthoracic echocardiographic demonstration of anomalous origin of left coronary artery from the pulmonary artery. (a) The arrowhead points to the orifice of the anomalous coronary artery, while the arrow shows the defect in the tunnel. (b, c) Color Doppler examination. In (b), flow signals (red, arrowhead) are seen moving into the orifice of the anomalous coronary artery from the tunnel (T). The arrow points to the tunnel-pulmonary artery shunt. In (c), the arrow points to color Doppler shunt flow signals visualized in three dimensions. (d) Coronary angiogram. The arrowhead points to fistula originating from the left anterior descending coronary artery (LAD) and draining into the pulmonary artery (PA) which is partially opacified. (e–g) Live 3D transthoracic echocardiography. (e) The arrowhead points to a small localized area of abnormal flow signals in the PA just distal to the pulmonary valve (PV) in both diastole (f) and systole (g) consistent with entrance of the fistula into the PA. The arrow in (f) points to mild pulmonary regurgitation. AO, aorta; AV, aortic valve; CX, circumflex coronary artery; LM, left main coronary artery; RPA, right pulmonary artery; RVOT, right ventricular outflow tract. ((a–c) Reproduced from Ilgenli *et al.* [31], with permission; (d–g) reproduced from Mehta *et al.* [32], with permission.)

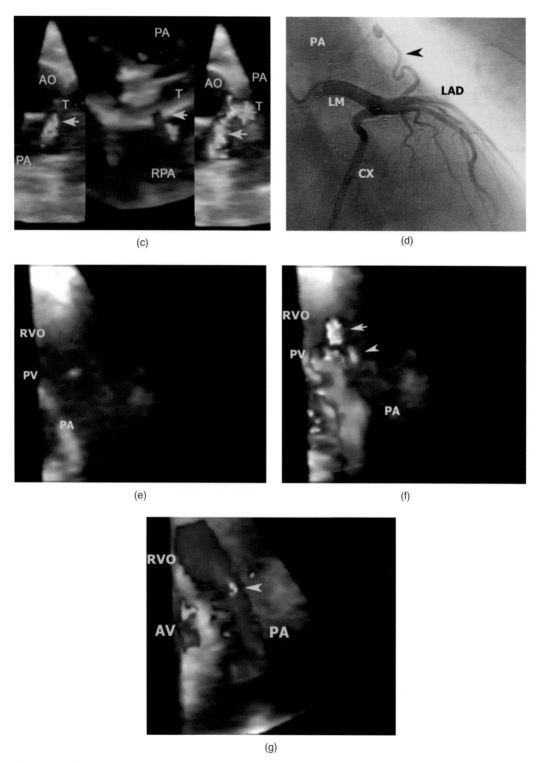

(c)

(d)

(e)

(f)

(g)

Figure 11.32 (*Continued*)

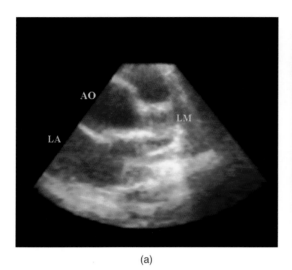
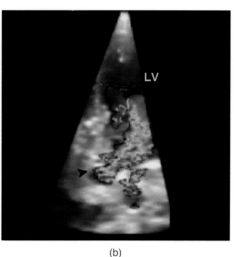

(a)   (b)

Figure 11.33 Live/real time 3D transthoracic echocardiographic detection of left main coronary artery (LM) fistula into the left ventricle (LV). (a, b) The arrowhead in (a) points to the enlarged LM. Its entrance into the LV is denoted by an arrowhead in (b). AO, aorta. Movie clips 11.33 A and 11.33 B.

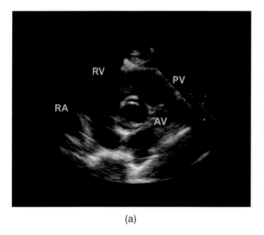
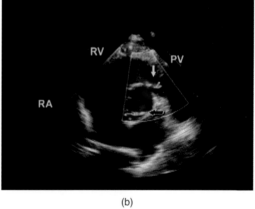

(a)   (b)

Figure 11.34 2D transthoracic echocardiography in an adult patient with bicuspid aortic valve and severe aortic regurgitation. (a) The bicuspid aortic valve (AV) is shown in systole in the open position with no evidence of stenosis. (b) Color Doppler examination shows an eccentric jet of aortic regurgitation originating posteriorly (horizontal arrow). The vertical arrow points to mild pulmonic regurgitation. PV, pulmonic valve; RA, right atrium; RV, right ventricle. Movie clips 11.34 A and 11.34 B. (Reproduced from Singh et al. [34], with permission.)

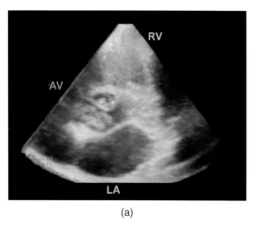

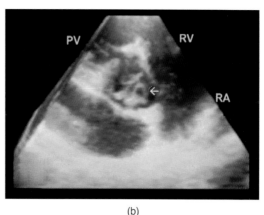

(a)   (b)

Figure 11.35 Live/real time 3D trasthoracic echocardiography in the same patient as Figure 11.34. (a) Note the presence of several folds in the bicuspid aortic valve (AV) in the closed position viewed from the ventricular side. (b) The arrow points to a well-circumscribed perforation in the posterior cusp of the aortic valve. LA, left atrium; PV, pulmonary artery; RV, right ventricle. Movie clips 11.35 A and 11.35 B. (Reproduced from Singh *et al.* [34], with permission.)

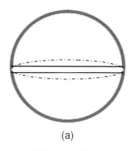

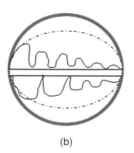

(a)   (b)

Figure 11.36 Bicuspid aortic valve. (a) Schematic illustrates a bicuspid aortic valve with equal-sized cusps and midline closure. Since the length of the free margins of the aortic cusps equals the diameter of the aortic root and the aortic lumen circumference is more than three times the diameter, this will result in markedly restricted opening of the valve leaflets in systole, leading to severe stenosis. (b) Same valve as in (a) but with multiple folds. The presence of these folds serves to substantially increase the length of the free margins of the leaflets resulting in a fully opened aortic valve in systole. (Reproduced from Singh *et al.* [34], with permission.)

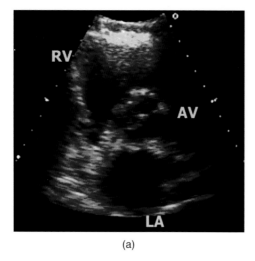

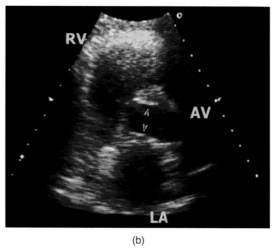

(a)   (b)

Figure 11.37 2D transthoracic echocardiography. (a, b) The aortic valve (AV) appears bicuspid. LA, left atrium; RV, right ventricle. Movie clip 11.37. (Reproduced from Burri *et al.* [35], with permission.)

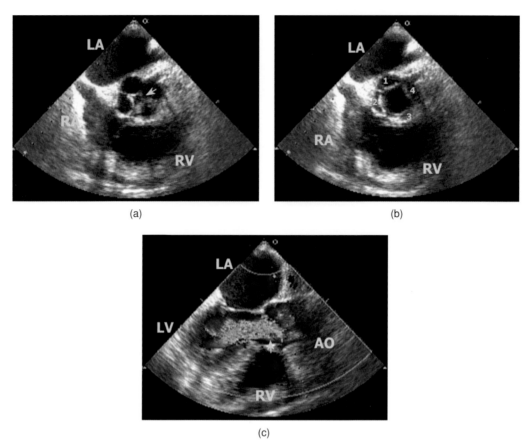

(a)　　　(b)

(c)

Figure 11.38 Multiplane 2D transesophageal echocardiography in a quadricuspid aortic valve. (a, b) Four aortic valve (AV) leaflets (numbered in (b)) are well seen. The arrow in (a) points to diastolic noncoaptation of AV leaflets which resulted in significant aortic regurgitation. (c) The arrow points to severe aortic regurgitation. AO, aorta; LA, left atrium; LV, left ventricle; RA, right atrium; RV, right ventricle. Movie clip 11.38 A–B. (Reproduced from Burri et al. [35], with permission.)

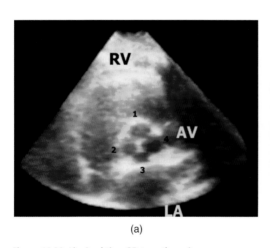

(a)

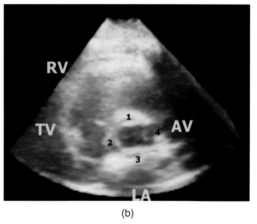

(b)

Figure 11.39 Live/real time 3D transthoracic echocardiography. (a, b) Shows a quadricuspid aortic valve with four numbered leaflets clearly visualized. AV, aortic valve; LA, left atrium; RV, right ventricle; TV, tricuspid valve. Movie clips 11.39 Part 1 and 11.39 Part 2. (Reproduced from Burri et al. [35], with permission.)

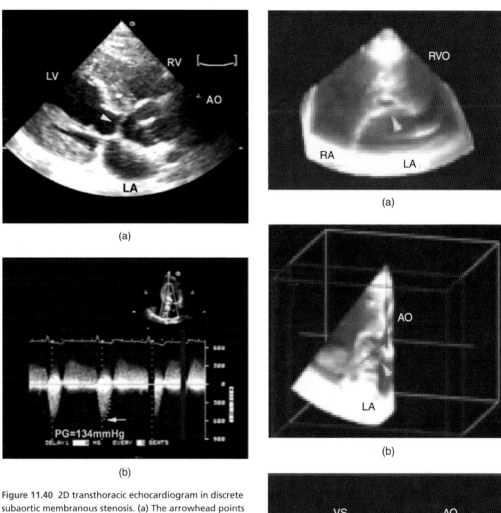

(a)

(b)

Figure 11.40 2D transthoracic echocardiogram in discrete subaortic membranous stenosis. (a) The arrowhead points to the subaortic membrane. (b) Using color Doppler-guided continuous wave Doppler, a peak gradient (PG) of 134 mmHg (arrow) was obtained across the left ventricular (LV) outflow tract. AO, aorta; LA, left atrium; RV, right ventricle; RVO, right ventricular outflow tract. (Reproduced from Agrawal *et al.* [40], with permission.)

(a)

(b)

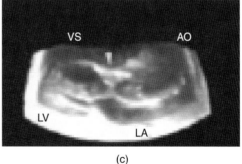

(c)

Figure 11.41 Live 3D transthoracic echocardiography in discrete subaortic membranous stenosis. (a, b) The arrowhead points to a narrow opening in the membrane imaged in short axis. (c) Membrane (arrowhead) viewed from the top showing its attachment to the ventricular septum (VS) and the anterior leaflet of the mitral valve. AO, aorta; LA, left atrium; LV, left ventricle; RA, right atrium. The arrowhead in Movie clip 11.41 points to the obstructing membrane. (Reproduced from Agrawal *et al.* [40], with permission.)

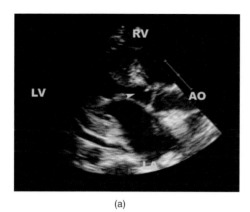

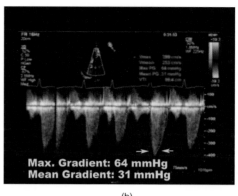

(a)   (b)

Figure 11.42 Discrete subaortic membrane. 2D transthoracic echocardiography. (a) The arrowhead points to the membrane imaged in the parasternal long-axis view. (b) Shows maximum and mean pressure gradients of 64 and 31 mmHg across the left ventricular outflow tract by continuous wave Doppler. AO, aorta; LA, left atrium; LV, left ventricle; RV, right ventricle. Movie clip 11.42. (Reproduced from Bandarupalli *et al.* [45], with permission.)

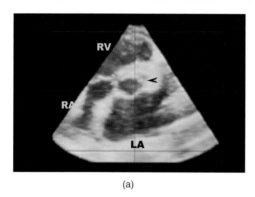

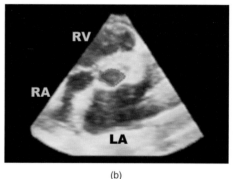

(a)   (b)

Figure 11.43 Discrete subaortic membrane. Live/real time 3D transthoracic echocardiography. (a, b) Subaortic membrane (arrowhead) and orifice viewed *en face*. The orifice measured 2.29 cm² by planimetry. LA, left atrium; RA, right atrium; RV, right ventricle. Movie clip 11.43. (Reproduced from Bandarupalli *et al.* [45], with permission.)

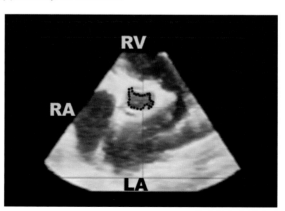

Figure 11.44 Discrete subaortic membrane. Live/real time 3D transthoracic echocardiography. Aortic valve orifice viewed *en face*. It measured 2.94 cm² by planimetry. LA, left atrium; RA, right atrium; RV, right ventricle. (Reproduced from Bandarupalli *et al.* [45], with permission.)

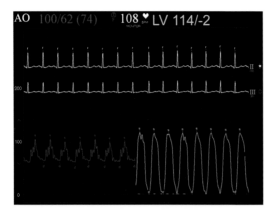

Figure 11.45 Discrete subaortic membrane. Cardiac catheterization pressure tracings showing no significant gradient across the left ventricular (LV) outflow tract. AO, aorta. (Reproduced from Bandarupalli *et al.* [45], with permission.)

that has a funnel shape area and extends from the free edges of the mitral leaflets to the aortic annulus. It is bounded anteriorly by the interventricular septum and posteriorly by the anterior mitral leaflet. Since the clinical presentation of patients with outflow obstruction share similar clinical presentations, subaortic stenosis should be suspected when Doppler examination reveals a high transaortic pressure gradient and the valve anatomy is normal. It is, therefore, not unusual that patients with discrete subaortic stenosis are misdiagnosed as hypertrophic cardiomyopathy [38]. Although 2DTEE can be useful for the diagnosis of this entity [39], a comprehensive examination of this lesion usually requires 3DTTE [40]. Using 3DTTE, the exact site and the full extent of the membrane can be identified and the orifice in the membrane can be delineated and planimetered to calculate its area and determine the severity of stenosis [40]. The attachment of the membrane to the ventricular septum and the anterior mitral leaflet can be easily visualized. In order to facilitate measuring the area of the orifice in the subaortic membrane, the 3D dataset can be rotated and cropped to view the orifice *en face*. In this view, the appearance of a "hole in a hole" is characteristic of subaortic stenosis. Therefore, 3DTTE has the advantage in assessing the severity of obstruction in subaortic stenosis over 2DTTE since the latter relies entirely on Doppler measurement of the gradi-

ent across the membrane which can be erroneous [41–44]. Indeed, we have recently reported on a patient with discrete subaortic stenosis who was erroneously diagnosed with significant subaortic obstruction by 2DTTE, but later found to have a large nonobstructive orifice by direct visualization with 3DTTE which was confirmed by invasive testing [45].

Complex and other abnormalities

3DTTE has been used for imaging a variety of CHDs and has shown its superiority over 2DTTE for a multitude of these conditions.

Cor triatriatum sinister (Figure 11.46)

3DTTE can be used to visualize cor triatriatum sinister, a rare congenital anomaly characterized by a fibromuscular membrane located in the left atrium superior to left atrial appendage, and to differentiate it from a supravalvular mitral membrane, which is located inferior to left atrial appendage [46]. The membrane can also be imaged *en face* which allows for assessment of the shape and an accurate measurement of the size of the opening in the membrane.

Ebstein's anomaly (Figures 11.47–11.50)

Although Ebstein's anomaly is classically diagnosed on 2DTTE by the familiar apparent displacement of the tricuspid valve toward the right ventricular apex, which suggests that the septal leaflet of the tricuspid valve is attached distally. In fact, this apparent displacement is due to the tethering of the tricuspid leaflet to the right ventricular wall. The tricuspid leaflets most commonly involved in this tethering process are the septal and posterior leaflets, but it is important to recognize that the tethering can be intermittent [47]. 3DTTE has shown value in evaluating patients with Ebstein's anomaly since 2DTTE is limited in the visualization of all three leaflets of the tricuspid valve which are often involved in this process [48,49]. Since 3DTTE is able to visualize all three leaflets of the tricuspid valve well, it is able to show the distribution and extent of the tethered and nontethered areas of the individual tricuspid valve leaflets much better than 2DTTE [50]. The bulging of the nontethered areas of the tricuspid valve leaflets produces a

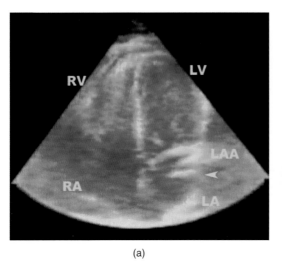
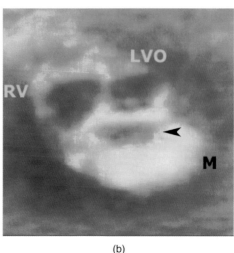

(a)   (b)

Figure 11.46 Live/real time 3D transthoracic echocardiography in cor triatriatum sinister. (a) The arrowhead points to cor triatriatum membrane (M), which is located superior to left atrial appendage (LAA). (b) The arrowhead points to a large opening in cor triatriatum membrane visualized *en face*. The dimensions were 3.06 1.03 cm and area 2.3 cm². LA, left atrium; LV, left ventricle; LVO, left ventricular outflow tract; RA, right atrium; RV, right ventricle. Movie clip 11.46. (Reproduced from Patel *et al.* [46], with permission.)

characteristic "bubble-like" appearance on 3DTTE and can be measured to estimate the free segments of the three leaflets of the tricuspid valve [50]. A full evaluation of the extent of leaflet tethering has important surgical implications [49,51]. 3DTTE can also be used to diagnose congenital or acquired Gerbode defect (left ventricular–right atrial communication), which is often missed or misdiagnosed as pulmonary hypertension with 2DTTE [52].

Transposition of the great arteries
(Figures 11.51–11.59)

Transposition of the great arteries (TGA) is a rare form of CHD. TGA occurs in two forms, dextro and levo (D-TGA and L-TGA, respectively). In D-TGA, there is ventriculo-arterial discordance in that the aorta arises from the morphological right ventricle and the pulmonary artery from the left ventricle [53]. In order for D-TGA to be compatible with life, it has to be accompanied by another lesion that allows for mixing of blood between the pulmonary and systemic circulations (ASD, VSD, or PDA).

D-TGA is one of the most common cyanotic defects seen in newborns. Multiple corrective surgeries have been developed over the years. The Senning and the Mustard procedures consist of an intra-atrial baffle that redirects deoxygenated blood from the vena cavae to the morphologic left ventricle. These procedures are accompanied by long-term complications such as baffle leaks, baffle obstructions, tricuspid valve regurgitation, arrhythmias, systemic right ventricular failure, and sudden death in the third to fourth decades of life. The more technically demanding arterial switch operation shows promise in addressing many of these complications [54]. In L-TGA, there is atrioventricular as well as ventriculo-atrial discordance. In these patients, the right atrium is connected to the morphological left ventricle, which gives rise to the pulmonary artery, and the left atrium is connected with the morphological right ventricle, which gives rise to the aorta [53]. Patients with L-TGA do not require corrective surgery and often do not get diagnosed until adulthood when they have failure of the systemic right ventricle.

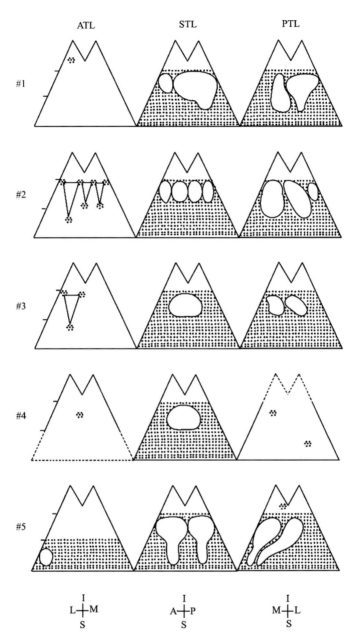

Figure 11.47 Schematic showing tethered (dotted areas) and nontethered (open areas) portions of all three leaflets of the tricuspid valve in patients with Ebstein's anomaly (#1–4). Break lines display poorly visualized areas of tricuspid valve leaflets. ATL, anterior tricuspid valve leaflet; STL, septal tricuspid valve leaflet; PTL, posterior tricuspid valve leaflet. Orientation symbols: A, anterior; I, inferior; L, lateral; M, medial; P, posterior; S, superior. (Reproduced from Patel *et al.* [46], with permission.)

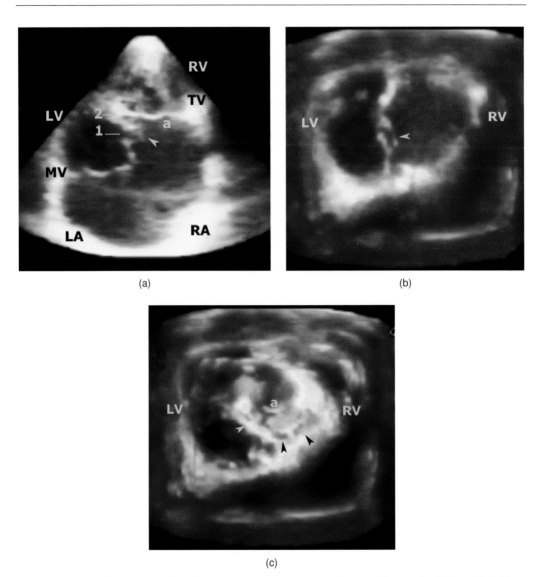

(a)

(b)

(c)

Figure 11.48 Live/real time 3D transthoracic echocardiography in Ebstein's anomaly associated with transposition of the great vessels. (a) Four-chamber view shows apparent displacement of the attachment of the septal leaflet of the tricuspid valve (TV) toward the apex. (b) Tethering of the septal leaflet of the TV results in a bubble-like appearance (yellow arrowhead) in the middle portion of the ventricular septum as the nontethered portion moves toward closure during systole. This transverse section was taken at a level denoted by #1 in (a). (c) Transverse section taken at a more inferior level (#2 in (a)) demonstrates bubble-like appearance of both septal (yellow arrowhead) and posterior (black arrowheads) TV leaflets produced by tethering. A, anterior TV leaflet; LA, left atrium; LV, left ventricle; MV, mitral valve; RA, right atrium; RV, right ventricle. (Reproduced from Patel *et al.* [46], with permission.)

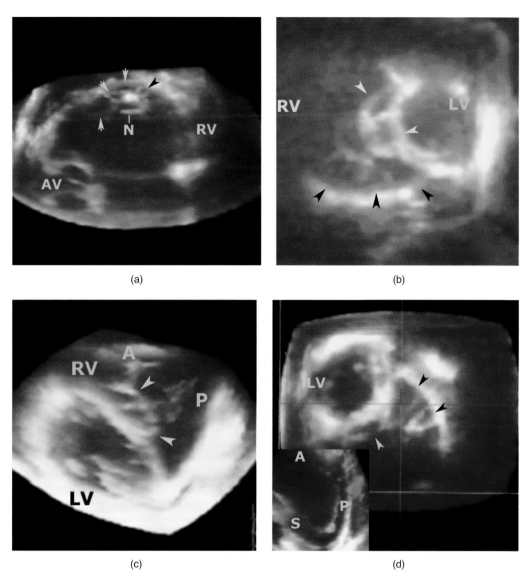

(a)

(b)

(c)

(d)

Figure 11.49 Live/real time 3D transthoracic echocardiography in isolated Ebstein's anomaly. (a) Transverse section taken at the apex of tricuspid valve (TV) shows a large area of noncoaptation (N) as well as tethering and bubble-like appearance of anterior (A; yellow arrows) and posterior (P; black arrowhead) TV leaflets. (b–d) Transverse sections taken more basally demonstrate multiple "bubbles" in the septal (S; yellow arrowheads) and posterior (P; black arrowheads) TV leaflets. Inset in (d) shows all three leaflets of the TV in the open position. (*Continued on next page*)

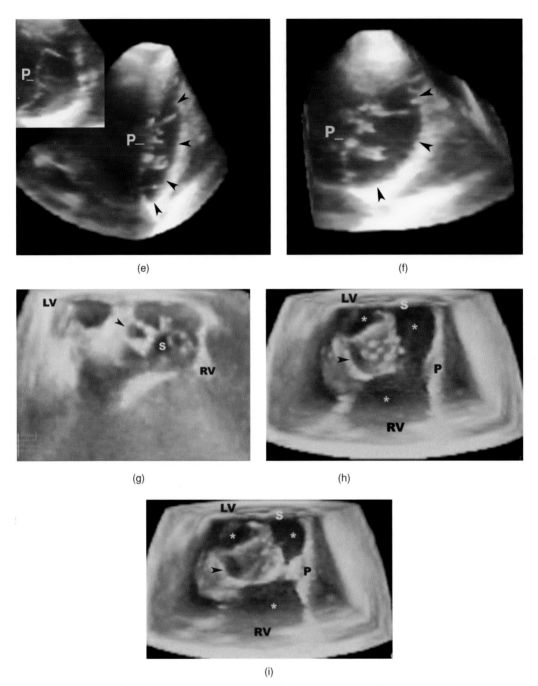

(e)

(f)

(g)

(h)

(i)

Figure 11.49 (*Continued*). (e) Oblique section shows multiple "bubbles" (black arrowheads) in the posterior (P) TV leaflet produced by tethering to right ventricular (RV) inferior wall. Inset in (e) shows a long snake-like posterior (P) TV leaflet. (f) The oblique section shown in (e) has been rotated to more optimally view the attachment of posterior (P) TV leaflet to the RV inferior wall. (g) The arrowhead in another patient with Ebstein's anomaly shows a bubble-like appearance resulting from tethering of the septal (S) TV leaflet to the ventricular septum. (h, i) The arrowhead points to a large defect in the anterior leaflet of the TV in a different patient with Ebstein's anomaly. Note also small, discrete nodular areas of thickening on the anterior tricuspid leaflet. Asterisks represent loss of TV tissue which is considerable in this patient. The septal leaflet of the TV was tethered to the ventricular septum. AV, aortic valve; LV, left ventricle; RV, right ventricle. Movie clips 11.49 B, 11.49 D, 11.49 D (Inset), 11.49 E (Inset) and F, 11.49 G, 11.49 H. ((a–f) Reproduced from Patel *et al.* [50], with permission; (g–i) reproduced from Pothineni *et al.* [57], with permission.)

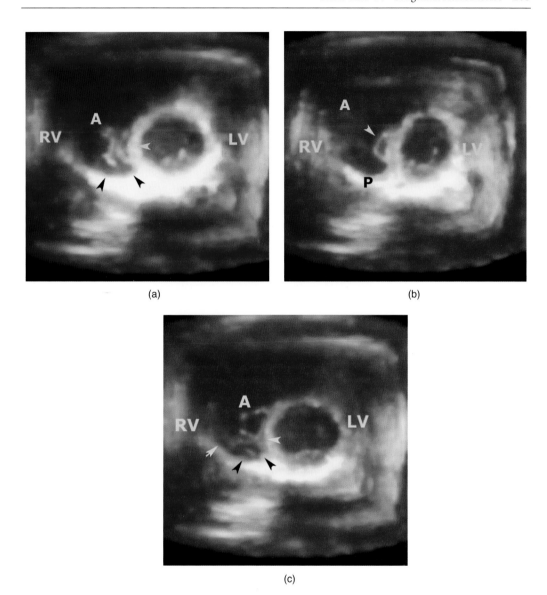

(a)   (b)

(c)

Figure 11.50 Isolated Ebstein's anomaly. (a–c) Shows tethering of all three tricuspid valve (TV) leaflets. The resulting "bubbles" are denoted by arrowheads for the septal (yellow) and posterior (P; black) TV leaflets and an arrow for the anterior (A) TV leaflet. LV, left ventricle; RV, right ventricle. (Reproduced from Patel *et al*. [50], with permission.)

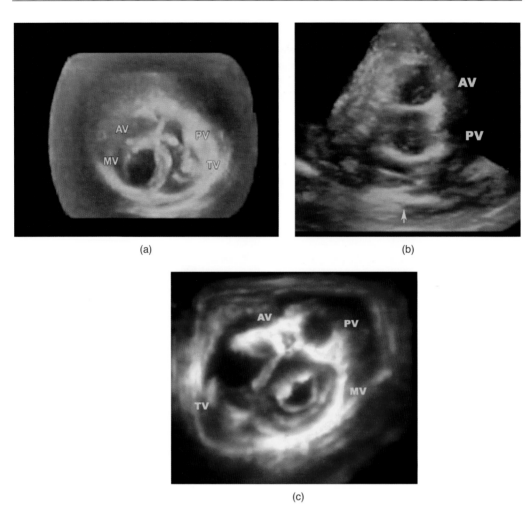

(a)

(b)

(c)

Figure 11.51 Dextro-transposition of the great arteries. In (a), the aortic valve (AV) and aorta are located anterior and to the right of the pulmonary valve (PV) and pulmonary artery. All four cardiac valves are visualized. In (b), the AV and aorta are located directly anterior to the PV and pulmonary artery. The arrow points to the intra-atrial baffle. (c) Shows normal relationship of the semilunar valves and the great arteries in a patient without transposition of the great arteries. The PV and the pulmonary artery are located anterior and to the left of the aorta and the AV. All four cardiac valves are visualized. MV, mitral valve; TV, tricuspid valve. Movie clips 11.51 A–C. (Reproduced from Enar et al. [55], with permission.)

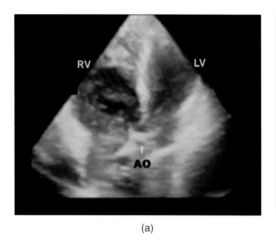

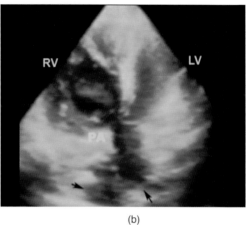

(a)   (b)

Figure 11.52 Dextro-transposition of the great arteries. (a) The aorta (AO) arises from the right ventricle (RV). (b) The pulmonary artery (PA) originates from the left ventricle (LV). The arrows point to left and right branches of the main PA. Movie clips 11.52 A and 11.52 B. (Reproduced from Enar et al. [55], with permission.)

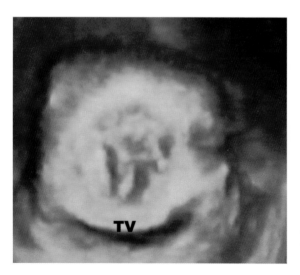

Figure 11.53 Dextro-transposition of the great arteries. Multiple anatomic defects are present in the tricuspid valve (TV), which is viewed *en face* in the closed position in systole. (Reproduced from Enar et al. [55], with permission.)

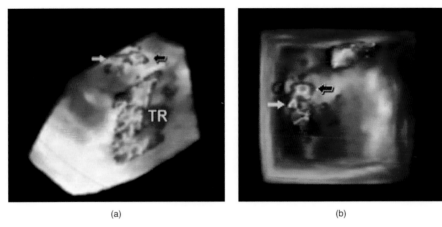

(a)   (b)

Figure 11.54 Levo-transposition (corrected transposition) of the great arteries. (a) The arrows point to two vena contractas of tricuspid regurgitation (TR) jets. (b) *En face* view of the two TR vena contractas (arrows). The Movie clips show cropping of the tricuspid regurgitation jet (arrow) to view the vena contracta (arrowhead) *en face* in another patient with levo-transposition (corrected transposition) of the great vessels. Movie clips 11.54 Part 1–3. (Reproduced from Enar *et al.* [55], with permission.)

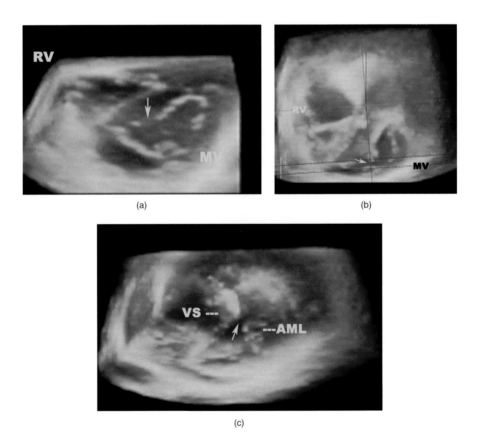

(a)   (b)

(c)

Figure 11.55 Dextro-transposition of the great arteries. (a, b) The arrow points to a cleft in the anterior mitral valve (MV) leaflet. (c) The arrow points to a narrow left ventricular outflow tract. Systolic anterior movement of the anterior mitral leaflet (AML) is also seen. The dataset was cropped from the top. RV, right ventricle; VS, ventricular septum. (Reproduced from Enar *et al.* [55], with permission.)

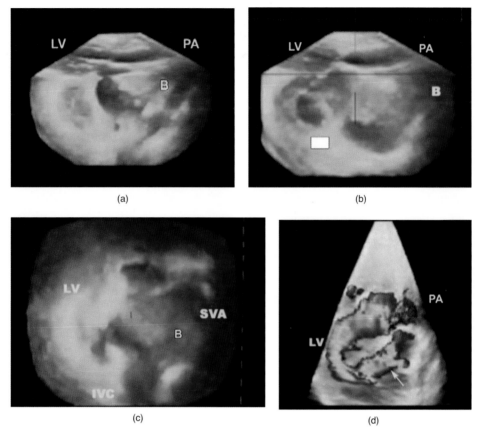

(a)

(b)

(c)

(d)

Figure 11.56 Dextro-transposition of the great arteries. (a, b) The intra-atrial baffle (B) appears as a shelf when viewed *en face* by cropping from the bottom. A defect in the baffle is not well seen in the illustration but it is clearly visualized (arrowhead) in the accompanying Movie clips which view the baffle *en face*. (c) Shows the relationship of the baffle to the inferior vena cava (IVC). (d) Color Doppler study shows systemic venous flow signals (arrow) moving through the left ventricle (LV) toward the pulmonary artery (PA). SVA, systemic venous atrium. Movie clips 11.56 Part 1 and 11.56 Part 2. (Reproduced from Enar *et al.* [55], with permission.)

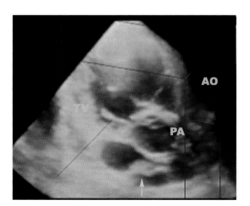

Figure 11.57 Dextro-transposition of the great arteries. The arrow points to a shelf-like intra-atrial baffle located behind the pulmonary artery (PA) in another patient. Note the anterior and leftward position of the aortic valve and aorta (AO) in relation to the pulmonary valve and pulmonary artery (PA). (Reproduced from Enar *et al.* [55], with permission.)

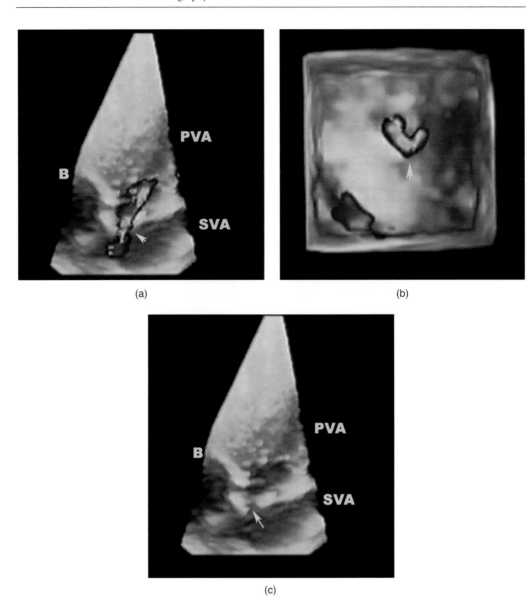

(a)

(b)

(c)

Figure 11.58 Dextro-transposition of the great arteries. (a) Color Doppler examination. The arrow points to a defect in the intra-atrial baffle (B). (b) *En face* view of the leak (arrow) at the origin (vena contracta). (c) The arrow points to the defect in the baffle seen after suppression of color Doppler flow signals. PVA, pulmonary venous atrium; SVA, systemic venous atrium. Movie clip 11.58. (Reproduced from Enar *et al.* [55], with permission.)

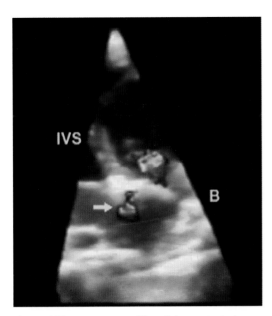

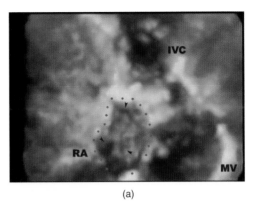

(a)

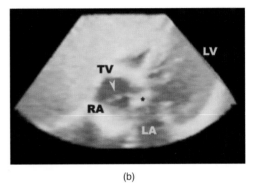

(b)

Figure 11.59 Dextro-transposition of the great arteries. The arrow points to a leak in the intra-atrial baffle (B) in another patient. IVS, interventricular septum. (Reproduced from Enar *et al.* [55], with permission.)

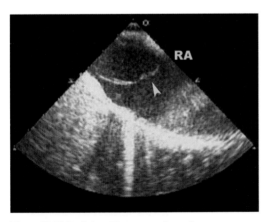

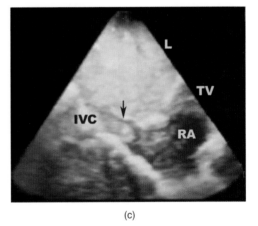

(c)

Figure 11.60 Real time 2D transesophageal echocardiography. The arrowhead points to a linear structure in the right atrium (RA) consistent with a Eustachian valve. Movie clips 11.60 Part 1 and 11.60 Part 2. (Movie clip 11.60 Part 2 arrow points to the tumor.) (Reproduced from Pothineni *et al.* [57], with permission.)

Figure 11.61 Live/real time 3D transthoracic echocardiography. (a, b) Chiari network. Small arrowheads in (a) point to some of the multiple openings in the large membrane, outlined by red dots. Attachment of the Chiari membrane (arrowhead) to the interatrial septum (*) is shown in (b). Movie clip 11.61 A arrowhead points to the Chiari membrane. (c) Renal cell carcinoma. Arrow points to the tumor in the inferior vena cava (IVC) at the right atrial (RA) junction. L, liver; LA, left atrium; LV, left ventricle; MV, mitral valve; TV, tricuspid valve. Movie clips 11.61 B and 11.61 C. (Reproduced from Pothineni *et al.* [57], with permission.)

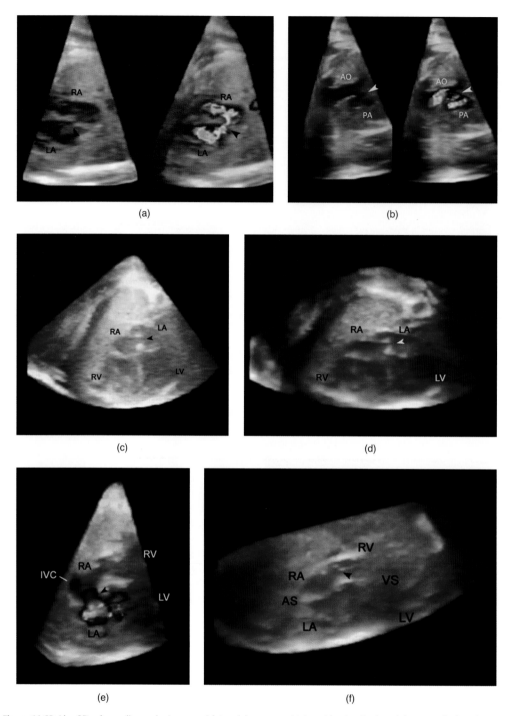

(a)

(b)

(c)

(d)

(e)

(f)

Figure 11.62 Live 3D echocardiography in normal fetus. (a) 31-week-old fetus. The arrowhead points to the foramen ovale. The arrowhead in (b) points to the ductus arteriosus connecting aorta (AO) to pulmonary artery (PA). (c–f) 19-week-old fetus. The arrowhead points to foramen ovale visualized in a four-chamber view (c) and from top (d). Color Doppler image shows physiological right to left shunting (arrowhead, (e)). The arrowhead in (f) points to a normal tricuspid valve. Both atrial septum (AS) and ventricular septum (VS) are viewed *en face* in this image. (g) 22-week-old fetus. Color Doppler image shows ascending aorta (AA), aortic arch (ACH), and descending thoracic aorta (DA). IVC, inferior vena cava; LA, left atrium; LV, left ventricle; RA, right atrium; RV, right ventricle. (Reproduced from Maulik *et al.* [61], with permission.)

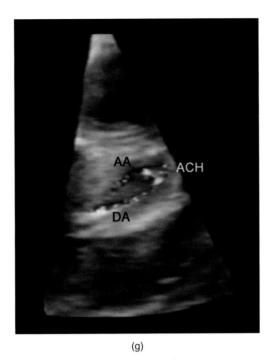

(g)

Figure 11.62 (*Continued*)

Conventionally, 2DTTE is used for the diagnosis of these entities as well as for clinical follow-up into adulthood. However, 3DTTE can be used to provide a more comprehensive evaluation of these patients [55]. 3DTTE is especially useful in the assessment of the systemic tricuspid valve which is most amenable to complications after an atrial baffle procedure. All three leaflets of this valve can be easily visualized in 3D, including the posterior leaflet which is difficult to see with 2DTTE, and areas of noncoaptation and prolapse identified. Severity of regurgitation can be assessed by measuring the vena contracta *en face*, as illustrated in previous chapters, to allow for the quantification of regurgitant volume. 3DTTE can be helpful in identifying other lesions that can be missed by 2DTTE such as a bicuspid pulmonary valve, clefts in the mitral valve leaflets, and chordal rupture of the mitral valve which are seen in these patients [55]. The atrial baffle can also be visualized well *en face* as a shelf which allows for the detection of the exact site and size of baffle leaks and obstructions that could be missed by 2DTTE [55]. This information allows for a comprehensive 3D evaluation and can be very helpful for surgical planning and substitute for the more invasive 2DTEE or MRI.

3DTTE is particularly valuable in patients who have implanted pacemakers [56].

Chiari network (Figures 11.60 and 11.61)

3DTTE can also be very useful for the visualization of the Chiari network, a large fenestrated membrane in the right atrium that has wide attachments in the right atrium at the crista terminalis and the interatrial septum. Using 3DTTE, a diagnosis of Chiari network can be made with certainty since it can be easily differentiated from other structures that can be seen in the right atrium such as the Eustachian and Thebesian valves, which are usually smaller and less extensive, and from cor triatriatum dexter, which is much thicker and has few or no fenestrations [57].

Fetal echocardiography (Figures 11.62 and 11.64)

Detection of CHD in utero is possible using fetal echocardiography [58,59]. However, due to the complexity of the fetal heart and its small size and rapid beating, it is fairly difficult to perform a comprehensive examination with 2D technology, and

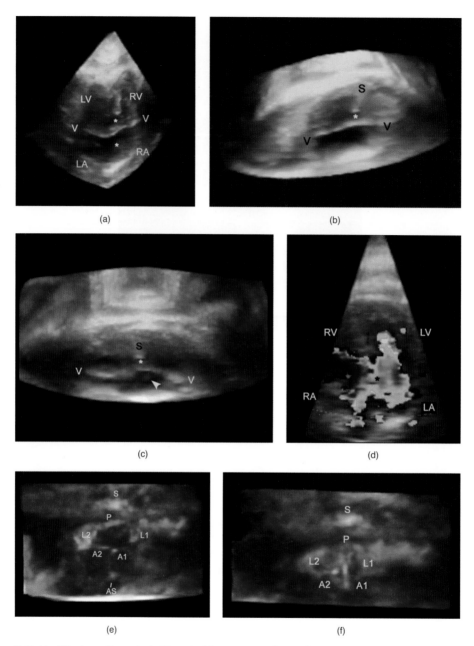

(a)

(b)

(c)

(d)

(e)

(f)

Figure 11.63 Live 3D echocardiography in 36-week-old fetus with complete atrioventricular septal defect. (a–d) Four-chamber views cropped to show the common atrioventricular valve (V) and the defect (asterisks). The arrowhead in (c) points to the atrial septum (AS). (e–f) The pyramidal section has been cropped from the top and rotated toward the examiner to display all five leaflets of V: posterior (P), left lateral (L1), left anterior (A1), right anterior (A2), and right lateral (L2). Small portions of the ventricular septum (S) and atrial septum (AS) have been retained to show their relationship to V. V is open in (d) and closed in (e). (*Continued on next page*)

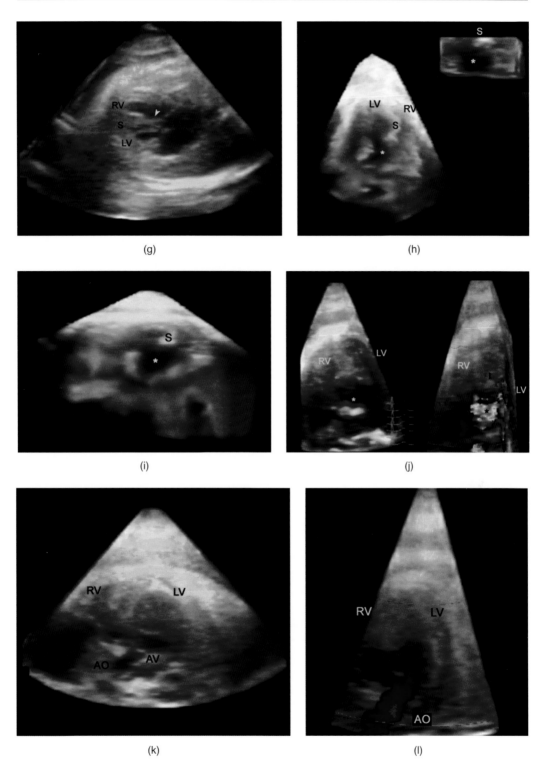

Figure 11.63 (*Continued*) (g) The arrowhead demonstrates multiple chordal attachments of V to S. (h–j) *En face* viewing of the defect (asterisk) from above (h), from the inferior aspect (i), and from the right side (j). (k–m) Five-chamber view shows the aorta (AO) arising from the left ventricle (LV).

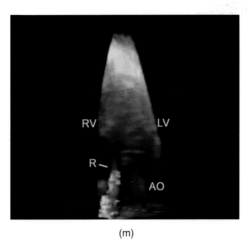

(m)

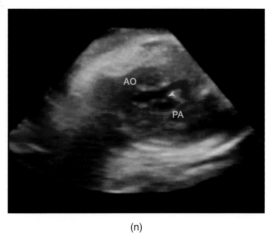

(n)

Figure 11.63 (*Continued*) In (m), the pyramidal section has been cropped to show regurgitation (R) from the right-sided component of V. (n) The arrowhead shows the ductus arteriosus. The arrowhead in Movie clips 11.63 Part 1–3 points to the common atrioventricular valve. AV, aortic valve; LA, left atrium; RA, right atrium; RV, right ventricle; S, ventricular septum. (Reproduced from Maulik *et al.* [61], with permission.)

3D technology can be quite useful in this setting [60]. Furthermore, 2D imaging in the fetus is limited by the fetal position which may not allow adequate imaging of a particular structure, and this is circumvented by a 3D examination in which cropping of the fetal heart will allow for visualization of the cardiac structures from any perspective [61]. Similar to adult 3DTTE, this technology allows for the visualization of atrial and ventricular septal walls as well as the valves *en face*, and therefore allow for greater confidence in the diagnosis of defects or valvular lesions [61]. Also, since defects are visualized *en face*, the extent of the defect can be easily measured. Using 3D examination with color Doppler, shunting can be detected as well as valvular regurgitation. It is therefore not surprising that this technology is being increasingly used for prenatal diagnosis of CHD [62].

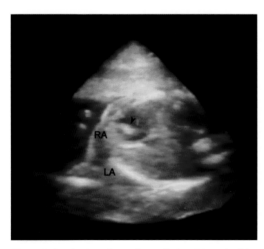

Figure 11.64 Live 3D echocardiography in a 20-week-old fetus. The arrowhead points to a markedly thickened tricuspid valve. LA, left atrium; RA, right atrium. (Reproduced from Maulik *et al.* [61], with permission.)

References

1. Gutierrez FR, Ho ML, Siegel MJ. Practical applications of magnetic resonance in congenital heart disease. *Magn Reson Imaging Clin N Am* 2008;16:403–35, v.
2. Valente AM, Powell AJ. Clinical applications of cardiovascular magnetic resonance in congenital heart disease. *Cardiol Clin* 2007;25:97–110, vi.
3. Nicol ED, Gatzoulis M, Padley SP, Rubens M. Assessment of adult congenital heart disease with multi-detector computed tomography: beyond coronary lumenography. *Clin Radiol* 2007;62:518–27.
4. Pacileo G, Di Salvo G, Limongelli G, Miele T, Calabro R. Echocardiography in congenital heart disease: usefulness, limits and new techniques. *J Cardiovasc Med* 2007;8:17–22.
5. Warnes CA, Williams RG, Bashore TM, *et al.* ACC/AHA 2008 Guidelines for the Management of Adults With Congenital Heart Disease: Executive Summary. A report of the American College of Cardiology/American

Heart Association Task Force on Practice Guidelines (Writing Committee to develop Guidelines for the Management of Adults With Congenital Heart Disease) developed in Collaboration with the American Society of Echocardiography, Heart Rhythm Society, International Society for Adult Congenital Heart Disease, Society for Cardiovascular Angiography and Interventions, and Society of Thoracic Surgeons. *J Am Coll Cardiol* 2008;52:1890–947.

6. Moake L, Ramaciotti C. Atrial septal defect treatment options. *AACN Clin Issues* 2005;16:252–66.

7. Chau AK, Leung MP, Yung T, Chan K, Cheung Y, Chiu S. Surgical validation and implications for transcatheter closure of quantitative echocardiographic evaluation of atrial septal defect. *Am J Cardiol* 2000;85:1124–30.

8. Mehmood F, Vengala S, Nanda NC, *et al.* Usefulness of live three-dimensional transthoracic echocardiography in the characterization of atrial septal defects in adults. *Echocardiography* 2004;21:707–13.

9. Dod H, Reddy VK, Bhardwaj R, *et al.* Embolization of atrial septal occluder device into the pulmonary artery: a rare complication and usefulness of live/real time three-dimensional transthoracic echocardiography. *Echocardiography* 2009;26:6

10. Sinha A, Nanda NC, Misra V, *et al.* Live three-dimensional transthoracic echocardiographic assessment of transcatheter closure of atrial septal defect and patent foramen ovale. *Echocardiography* 2004;21:749–53.

11. Panwar SR, Perrien JL, Nanda NC, Anurag S, Rajdev S. Real time/three-dimensional transthoracic echocardiographic visualization of the valve of foramen ovale. *Echocardiography* 2007;24:1105–7.

12. Berdat PA, Chatterjee T, Pfammatter JP, Windecker S, Meier B, Carrel T. Surgical management of complications after transcatheter closure of an atrial septal defect or patent foramen ovale. *J Thorac Cardiovasc Surg* 2000;120:1034–9.

13. Rastelli G, Kirklin JW, Titus JL. Anatomic observations on complete form of persistent common atrioventricular canal with special reference to atrioventricular valves. *Mayo Clin Proc* 1966;41:296–308.

14. Suzuki K, Ho SY, Anderson RH, *et al.* Morphometric analysis of atrioventricular septal defect with common valve orifice. *J Am Coll Cardiol* 1998;31:217–23.

15. Smallhorn JF. Cross-sectional echocardiographic assessment of atrioventricular septal defect: basic morphology and preoperative risk factors. *Echocardiography* 2001;18:415–32.

16. Singh A, Romp RL, Nanda NC, *et al.* Usefulness of live/real time three-dimensional transthoracic echocardiography in the assessment of atrioventricular septal defects. *Echocardiography* 2006;23:598–608.

17. Reeder GS, Danielson GK, Seward JB, Driscoll DJ, Tajik AJ. Fixed subaortic stenosis in atrioventricular canal defect: a Doppler echocardiographic study. *J Am Coll Cardiol* 1992;20:386–94.

18. Sinha A, Kasliwal RR, Nanda NC, *et al.* Live three-dimensional transthoracic echocardiographic assessment of isolated cleft mitral valve. *Echocardiography* 2004;21:657–61.

19. Hoffman JI, Kaplan S. The incidence of congenital heart disease. *J Am Coll Cardiol* 2002;39:1890–900.

20. Butera G, Chessa M, Carminati M. Percutaneous closure of ventricular septal defects. State of the art. *J Cardiovasc Med* 2007;8:39–45.

21. Pedra CA, Pedra SR, Esteves CA, *et al.* Percutaneous closure of perimembranous ventricular septal defects with the Amplatzer device: technical and morphological considerations. *Catheter Cardiovasc Interv* 2004;61:403–10.

22. Mehmood F, Miller AP, Nanda NC, *et al.* Usefulness of live/real time three-dimensional transthoracic echocardiography in the characterization of ventricular septal defects in adults. *Echocardiography* 2006;23:421–7.

23. Chen FL, Hsiung MC, Nanda N, Hsieh KS, Chou MC. Real time three-dimensional echocardiography in assessing ventricular septal defects: an echocardiographic-surgical correlative study. *Echocardiography* 2006;23:562–8.

24. Singh A, Mehmood F, Romp RL, Nanda NC, Mallavarapu RK. Live/real time three-dimensional transthoracic echocardiographic assessment of aortopulmonary window. *Echocardiography* 2008;25:96–9.

25. Campbell M. Natural history of persistent ductus arteriosus. *Br Heart J* 1968;30:4–13.

26. Grifka RG. Transcatheter closure of the patent ductus arteriosus. *Catheter Cardiovasc Interv* 2004;61:554–70.

27. Sharma S, Mehta AC, O'Donovan PB. Computed tomography and magnetic resonance findings in long-standing patent ductus. Case reports. *Angiology* 1996;47:393–8.

28. Sinha A, Nanda NC, Khanna D, *et al.* Live three-dimensional transthoracic echocardiographic delineation of patent ductus arteriosus. *Echocardiography* 2004;21:443–8.

29. Hlavacek A, Lucas J, Baker H, Chessa K, Shirali G. Feasibility and utility of three-dimensional color flow echocardiography of the aortic arch: the "echocardiographic angiogram." *Echocardiography* 2006;23:860–864.

30. Patel S. Normal and anomalous anatomy of the coronary arteries. *Semin Roentgenol* 2008;43:100–112.

31. Ilgenli TF, Nanda NC, Sinha A, Khanna D. Live three-dimensional transthoracic echocardiographic assessment of anomalous origin of left coronary artery from the pulmonary artery. *Echocardiography* 2004;21:559–62.

32. Mehta D, Nanda NC, Vengala S, Mehmood F, Taylor J. Live three-dimensional transthoracic echocardiographic demonstration of coronary artery to pulmonary artery fistula. *Am J Geriatr Cardiol* 2005;14:42–4.

33. Friedman T, Mani A, Elefteriades JA. Bicuspid aortic valve: clinical approach and scientific review of a common clinical entity. *Expert Rev Cardiovasc Ther* 2008;6:235–48.

34. Singh P, Dutta R, Nanda NC. Live/real time three-dimensional transthoracic echocardiographic assessment of bicuspid aortic valve morphology. *Echocardiography* 2009;26:478–80.

35. Burri MV, Nanda NC, Singh A, Panwar SR. Live/real time three-dimensional transthoracic echocardiographic identification of quadricuspid aortic valve. *Echocardiography* 2007;24:653–5.

36. Aboulhosn J, Child JS. Left ventricular outflow obstruction: subaortic stenosis, bicuspid aortic valve, supravalvar aortic stenosis, and coarctation of the aorta. *Circulation* 2006;114:2412–22.

37. Tentolouris K, Kontozoglou T, Trikas A, *et al.* Fixed subaortic stenosis revisited. Congenital abnormalities in 72 new cases and review of the literature. *Cardiology* 1999;92:4–10.

38. Bruce CJ, Nishimura RA, Tajik AJ, Schaff HV, Danielson GK. Fixed left ventricular outflow tract obstruction in presumed hypertrophic obstructive cardiomyopathy: implications for therapy. *Ann Thorac Surg* 1999;68:100–104.

39. Alboliras ET, Gotteiner NL, Berdusis K, Webb CL. Transesophageal echocardiographic imaging for congenital lesions of the left ventricular outflow tract and the aorta. *Echocardiography* 1996;13:439–46.

40. Agrawal GG, Nanda NC, Htay T, Dod HS, Gandhari SR. Live three-dimensional transthoracic echocardiographic identification of discrete subaortic membranous stenosis. *Echocardiography* 2003;20:617–19.

41. Baumgartner H, Stefenelli T, Niederberger J, Schima H, Maurer G. "Overestimation" of catheter gradients by Doppler ultrasound in patients with aortic stenosis: a predictable manifestation of pressure recovery. *J Am Coll Cardiol* 1999;33:1655–61.

42. Sakthi C, Yee H, Kotlewski A. Overestimation of aortic valve gradient measured by Doppler echocardiography in patients with aortic stenosis. *Catheter Cardiovasc Interv* 2005;65:176–9.

43. Garcia D, Dumesnil JG, Durand LG, Kadem L, Pibarot P. Discrepancies between catheter and Doppler estimates of valve effective orifice area can be predicted from the pressure recovery phenomenon: practical implications with regard to quantification of aortic stenosis severity. *J Am Coll Cardiol* 2003;41:435–42.

44. Aghassi P, Aurigemma GP, Folland ED, Tighe DA. Catheterization-Doppler discrepancies in nonsimultaneous evaluations of aortic stenosis. *Echocardiography* 2005;22:367–73.

45. Bandarupalli N, Faulkner M, Nanda NC, Pothineni KR. Erroneous diagnosis of significant obstruction by Doppler in a patient with discrete subaortic membrane: correct diagnosis by 3D-transthoracic echocardiography. *Echocardiography* 2008;25:1004–6.

46. Patel V, Nanda NC, Arellano I, Yelamanchili P, Rajdev S, Baysan O. Cor triatriatum sinister: assessment by live/real time three-dimensional transthoracic echocardiography. *Echocardiography* 2006;23:801–2.

47. Anderson KR, Zuberbuhler JR, Anderson RH, Becker AE, Lie JT. Morphologic spectrum of Ebstein's anomaly of the heart: a review. *Mayo Clin Proc* 1979;54:174–80.

48. Ports TA, Silverman NH, Schiller NB. Two-dimensional echocardiographic assessment of Ebstein's anomaly. *Circulation* 1978;58:336–43.

49. Shiina A, Seward JB, Edwards WD, Hagler DJ, Tajik AJ. Two-dimensional echocardiographic spectrum of Ebstein's anomaly: detailed anatomic assessment. *J Am Coll Cardiol* 1984;3:356–70.

50. Patel V, Nanda NC, Rajdev S, *et al.* Live/real time three-dimensional transthoracic echocardiographic assessment of Ebstein's anomaly. *Echocardiography* 2005;22:847–54.

51. Danielson GK, Driscoll DJ, Mair DD, Warnes CA, Oliver WC, Jr. Operative treatment of Ebstein's anomaly. *J Thorac Cardiovasc Surg* 1992;104:1195–202.

52. Hansalia S, Manda J, Pothineni KR, Nanda NC. Usefulness of live/real time three-dimensional transthoracic echocardiography in diagnosing acquired left ventricular-right atrial communication misdiagnosed as severe pulmonary hypertension by two-dimensional transthoracic echocardiography. *Echocardiography* 2009;26:224–7.

53. Warnes CA. Transposition of the great arteries. *Circulation* 2006;114:2699–709.

54. Skinner J, Hornung T, Rumball E. Transposition of the great arteries: from fetus to adult. *Heart* 2008;94:1227–35.

55. Enar S, Singh P, Douglas C, *et al.* Live/real time three-dimensional transthoracic echocardiographic assessment of transposition of the great arteries in the adult. *Echocardiography* 2009;26:1095–104.

56. Therrien J, Webb G. Clinical update on adults with congenital heart disease. *Lancet* 2003;362:1305–13.

57. Pothineni KR, Nanda NC, Burri MV, Singh A, Panwar SR, Gandhari S. Live/real time three-dimensional transthoracic echocardiographic visualization of Chiari network. *Echocardiography* 2007;24:995–7.

58. Allan L. Technique of fetal echocardiography. *Pediatr Cardiol* 2004;25:223–33.

59. Small M, Copel JA. Indications for fetal echocardiography. *Pediatr Cardiol* 2004;25:210–222.

60. Deng J, Rodeck CH. Current applications of fetal cardiac imaging technology. *Curr Opin Obstet Gynecol* 2006;18:177–84.

61. Maulik D, Nanda NC, Singh V, *et al.* Live three-dimensional echocardiography of the human fetus. *Echocardiography* 2003;20:715–21.

62. Tutschek B, Sahn DJ. Three-dimensional echocardiography for studies of the fetal heart: present status and future perspectives. *Cardiol Clin* 2007;25:341–55.

CHAPTER 12

Tumors and Other Mass Lesions

Introduction

Echocardiography is the diagnostic test of choice for cardiac masses, traditionally using 2D trasthoracic echocardiography (2DTTE) [1,2]. This advantage has been deserved due to the noninvasive and portable nature of this modality and the ability not only to uncover the presence of cardiac masses, but also to identify their location and attachment, identify their shape and size, and determine the nature of their mobility [1]. More recently, 3DTTE has been utilized to further assess cardiac masses. The most commonly encountered cardiac masses include thrombi, tumors, and vegetations, and all can be well characterized using echocardiography. The additive value of 3DTTE over 2DTTE lies in its ability to better characterize irregular cardiac masses, and since a full-volume dataset is obtained of the mass, even the interior of these masses [2].

Most cardiac tumors are benign. In adults, myxoma is the most frequent tumor, while in the pediatric population, the most common tumor is the rhabdomyoma. Among the malignant tumors, sarcomas are the most frequent, including angiosarcoma, rhabdomyosarcoma, and fibrosarcoma [1]. Neoplasms extrinsic to the heart have also been known to metastasize to the heart, including primary lung, breast, ovarian, renal, and skin cancers, among others. Thrombi in the heart generally occur in areas of blood stasis. In the left ventricle, most thrombi occur at the apex in patients with aneurysms or at sites of previous infarcts. Thrombi also occur in the left atrium, mostly in the left atrial appendage, in patients with atrial arrhythmias or those with mitral valve pathologies. Although thrombi occur in the right atrium and right ventricle, these are generally rare. Other sites for cardiac thrombi include diseased valves, prosthetic valves, cardiac tumors, and other prosthetic devices, including pacemaker wires and vascular catheters. In general, 2DTTE is adequate for the assessment of thrombi in the left ventricular apex but until recently has proven limited in the evaluation of left atrial appendage, and 2DTEE has been mostly utilized for that purpose with the disadvantage of the necessity of esophageal intubation [3]. Vegetations, on the other hand, generally occur on cardiac valves, prosthetic devices, or at the site of previous trauma.

Classification of cardiac mass lesions into tumors, thrombi, or vegetations has, on occasions, proven difficult, even with 2DTTE and 2DTEE. More rigorous evaluation with 3DTTE might prove helpful in the care of these patients.

Thrombi

The identification of thrombi in the heart can have major implications for the clinical care of patients. 2DTTE is generally requested to evaluate for the presence of thrombi in patients with atrial fibrillation/flutter, after myocardial infarction, especially in patients with left ventricular aneurysms, and in patients with signs or symptoms of systemic embolization such as cerebrovascular accidents.

In the case of left ventricular thrombi, 3DTTE can provide additive information to the 2DTTE examination by allowing for more precise identification of the clot's point of attachment to the myocardium. Furthermore, since the entire left ventricular apex can be contained within one pyramidal 3D dataset, meticulous cropping of this single dataset should be enough for a comprehensive evaluation. Thus, we have shown that such an

Live/Real Time 3D Echocardiography, 1st edition.
By Navin C. Nanda, Ming Chon Hsiung, Andrew P. Miller, and Fadi G. Hage. Published 2010 by Blackwell Publishing Ltd.

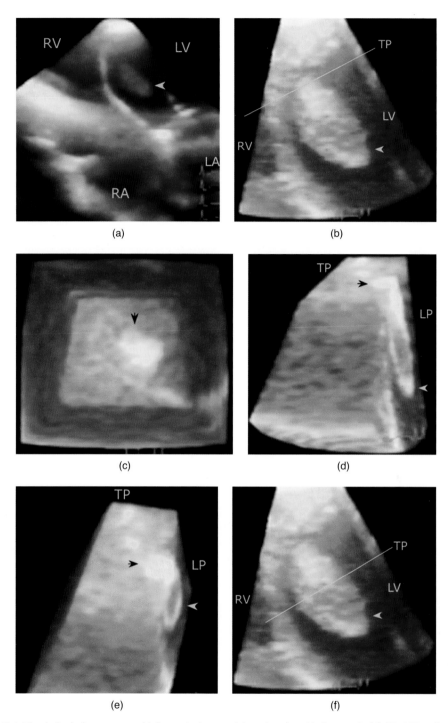

(a)

(b)

(c)

(d)

(e)

(f)

Figure 12.1 Morphological assessment of left ventricular thrombus by live 3D transthoracic echocardiography in a young female with post-partum cardiomyopathy. (a) The arrowhead points to the thrombus attached to left ventricular apex. (b, c) Transverse plane (TP, horizontal plane or short-axis) section at the attachment point of the thrombus (arrowhead) shows it to be highly echogenic (viewed *en face*, black arrow in (c)). (d, e) TP and longitudinal plane (LP, vertical plane or long-axis) sections through the thrombus (arrowhead) showing the echogenic attachment (black arrow) and a large echolucency within the thrombus consistent with lysis. (f–h) TP and both TP and LP sections at mid-thrombus level showing clot lysis. (*Continued on next page*)

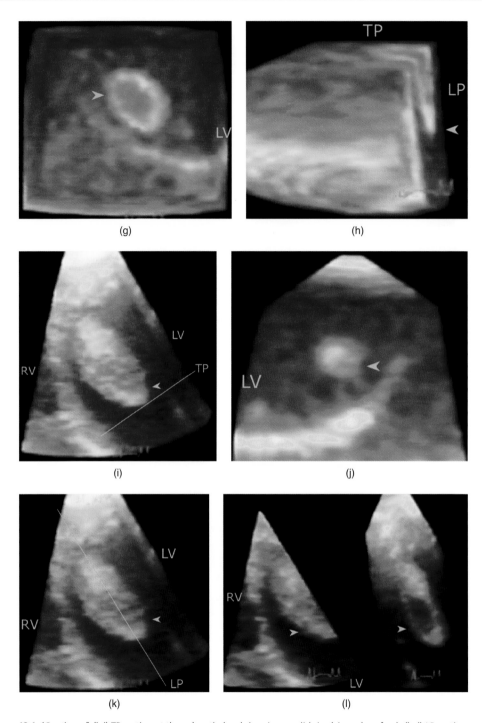

Figure 12.1 (*Continued*) (i, j) TP section at thrombus tip level showing a solid rim (viewed *en face*). (k, l) LP section through thrombus showing clot lysis.

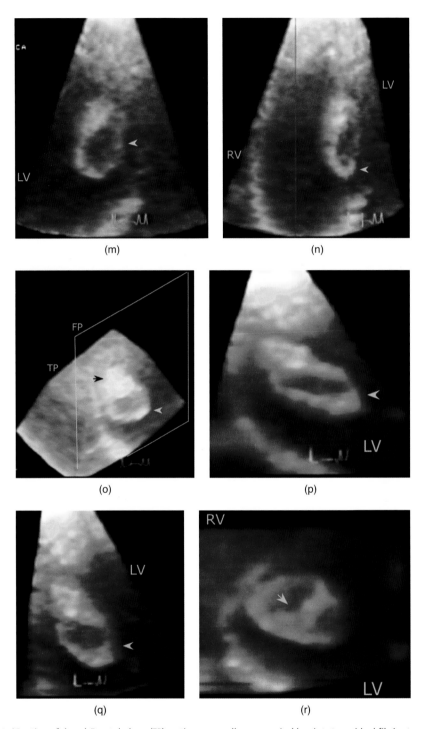

Figure 12.1 (*Continued*) (m, n) Frontal plane (FP) section through the thrombus viewed *en face* (m) and after tilting (n). (o) TP and LP sections through the thrombus. The dataset has been tilted and rotated to show the position of the FP. (p–r) Oblique sections through the thrombus. The yellow arrow in (r) points to residual fibrin strands within the lytic area of the thrombus. LA, left atrium; LV, left ventricle; RA, right atrium, RV, right ventricle. Movie clip 12.1. (Reproduced from Sinha *et al*. [19], with permission.)

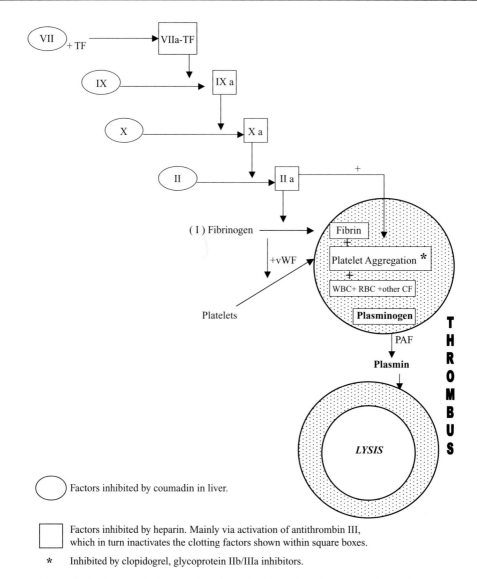

Figure 12.2 Schematic showing coagulation cascade and thrombus lysis. Plasminogen activating factor (PAF) is secreted by endothelialized mesenchymal cells lining the microscopic crypts which develop within the thrombus. PAF activates plasminogen to plasmin which digests fibrin leading to thrombus lysis. CF, clotting factor; RBC, red blood cell; TF, tissue factor; vWF, von Willibrand factor; WBC, white blood cell. (Reproduced from Sinha *et al.* [19], with permission.)

examination can be performed in a timely manner, even without breath holding, in not fully cooperative patients [4]. 3DTTE is superior to 2DTTE in its ability to visualize the interior of these thrombi and identifying the presence of areas of echolucency within the clot. The presence of such focal areas of echolucency are indicative of the presence and extent of clot lysis and can have therapeutic as well as prognostic implications [4]. Other beneficial aspects of 3DTTE include its ability to define clot mobility in a manner that is not always possible with 2DTTE, and this could be a sign of increased propensity of the clot to embolize [4–6]. Subsequently, these thrombi can be followed over

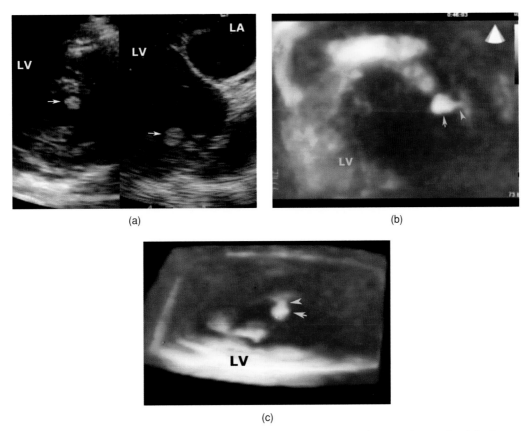

(a)

(b)

(c)

Figure 12.3 (a) Real time 2D transthoracic (left) and transesophageal (right) echocardiogram. The arrow indicates thrombus in left ventricle (LV). Attachment point to LV wall is not delineated. (b, c) Live/real time 3D transthoracic echocardiogram. The arrowhead clearly demonstrates attachment of thrombus (arrow) to LV wall. LA, left atrium. Movie clip 12.3. (Reproduced from Duncan *et al.* [4], with permission.)

time using 3DTTE for monitoring of the progression in these characteristics and their response to therapy (Figures 12.1–12.4). More recently, 3DTTE has been evaluated for the assessment of right ventricular thrombi [7]. In a manner very similar to left ventricular thrombi, 3DTTE offered incremental value over 2DTTE in allowing for a more certain diagnosis, in determining the number of thrombi present, the precise location where the thrombi attach to the ventricular wall, the measurement of thrombi volume, and finally, by visualizing echolucencies within the thrombi that signify clot lysis (Figure 12.5) [7].

An important limitation of 2DTTE has been its inability to fully evaluate the left atrial appendage in most patients in order to reliably exclude the presence of a thrombus in patients who present with neurological events or alternatively in those who have atrial arrhythmias and are at high risk of developing thrombi. Historically, 2DTEE has been utilized to augment the diagnostic capability of 2DTTE. This approach has been proven useful over the years due to the high quality of images that can be obtained with the probe situated in the esophagus in close proximity to the appendage. The only drawback is the necessity for esophageal intubation which is uncomfortable to the patient and not without risk [8]. We examined the utility of a combined approach with 2DTTE and 3DTTE in comparison to 2DTEE. In this study, 92 patients underwent 2DTTE, 3DTTE, as well as 2DTEE for various indications, while 20 patients underwent

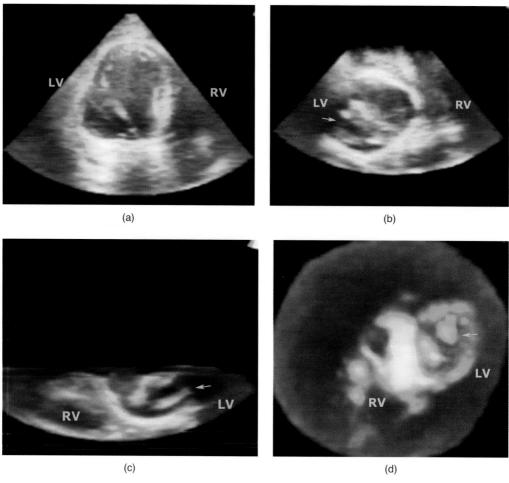

(a)

(b)

(c)

(d)

Figure 12.4 Live/real time 3D transthoracic echocardiogram. (a) Four-chamber view showing no thrombus or aneurysm in the left ventricle (LV). (b) Anterior–posterior cropping displays the large aneurysm containing thrombus (arrow). (c, d) Sectioning of thrombus (c) and viewing it *en face* (d) shows no evidence of lysis or liquefaction. RV, right ventricle. Movie clip 12.4 C. (Reproduced from Duncan *et al.* [4], with permission.)

only 2DTTE and 2DTEE due to the inability to perform 2DTEE (contraindications or other considerations). The left atrial appendage was well visualized in all patients with 2DTEE, 2DTTE, as well as 3DTEE, thus showing that with newer technologies and experienced sonographers, the appendage can be evaluated from the transthoracic approach in most patients. In 7 patients, a thrombus was seen in the appendage by 2DTEE as well as by 3DTTE. There was no evidence of clot lysis in these thrombi by 3DTTE. In 11 patients, a thrombus was thought to be present on 2DTEE, but on 3DTTE these

were determined to have prominent transversely oriented pectinate muscles. In the 20 patients who could not have 2DTEE, 3DTTE showed a thrombus in the left atrial appendage in one patient which resolved on a follow-up examination. The other 19 patients with no evidence of clots by 3DTTE underwent cardioversion for atrial fibrillation and had no complications during the procedure. Therefore, in this circumstance, a combined 2DTTE and 3DTTE is not only convenient to perform but also provides additional information to 2DTEE and can, in a significant percentage of patients, provide a better

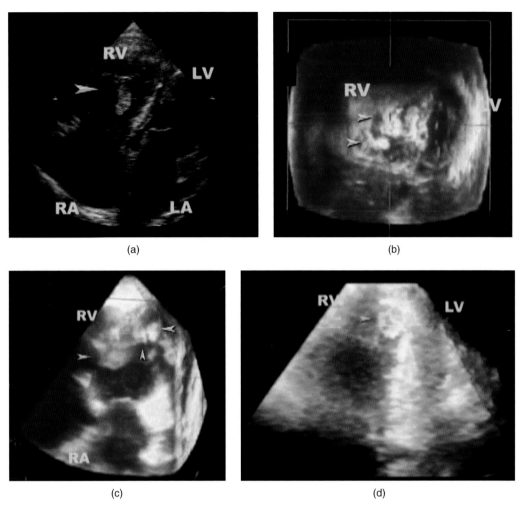

(a)

(b)

(c)

(d)

Figure 12.5 Real time 2D and 3D transthoracic echocardiography in right ventricular thrombus. (a) 2D study. The arrowhead points to one bifid or possibly two clots in the right ventricle (RV). (b, c) 3D study. Cropping the 3D dataset demonstrates three separate clots in the RV (arrowheads). (d) Another patient with clot in RV showing central lysis in a cropped 3D image. LA, left atrium; LV, left ventricle; RA, right atrium. Movie clips 12.5 A, 12.5 B–C Part 1–4, 12.5 D. (Reproduced from Reddy *et al.* [7], with permission.)

assessment of the presence of thrombi. This is mostly because on 2DTEE, the mass lesion is seen in only one or two planes and, therefore, mistaken for a thrombus, whereas by 3DTTE careful sectioning can reveal that this "mass lesion" is merely a prominent pectinate muscle. It might be a prudent strategy, therefore, to evaluate patients who have a "positive" 2DTEE for a clot in the left atrial appendage with a 3DTTE [9]. Also, a negative 2DTEE, because of its inherent limitation of using a single-plane technique, may not preclude a thrombus in

one of the lobes of the left atrial appendage. On the other hand, with an adequate quality 3DTTE, multiple sections at various angulations can be taken to comprehensively examine the left atrial appendage for the presence or absence of thrombi and to differentiate a thrombus from a pectinate muscle (Figures 12.6–12.10). This same approach can also be used to evaluate the right atrium for the presence of free-floating thrombi [10], or more commonly, thrombi attached to pacemaker leads or vascular catheters [11]. Since 3DTTE is able to visualize the

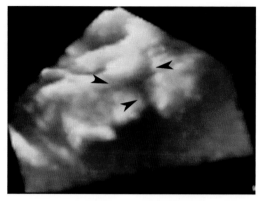

Figure 12.6 3D transthoracic echocardiographic image of left atrial appendage. The arrowheads point individual lobes as visualized by cropping a 3D dataset of left atrial appendage. (Reproduced with permission from Karakus *et al.* [9], with permission)

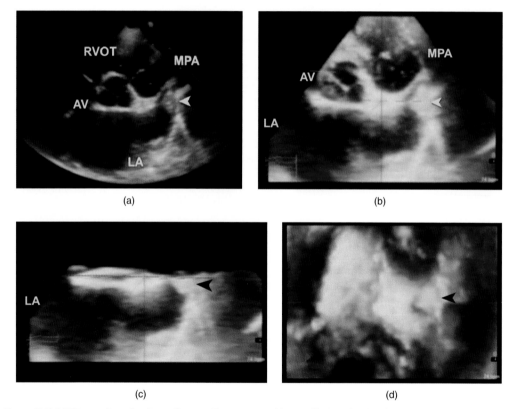

(a)   (b)   (c)   (d)

Figure 12.7 (a) 2D transthoracic echocardiogram. The arrowhead points to a thrombus within the LAA. (b–d) Live/real time 3D transthoracic echocardiogram. The thrombus (arrowhead) was cropped from the top and rotated to view it *en face* in short axis. There was no evidence of lysis within the thrombus. AV, aortic valve; LA, left atrium; LAA, left atrial appendage; MPA, main pulmonary artery; RVOT, right ventricular outflow tract. (Reproduced from Karakus *et al.* [9], with permission.) Movie clip 12.7 A–D.

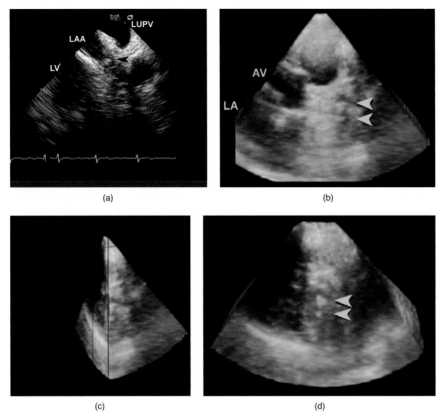

Figure 12.8 (a) 2D transesophageal echocardiogram. The arrowhead points to an echo dense mass within the left atrial appendage (LAA) consistent with a thrombus. (b–d) Live/real time 3D transthoracic echocardiogram. Within the LAA there are two echo densities noted. Sequential cropping shows both to be parts of pectinate muscles which traverse the LAA. The upper echo density (upper arrowhead) is larger because it represents a short axis cut through two pectinate muscles virtually in contact with each other. This most likely represents the "thrombus" seen on the transesophageal echocardiogram. The second echo density (bottom arrowhead) is smaller because only one pectinate muscle is involved. AV, aortic valve; LV, left ventricle; LUPV, left upper pulmonary vein. (Reproduced from Karakus *et al.* [9], with permission.) Movie clip 12.8 B–D.

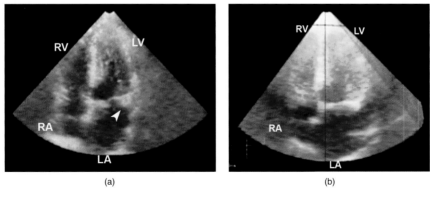

Figure 12.9 3D transthoracic echocardiogram. (a) The arrowhead points to a thrombus in the left atrial appendage (LAA) with an echolucency in the center suggestive of clot lysis. (b) Repeat study in the same patient 54 days later. LAA (magnified) is free of thrombus. LA, left atrium; LV, left ventricle, RA, right atrium, RV, right ventricle. (Reproduced from Karakus *et al.* [9], with permission.)

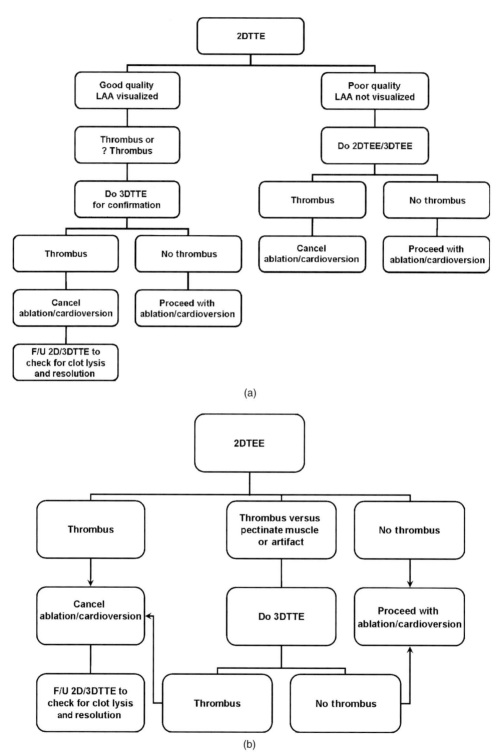

Figure 12.10 Suggested algorithm to evaluate the left atrial appendage (LAA) for thrombus using echocardiography. (a) Initial test: 2D transthoracic echocardiography (2DTTE). (b) Initial test: 2D transesophageal echocardiography (2DTEE). (Reproduced from Karakus *et al*. [9], with permission.) (Reproduced from Upendram *et al*. [10], with permission.)

right atrium and its junction with the superior vena cava well (right parasternal approach), 2DTEE can potentially be avoided for this purpose. In some patients, the right atrial appendage may also be visualized by 3DTTE, especially using the right parasternal approach. In addition, right and left supraclavicular approaches can be utilized to image the right and left innominate veins, the proximal superior vena cava, azygos vein, and inferior thyroid vein and clots can be easily differentiated from venous valves by 3DTTE. We have used 3DTTE to detect a thrombus on a catheter placed in the superior vena cava for hemodialysis [11]. The thrombus protruded into the right atrium and involved the right innominate vein and exhibited multiple echolucent areas suggesting that clot lysis had already begun [11]. 3DTTE is not only important in providing a comprehensive evaluation of the size and extent of the thrombus, including measurement of its volume, but is also useful in following the course of the patient during treatment with anticoagulation to demonstrate clot lysis and eventually the regression and resolution of the clot [11]. A distinct advantage of 3DTTE is that the dataset may be sequentially cropped and the images viewed from any plane, thereby allowing the examiner to further assess the inner portions of a mass. One can, therefore, crop the image into sections which provides "a unique look inside the thrombus" [4,10]. When 3DTTE images are cropped and sectioned, the examiner may note the presence of echolucent areas within the clot. This finding should help the sonographer in determining the time course of clot lysis, i.e., when echolucencies are present, this finding suggests that clot lysis has begun (Figures 12.11–12.16) [4,11].

In summary, 3DTTE is useful in examining cardiac thrombi because it can further clarify the number of thrombi, the location of attachment to the myocardium, and the presence of echolucencies that would indicate clot lysis (which has important therapeutic implications). Another potential advantage that is worth mentioning is that a combination of 2DTTE and 3DTTE in the evaluation of thrombi has been shown to have comparable accuracy to that of transesophageal echocardiography in the evaluation of left atrial and left atrial appendage thrombi. Furthermore, in the case of left ventricular noncompaction, 3DTTE is able to differentiate trabeculations from thrombi better than 2DTTE, as discussed elsewhere in this book [12].

Tumors

3DTTE has been shown to be of great benefit in the evaluation of cardiac tumors, specifically because of its ability to locate the precise attachment of a mass to the myocardium, the ability to section the mass and view it from any plane, its ability to calculate the volume of a mass and follow this volume over time, and the spatial relationship of the mass to other structures [2,13,14]. Since cardiac tumors can have complex geometric shapes, 3DTTE has an important advantage over 2DTTE in its ability to show 3D structures rather than the need to conceptualize these complex shapes from multiple cross-sectional 2D images [15].

The assessment of cardiac tumors by 3DTTE has another advantage that is very similar to what we discussed for cardiac thrombi, namely that the images obtained by 3DTTE can be sectioned and viewed from any angle, providing the examiner a more detailed assessment of the mass even from within. This is important as certain masses have specific identifying characteristics by 3DTTE. For example, fibromas and lipomas typically are dense, very bright homogeneous masses; their brightness relates to the presence of fibrous tissue (collagen). Myxomas, on the other hand, demonstrate localized areas of large echolucencies consistent with necrosis or hemorrhage as well as very bright punctate areas of calcifications pointing to their chronicity [7,13]. Hemangiomas are highly vascular tumors which demonstrate more extensive and closely packed vascular (echolucent) areas that extend all the way to the periphery with little solid tissue as compared to myxomas [13,16]. Chordomas, metastatic to the heart, demonstrate multiple echodense areas consistent with fibrotic bands and scattered echolucencies [17]. High grade sarcomas may demonstrate areas of necrosis with dilated vasculature (echolucencies) surrounded by dense hyperechoic band-like tissue consistent with fibrosis, thus giving the appearance of a "doughnut" [7,18]. 3DTTE can also visualize hydatid cysts well and can complement the 2DTTE exam by showing the granddaughter cysts budding from the daughter cysts as well as great-granddaughter cysts from granddaughter

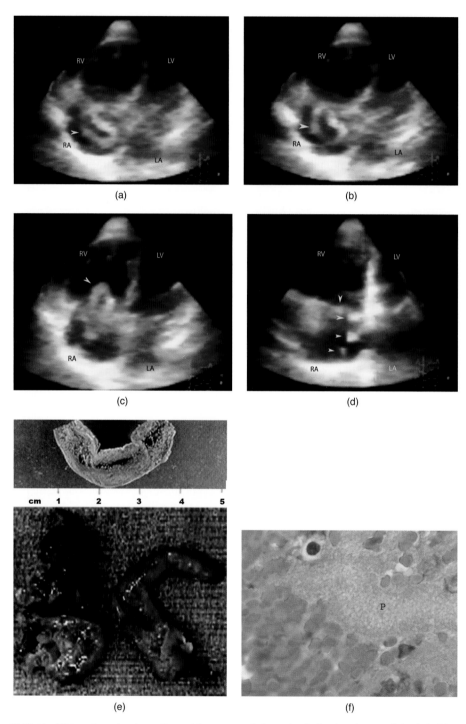

(a)

(b)

(c)

(d)

(e)

(f)

Figure 12.11 Live 3D transthoracic echocardiographic assessment of right atrial thrombus. (a–c) The arrowhead points to a large mobile serpiginous thrombus in the right atrium (RA) prolapsing into the right ventricle (RV). (d) Cropped segments of the thrombus (arrowheads) demonstrate a homogenous appearance with no echolucencies, indicating absence of clot lysis. (e) Resected thrombus. Note absence of lysis. (f) Microscopic section shows presence of intact platelets (P) indicating that the thrombus is of recent origin. LA, left atrium; LV, left ventricle. Movie clip 12.11.

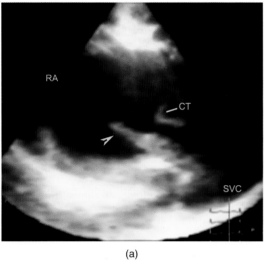
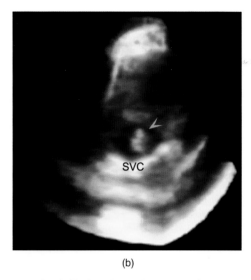

(a)   (b)

Figure 12.12 Live 3D transthoracic echocardiographic assessment of thrombus in the innominate veins and superior vena cava utilizing the right parasternal approaches. (a) The arrowhead shows a large thrombus protruding into the right atrium (RA) from the superior vena cava (SVC). (b) Thrombus in the SVC viewed in short axis. CT, crista terminalis. Movie clips 12.12 A, 12.12 B Part 1–2. (Reproduced from Upendram *et al.* [11], with permission.)

cysts [19]. Therefore, on 3DTTE various masses have distinctive and characteristic appearances that can aid in making the diagnosis.

Some tumors are attached to the cardiac valves and may resemble vegetations or thrombi on 2DTTE. Most of these tumors are benign, and they include myxomas, fibroelastomas, lipomas, and Lambl's excrescences. On 3DTTE papillary fibroelastomas show a central echo density which corresponds to their fibrocollagenous core, and finger-like projections which represent the multiple fronds [20,21]. The stalk by which this tumor attaches to the valve can also be well seen. In contrast, Lambl's excrescences are attached to the tip of the valve and usually present as multiple strands on multiple valves [20]. On the right side of the heart, 3DTTE can visualize all three leaflets of the tricuspid valve, the right atrium and ventricle and any indwelling catheters to assess for the presence of vegetations. Therefore, when 2DTTE and 2DTEE cannot provide definitive answers regarding presence or absence of vegetations, a 3DTTE might prove useful [22].

3DTTE can also be used to provide a more comprehensive evaluation of a hiatal hernia which can be seen on 2DTTE [23]. *Hiatal hernia* refers to the herniation of abdominal cavity contents into the thoracic cavity through the hiatus of the diaphragm, and can usually be seen on echocardiography behind the left ventricular posterior wall. A definitive diagnosis can be obtained by letting the patient drink a carbonated beverage while lying supine for the echocardiographic study. The appearance of contrast microbubbles in the lesion is diagnostic for a hiatal hernia. 3DTTE can provide incremental information on top of 2DTTE with respect to the extent and size of the hernia and its wall thickness which has clinical implications on patient management (Figures 12.17–12.41) [23].

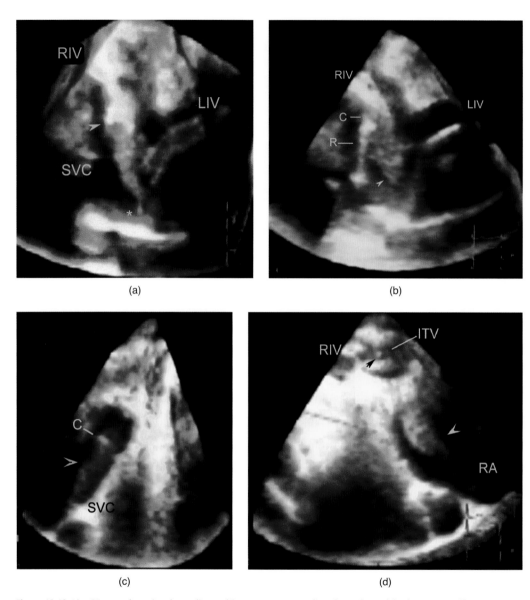

(a)

(b)

(c)

(d)

Figure 12.13 Live 3D transthoracic echocardiographic assessment of thrombus in the innominate veins and superior vena cava (SVC) utilizing supraclavicular approaches. (a–c) Long-axis views. The arrowhead points to a large thrombus occupying the right innominate vein (RIV) and SVC. Asterisk in (a) points to a mobile component of the thrombus. No thrombus is visualized in the left innominate vein (LIV) in (b). (d) No thrombus is noted in the inferior thyroid vein (ITV) and the RIV further upstream from RIV–SVC junction. The arrow points to a venous valve in the ITV. (e–h) Short-axis views. (e) Short-axis view of SVC showing the thrombus surrounding the catheter (C). The arrow in (f) points to an area of lysis in the thrombus. The arrowhead in (g) points to the thrombus, which occupies about 50% of the SVC. The short-axis section was taken near SVC entrance into right atrium (RA). (h) No thrombus is visualized in the azygos vein (AZ) and LIV. V is a venous valve at the junction of innominate veins and SVC. V1 is a venous valve at the junction of AZ and SVC. ACH, aortic arch; LIJ, left internal jugular vein; LSV, left subclavian vein; R, reverberation from the catheter. Movie clips 12.13 A Parts 1–2, 12.13 E–H. (Reproduced from Upendram *et al.* [11], with permission.)

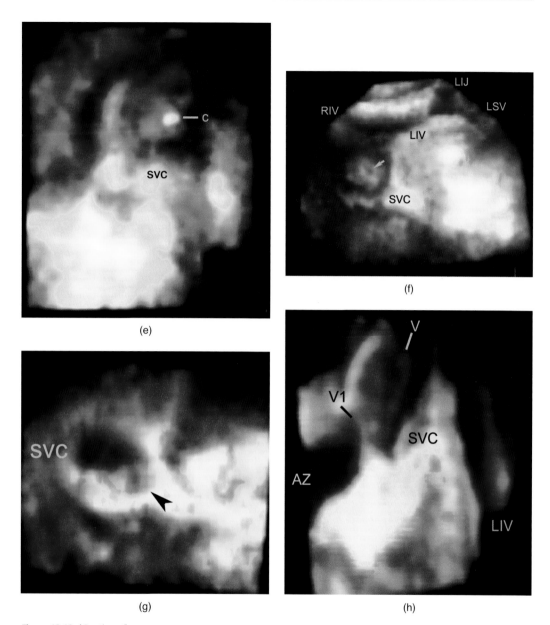

(e)

(f)

(g)

(h)

Figure 12.13 (*Continued*).

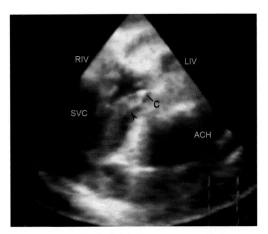

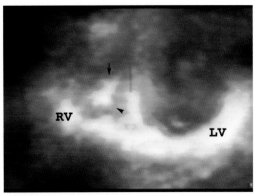

Figure 12.16 Live/real time 3D transthoracic echocardiographic detection of a vegetation on pacemaker/defibrillator lead. The arrow points to a mobile vegetation on the pacemaker/defibrillator lead (arrowhead) in the right ventricle (RV). LV, left ventricle. (Reproduced from Pothineni et al. [22], with permission.)

Figure 12.14 Live 3D transthoracic echocardiographic assessment of thrombus in the innominate veins and superior vena cava (SVC) utilizing supraclavicular approaches. The arrowhead points to a portion of the thrombus extending to involve the left innominate vein (LIV). ACH, aortic arch; C, catheter; RIV, right innominate vein. Movie clip 12.9 shows thrombus extending to involve catheter in the LIV (black arrow). Movie clip 12.14. (Reproduced from Upendram et al. [11], with permission.)

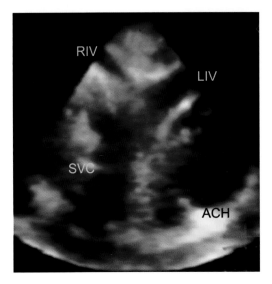

Figure 12.15 Live 3D transthoracic echocardiographic assessment of thrombus in the innominate veins and superior vena cava (SVC) utilizing supraclavicular approaches. No thrombus is visualized in the left innominate vein (LIV), right innominate vein (RIV), and SVC; ACH, aortic arch. (Reproduced from Upendram et al. [11], with permission.)

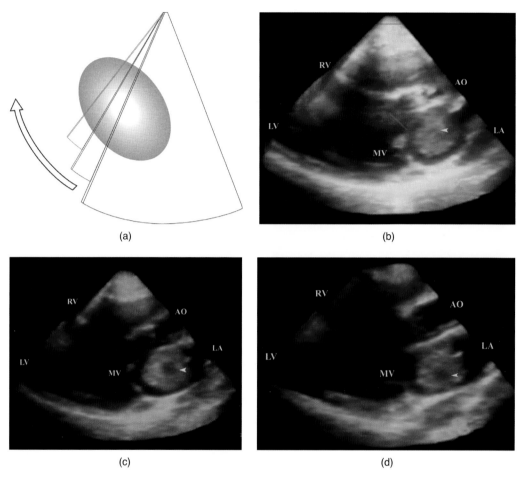

(a)

(b)

(c)

(d)

Figure 12.17 Live 3D transthoracic echocardiographic assessment of left atrial myxoma. (a–d) Frontal plane sections taken at three different sequential levels in the 3D dataset demonstrate echolucencies (arrowhead) within the tumor consistent with hemorrhage, which is largest in the middle section (c). (*Continued on next page*)

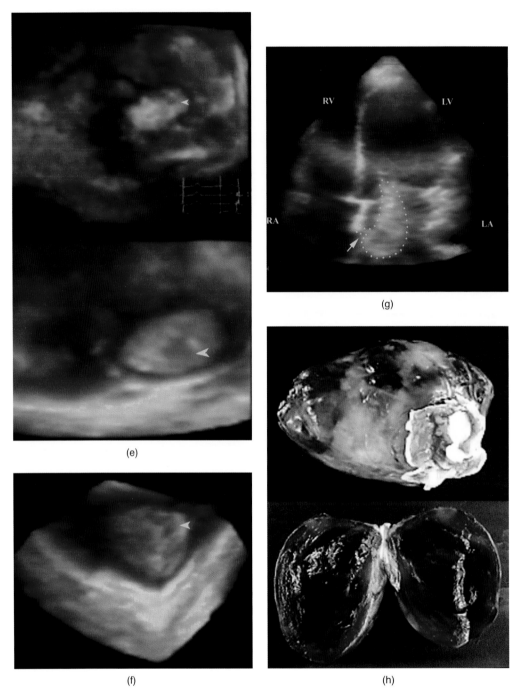

(e)

(f)

(g)

(h)

Figure 12.17 (*Continued*) (e) Transverse plane sections of the tumor viewed *en face*, also demonstrating hemorrhage (arrowhead). (f) Frontal plane, transverse plane, and vertical plane sections of the tumor showing extensive hemorrhage (arrowhead). (g) The arrow points to the tumor stalk. (h) Resected specimen showing a large hemorrhage. Arrows in Movie clip 12.17 point to large areas of hemorrhage which correspond with the surgical specimen. AO, aortic valve; LA, left atrium; LV, left ventricle; MV, mitral valve; RA, right atrium; RV, right ventricle. (Reproduced from Mehmood *et al.* [13], with permission.)

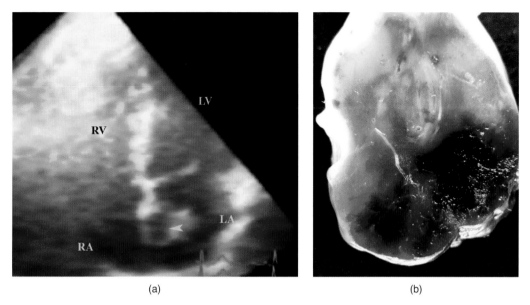

(a)   (b)

Figure 12.18 Live 3D tranthoracic echocardiographic assessment of left atrial myxoma. (a) The arrowhead points to a large echolucency consistent with a large hemorrhage. (b) Resected specimen showing a large hemorrhage. LA, left atrium; LV, left ventricle; RA, right atrium; RV, right ventricle. (Reproduced from Mehmood *et al.* [13], with permission.)

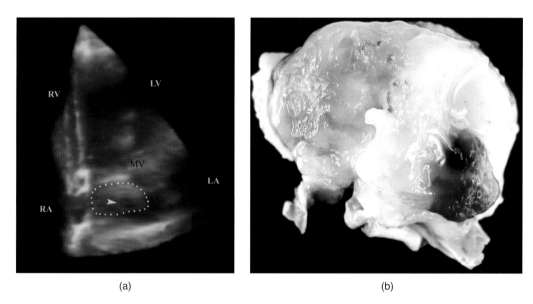

(a)   (b)

Figure 12.19 Live 3D transthoracic echocardiographic assessment of left atrial myxoma. (a) The arrowhead points to a large echolucency which corresponds closely to the hemorrhage, seen in the resected specimen (b). LA, left atrium; LV, left ventricle; MV, mitral valve; RA, right atrium; RV, right ventricle. (Reproduced from Mehmood *et al.* [13], with permission.)

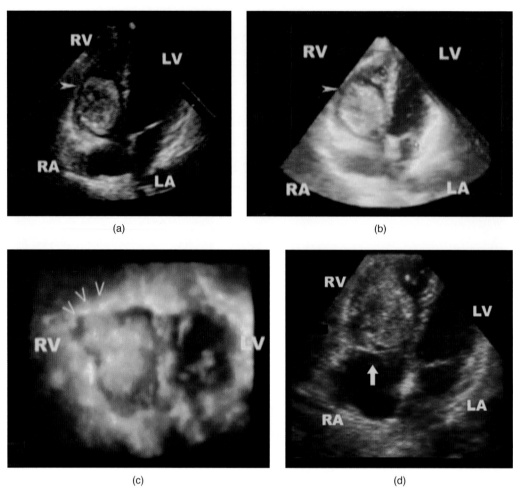

(a)

(b)

(c)

(d)

Figure 12.20 Real time 2D and 3D transthoracic echocardiography in right ventricular myxoma. (a) 2D study. The arrowhead points to a large myxoma in the right ventricle (RV) visualized in the apical four-chamber view. Tumor attachment is not visualized. (b–d) 3D study. The arrowhead in (b) points to the large myxoma. The arrowheads in (c) show attachments of the myxoma to the right ventricular inferior wall. (d) Shows one of the attachments (arrow) of the tumor to the tricuspid valve using the QLAB on the system. LA, left atrium; LV, left ventricle; RA, right atrium. Movie clips 12.20 B–D Parts 1–2. (Reproduced from Reddy *et al.* [7], with permission.)

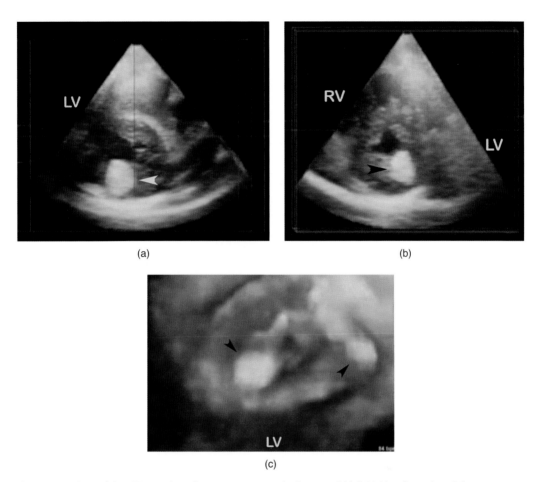

(a)　　　　　　　　　　　　　　　　　　(b)

(c)

Figure 12.21 Live/real time 3D transthoracic echocardiographic assessment of left ventricular lipoma. The arrowheads in (a) and (b) point to a highly echogenic mass in the left ventricle (LV). Further cropping of the 3D dataset shows the presence of two lipomas (arrowheads in (c)) in the LV. The arrow in Movie clip 12.21 A–B points to the lipoma, which is highly echogenic and shows no echolucencies on cropping. Movie clip 12.21 C shows another patient with a left ventricular lipoma (arrow) together with the surgically resected specimen. A few trabeculations are also present adjoining the lipoma in the left ventricular apex. RV, right ventricle.

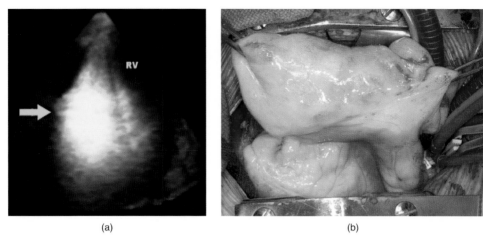

(a)   (b)

Figure 12.22 Real time 3D transthoracic echocardiography in right ventricular lipoma. (a) The arrow points to a large markedly echogenic lipoma interdigitating and infiltrating the right ventricular free wall. (b) Surgical specimen. RV, right ventricle. Movie clips 12.22 Part 1–12.22 Part 1–3. (Reproduced from Reddy *et al.* [7], with permission.)

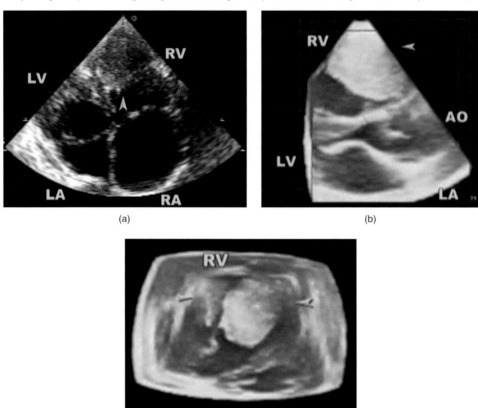

(a)   (b)

(c)

Figure 12.23 Real time 2D and 3D transthoracic echocardiography in right ventricular fibroma. (a) 2D study. The arrowhead points to a single mass in the right ventricle (RV). (b, c) 3D study. The arrowhead in (b) points to a highly echogenic mass occupying right ventricular cavity and outflow tract. Sectioning the mass and viewing it *en face* demonstrates two separate tumors (arrowheads in (c)). AO, aorta; LA, left atrium; LV, left ventricle; RA, right atrium. Movie clips 12.23 Parts 1–3. (Reproduced from Reddy *et al.* [7], with permission.)

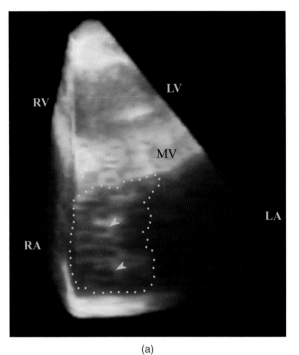

(a)

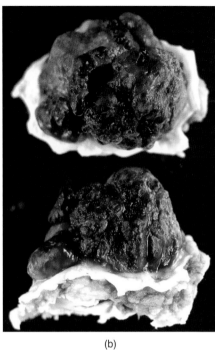

(b)

Figure 12.24 Live 3D transthoracic echocardiographic assessment of left atrial hemangioma. (a) The arrowheads (arrow in Movie clip 12.19) point to two of the large number of closely packed echolucencies in the tumor mass with sparse solid tissue. (b) Resected specimen showing multiple vascular areas. LA, left atrium; LV, left ventricle; MV, mitral valve; RA, right atrium; RV, right ventricle. Movie clip 12.24. (Reproduced from Mehmood *et al.* [13], with permission.)

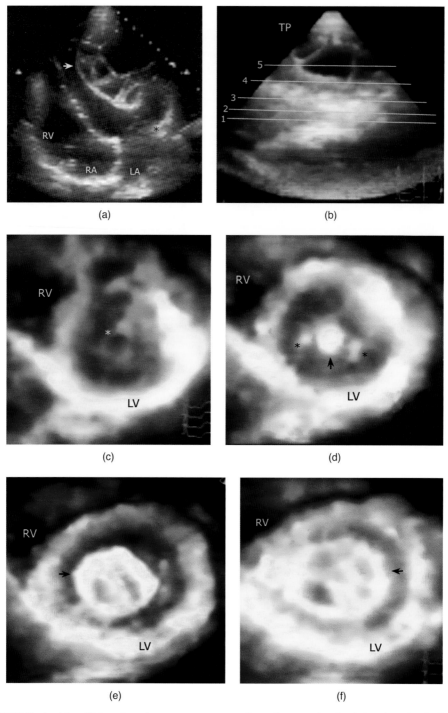

(a)

(b)

(c)

(d)

(e)

(f)

Figure 12.25 Live/real time 3D transthoracic echocardiographic assessment of hydatid cyst in the left ventricle (LV). (a) The arrow points to the large hydatid cyst in the LV seen on the 2D transthoracic echocardiogram. (b–h) Sequential transverse plane (TP) sections taken at various levels (numbered 1–5) of the 3D dataset. The cyst is not visualized at the level of the body of the mitral valve (c, ∗), but its basal tip (arrow) comes into view when the section is taken further down at the mitral valve leaflet tips (d).

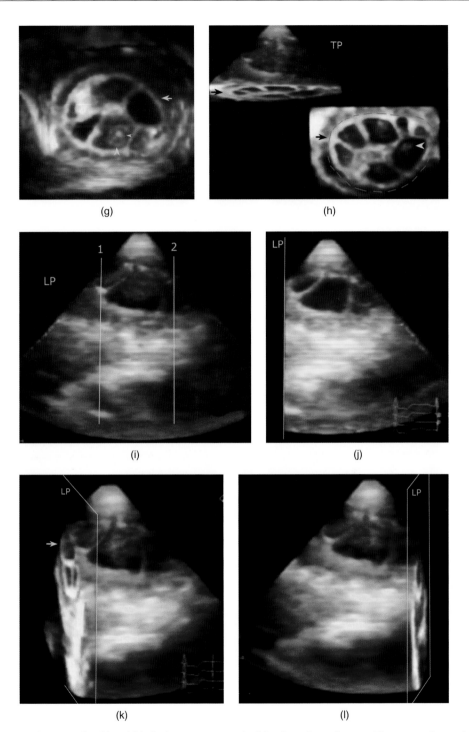

Figure 12.25 (*Continued*) In (g) and (h), the large arrowhead points to a tertiary or granddaughter cyst located within the secondary or daughter cyst. The small arrowhead in (g) shows a small great-granddaughter cyst budding from the tertiary cyst. The arrow points to the parent hydatid cyst. (i–l) Longitudinal plane (LP) sections (numbered 1 and 2) through the hydatid cyst (arrow).

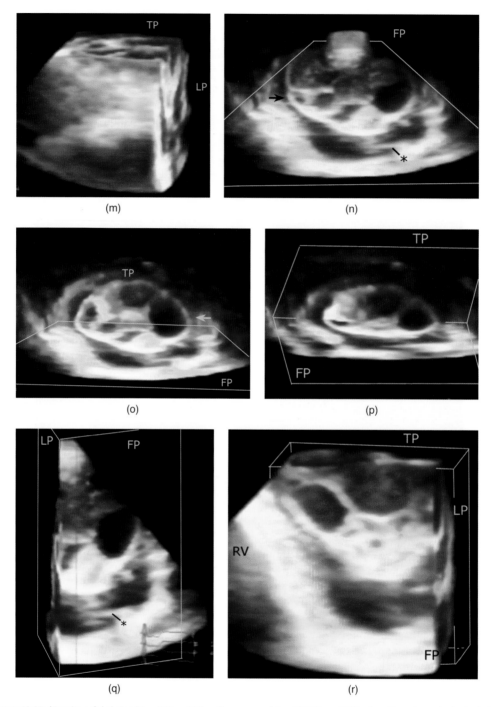

Figure 12.25 (*Continued*) (m) Combined TP and LP sections through the hydatid cyst. (n–s) Only frontal plane (FP) (n), combined FP and TP (o, p), combined FP and LP (q), and combined FP, TP, and LP (r, s) sections through the hydatid cyst.

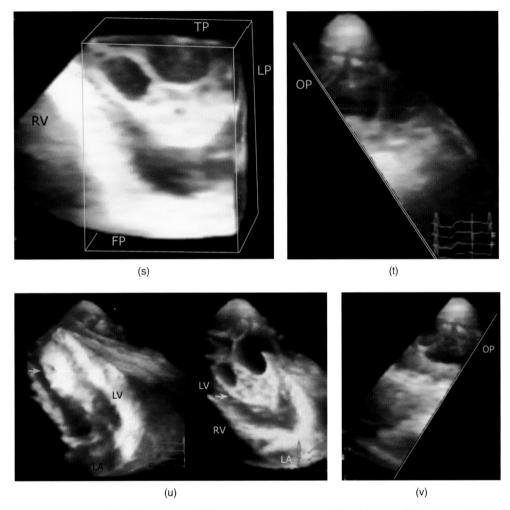

(s)

(t)

(u)

(v)

Figure 12.25 (*Continued*) (t–x) Oblique plane (OP) sections through the hydatid cyst. In (x), the OP section is rotated to view the cyst *en face*. The large arrowhead points to the tertiary or granddaughter cyst, which is shown attached to the secondary or daughter cyst by a stalk (small double arrowheads).

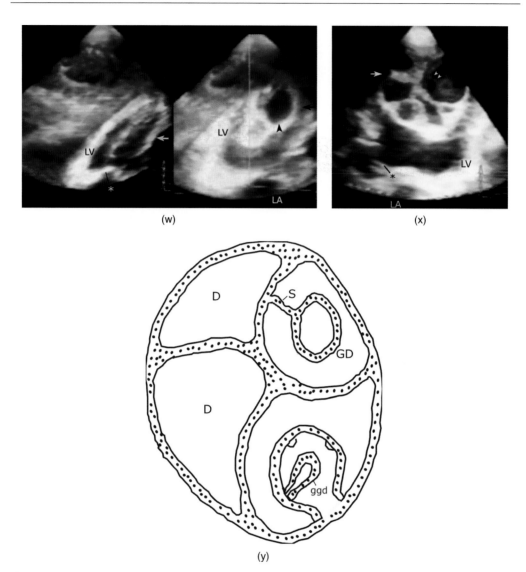

(w)   (x)

(y)

Figure 12.25 (*Continued*) (y) Schematic of hydatid cyst. D, daughter cyst; GD, granddaughter cyst; ggd, great granddaughter cyst; LA, left atrium; RA, right atrium; RV, right ventricle; S, stalk. Movie clip 12.25. (Reproduced from Sinha *et al.* [19], with permission.)

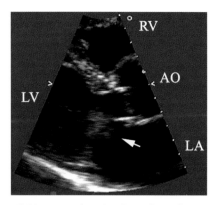

Figure 12.26 2D transthoracic echocardiography in epithelioid hemangioma involving the mitral valve. Left parasternal long-axis view. The arrow points to the mass attached to the anterior mitral leaflet, with a few echolucencies within it. AO, aorta; LA, left atrium; LV, left ventricle; RV, right ventricle. (Reproduced from Dod *et al.* [16], with permission.)

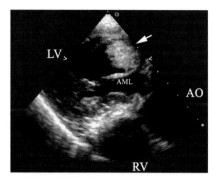

Figure 12.28 Transesophageal echocardiography in epithelioid hemangioma involving the mitral valve. Low esophageal modified five-chamber view. The arrow points to the mass on the anterior mitral leaflet (AML), with a few scattered echolucencies within it. AO, aorta; LV, left ventricle; RV, right ventricle. (Reproduced from Dod *et al.* [16], with permission.)

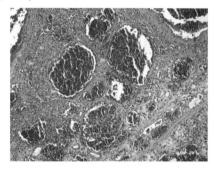

Figure 12.29 Histopathology. H&E stain 10 . In addition to the sheet-like areas of "epithelioid" endothelial cells with small vascular spaces typical of epithelioid hemangioma (arrows), this lesion contains larger more cavernous vascular spaces (arrowheads). (Reproduced from Dod *et al.* [16], with permission.)

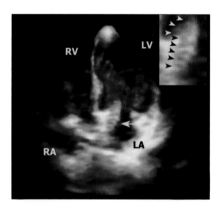

Figure 12.27 Live/real time 3D transthoracic echocardiography in epithelioid hemangioma involving the mitral valve. Apical four-chamber view. The arrow points to a mass attached to the mitral valve. The presence of multiple echolucencies (arrowheads in the inset) within the mass is consistent with a hemangioma. LA, left atrium; LV, left ventricle; RA, right atrium; RV, right ventricle. Movie clip 12.27. (Reproduced from Dod *et al.* [16], with permission.)

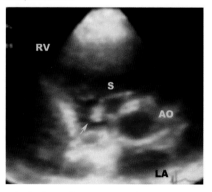

Figure 12.30 Live/real time 3D transthoracic echocardiographic evaluation of tricuspid valve fibroelastoma. The arrow shows a fibroelastoma attached to the septal leaflet (S) of the tricuspid valve. AO, aorta; LA, left atrium; RV, right ventricle. Movie clip 12.30. (Reproduced from Pothineni *et al.*, *Echocardiography* 2007;24:541–52, with permission.)

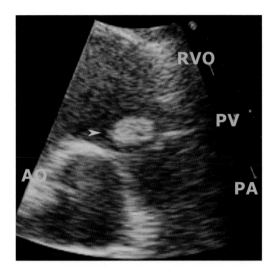

Figure 12.31 Real time 2D transthoracic echocardiographic findings in pulmonary valve fibroelastoma. The arrowhead points to finger-like projections on the fibroelastoma. AO, aorta; PA, pulmonary artery; PV, pulmonary valve; RVO, right ventricle outflow tract. (Reproduced from Singh *et al.* [20], with permission.)

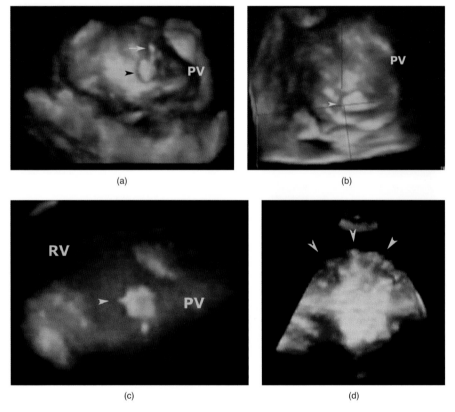

(a)

(b)

(c)

(d)

Figure 12.32 Live/real time 3D transthoracic echocardiographic findings in pulmonary valve fibroelastoma. (a) The arrowhead points to fibroelastoma and the arrow to the echogenic stalk attaching it to the pulmonary valve (PV). (b) Cropping and sectioning the tumor and viewing it *en face* shows no evidence of echolucency. (c) The arrowhead points to finger-like projections (fronds) on the fibroelastoma. (d) Ex vivo imaging of the resected fibroelastoma shows a dense central core and multiple finger-like projections (arrowheads). RV, right ventricle. Movie clips 12.32 A, 12.32 B Part 1–2, 12.32 D. (Reproduced from Singh *et al.* [20], with permission.)

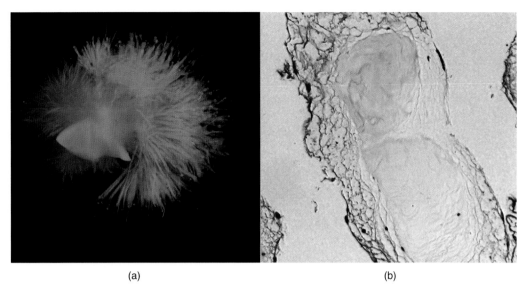

(a)   (b)

Figure 12.33 Gross pathological specimen of fibroelastoma showing multiple frond-like structures resembling a sea anemone (a) and histopathology of the surgical specimen demonstrating a central core of collagen and elastin covered by a single layer of endothelial cells (b). (Reproduced from Singh *et al.* [20], with permission.)

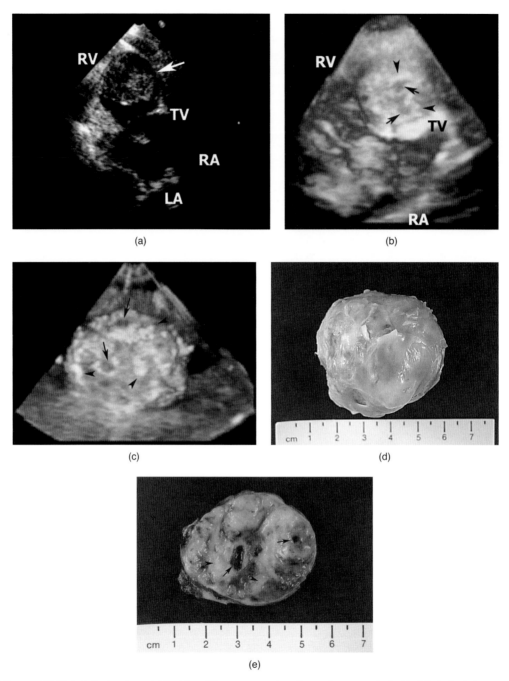

Figure 12.34 Metastatic chordoma. (a) Real time 2D transthoracic echocardiography. The arrow points to the chordoma in the right ventricle (RV). (b, c) Live/real time 3D transthoracic echocardiography. The arrows point to echolucencies consistent with hemorrhages and cystic areas and the arrowheads denote echodense areas produced by fibrotic bands. The less intense areas represent the myxoid stroma. (b) and (c) represent in vivo and ex vivo studies, respectively. (d, e) Pathological specimen showing the lobulated resected tumor (d). The cut surface (e) shows hemorrhagic and cystic areas (arrows) and dense fibrotic bands (arrowheads). LA, left atrium; RA, right atrium; TV, tricuspid valve. Movie clips 12.34 A and 12.34 B. (Reproduced from Pothineni *et al.* [17], with permission.)

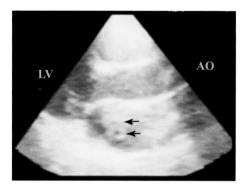

Figure 12.35 Live/real time 3D transthoracic echocardiographic findings in primary left atrial leiomyosarcoma. The arrows point to a "doughnut"-like appearance of the tumor mass located in the left atrium. AO, aorta; LV, left ventricle. Movie clip 12.35. (Reproduced from Suwanjutah *et al.* [18], with permission.)

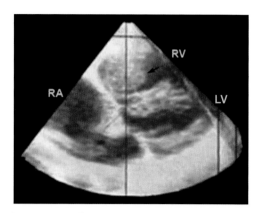

Figure 12.37 Real time 3D transthoracic echocardiography in right ventricular sarcoma. The arrow points to a mass in the right ventricle (RV) showing large echolucencies surrounded by echogenic band-like tissue giving "doughnut" appearance (see Movie clip 12.37). Movie clip 12.37 A shows, in a different patient, renal cell carcinoma invading the inferior vena cava (IV) and the proximal right atrium (RA). Cut section demonstrates a solid tumor with no evidence of necrosis. Surgically resected specimen is also shown. LV, left ventricle. (Reproduced from Reddy *et al.* [7], with permission.)

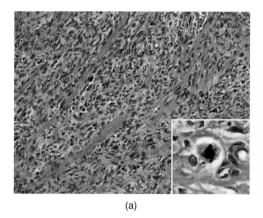

(a)

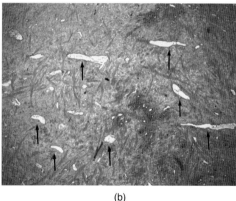

(b)

Figure 12.36 (a) Intermediate and high-power microscopic appearances of the leiomyosarcoma. The tumor is composed of pleomorphic spindle cells arranged in a fascicular pattern. Abnormal mitotic activity (inset) was easily identified. (b) Low-power microscopic appearance of necrotic tumor. The periphery of a necrotic area within the tumor showed acellular stroma and dilated/ectatic blood vessels (arrows) consistent with the echocardiographic findings. (Reproduced from Suwanjutah *et al.* [18], with permission.)

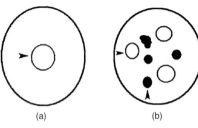

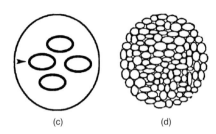

(a)   (b)   (c)   (d)

Figure 12.38 Schematics of (a) clot, (b) myxoma, (c) sarcoma/chordoma, and (d) hemangioma. The horizontal arrowhead in (a) points to central lysis in a clot, in (b) it points to an area of hemorrhage/necrosis in a myxoma, and in (c) to an area of necrosis surrounded by thick, band-like tissue containing collagen, giving a doughnut-like appearance seen with chordoma and sarcoma. The vertical arrowhead in (b) points to dense calcification in the myxoma. (d) Demonstrates a hemangioma which is completely vascular and the echolucencies involve the whole tumor, including periphery. (Reproduced from Reddy et al. [7], with permission.)

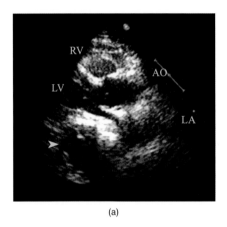

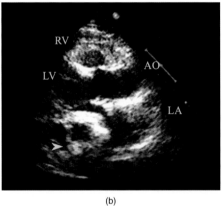

(a)   (b)

Figure 12.39 2D transthoracic echocardiography in a patient with a hiatal hernia. (a) The arrowhead points to the hiatal hernia located behind the left atrioventricular junction and left ventricular posterior wall. (b) Contrast bubbles (arrowhead) appear in the hernia after oral administration of a carbonated beverage. AO, aorta; LA, left atrium; LV, left ventricle; RV, right ventricle. Movie clips 12.39 A and 12.39 B. (Reproduced from Gupta et al. [23], with permission.)

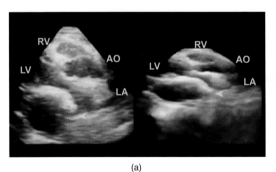

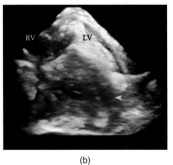

(a)   (b)

Figure 12.40 Live/real time 3D transthoracic echocardiography in a patient with a hiatal hernia. (a) The arrowhead shows a large hiatal hernia located behind the left atrioventricular junction and left ventricular posterior wall. The walls of the hernia are thick. Echo densities of various shapes and sizes consistent with stomach contents are present within the hernia. (b) Cropping of the 3D echo dataset demonstrates a large hiatal hernia (arrowhead) which measured at least 7   4.8 cm in size. (c) The arrowhead points to contrast echoes in the hernia. (d) Real time 3D image showing the initial appearance of contrast echoes (arrowhead) in the hiatal hernia. AO, aorta; LA, left atrium; LV, left ventricle; RV, right ventricle. Movie clips 12.40 A–D. (Reproduced from Gupta et al. [23], with permission.)

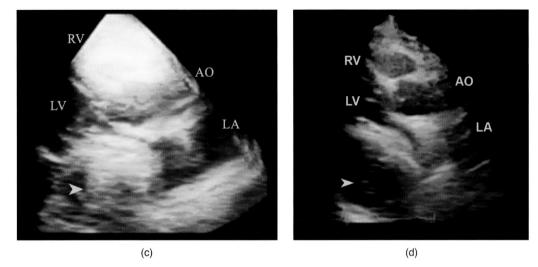

(c)   (d)

Figure 12.40 (*Continued*).

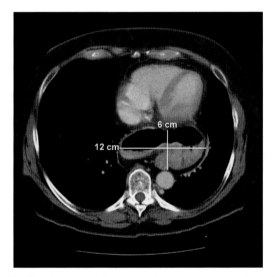

Figure 12.41 CT scan image of the hiatal hernia, in the same patient, seen in cross section at its maximal dimensions. Measurements are as labeled. (Reproduced from Gupta *et al.* [23], with permission.)

Acknowledgement

We are most grateful to Dr. Michael Faulkner, Internal Medicine Resident, for his help in writing the text portion of Chapter 12.

References

1. Peters PJ, Reinhardt S. The echocardiographic evaluation of intracardiac masses: a review. *J Am Soc Echocardiogr* 2006;19(2):230–240.

2. Asch FM, Bieganski SP, Panza JA, Weissman NJ. Real-time 3-dimensional echocardiography evaluation of intracardiac masses. *Echocardiography* 2006;23(3):218–24.

3. Ragland MM, Tak T. The role of echocardiography in diagnosing space-occupying lesions of the heart. *Clin Med Res* 2006;4(1):22–32.

4. Duncan K, Nanda NC, Foster WA, Mehmood F, Patel V, Singh A. Incremental value of live/real time three-dimensional transthoracic echocardiography in the assessment of left ventricular thrombi. *Echocardiography* 2006;23(1):68–72.

5. Stratton JR, Resnick AD. Increased embolic risk in patients with left ventricular thrombi. *Circulation* 1987;75(5):1004–11.

6. Jugdutt BI, Sivaram CA. Prospective two-dimensional echocardiographic evaluation of left ventricular thrombus and embolism after acute myocardial infarction. *J Am Coll Cardiol* 1989;13(3):554–64.

7. Reddy VK, Faulkner M, Bandarupalli N, et al. Incremental value of live/real time three-dimensional transthoracic echocardiography in the assessment of right ventricular masses. *Echocardiography* 2009;26(5):598–609.

8. Ellis K, Ziada KM, Vivekananthan D, et al. Transthoracic echocardiographic predictors of left atrial appendage thrombus. *Am J Cardiol* 2006;97(3):421–5.

9. Karakus G, Kodali V, Inamdar V, Nanda NC, Suwanjutah T, Pothineni K. Comparative assessment of left atrial appendage by transesophageal and combined two and three-dimensional transthoracic echocardiography. *Echocardiography* 2008;25: 918–24.

10. Upendram S, Nanda NC, Mehmood F, et al. Images in geriatric cardiology: live three-dimensional transthoracic echocardiographic assessment of right atrial thrombus. *Am J Geriatr Cardiol* 2004;13(6):330–331.

11. Upendram S, Nanda NC, Vengala S, et al. Live three-dimensional transthoracic echocardiographic assessment of thrombus in the innominate veins and superior vena cava utilizing right parasternal and supraclavicular approaches. *Echocardiography* 2005;22(5):445–9.

12. Yelamanchili P, Nanda NC, Patel V, et al. Live/real time three-dimensional echocardiographic demonstration of left ventricular noncompaction and thrombi. *Echocardiography* 2006;23(8):704–6.

13. Mehmood F, Nanda NC, Vengala S, et al. Live three-dimensional transthoracic echocardiographic assessment of left atrial tumors. *Echocardiography* 2005;22(2):137–43.

14. Muller S, Feuchtner G, Bonatti J, et al. Value of transesophageal 3D echocardiography as an adjunct to conventional 2D imaging in preoperative evaluation of cardiac masses. *Echocardiography* 2008;25(6):624–31.

15. Lokhandwala J, Liu Z, Jundi M, Loyd A, Strong M, Vannan M. Three-dimensional echocardiography of intracardiac masses. *Echocardiography* 2004;21(2):159–63.

16. Dod HS, Burri MV, Hooda D, et al. Two- and three-dimensional transthoracic and transesophageal echocardiographic findings in epithelioid hemangioma involving the mitral valve. *Echocardiography* 2008;25(4):443–5.

17. Pothineni KR, Nanda NC, Burri MV, Bell WC, Post JD. Live/real time three-dimensional transthoracic echocardiographic description of chordoma metastatic to the heart. *Echocardiography* 2008;25(4):440–442.

18. Suwanjutah T, Singh H, Plaisance BR, Hameed O, Nanda NC. Live/real time three-dimensional transthoracic echocardiographic findings in primary left atrial leiomyosarcoma. *Echocardiography* 2008;25(3):337–9.

19. Sinha A, Nanda NC, Panwar RB, et al. Live three-dimensional transthoracic echocardiographic assessment of left ventricular hydatid cyst. *Echocardiography* 2004;21(8):699–705.

20. Singh A, Miller AP, Nanda NC, Rajdev S, Mehmood F, Duncan K. Papillary fibroelastoma of the pulmonary valve: assessment by live/real time three-dimensional transthoracic echocardiography. *Echocardiography* 2006;23(10):880–883.

21. Le Tourneau T, Pouwels S, Gal B, et al. Assessment of papillary fibroelastomas with live three-dimensional transthoracic echocardiography. *Echocardiography* 2008;25(5):489–95.

22. Pothineni KR, Nanda NC, Patel V, Madadi P. Live/real time three-dimensional transthoracic echocardiographic detection of vegetation on a pacemaker/defibrillator lead. *Am J Geriatr Cardiol* 2006;15(1):62–3.

23. Gupta M, Nanda NC, Inamdar V. Two- and three-dimensional transthoracic echocardiographic assessment of hiatal hernia. *Echocardiography* 2008;25(7):790–793.

CHAPTER 13

Pericardial Disorders

Real time 2D transthoracic echocardiography (2DTTE) represents the most useful and popular noninvasive technique for the diagnosis of pericardial effusion. In addition, 2DTTE provides an estimate of the size of the effusion, and several indicators on the echocardiogram can lead one to suspect cardiac tamponade or impending tamponade [1–5]. However, as emphasized elsewhere in the book, there are many limitations of the 2D technique [6–10]. Each 2D view represents only a thin section through the heart, and the findings displayed, such as pericardial layers and effusion, lack a 3D perspective. Live/real time 3DTTE overcomes some of these limitations of 2D imaging. In our experience, it supplements 2DTTE by providing additional clinically useful information in patients with various pericardial disorders [11] (Figures 13.1–13.11).

First of all, since the acquired 3D datasets can be cropped and viewed from any desired angulation and viewing perspective, the full extent of pericardial effusion, including extension behind atrial walls, can be fully delineated. Because of this, a more accurate estimation of the size of pericardial effusions is possible with 3DTTE. Another important advantage of 3DTTE is the ability to view *en face* both visceral and parietal layers of pericardium, thus facilitating the inspection for any abnormalities. The presence and distribution of fibrin can be very well appreciated. Both ventricles and both atria can be systematically cropped to practically view the entire visceral pericardium covering them. The parietal pericardium can also be studied in a

similar manner. Fibrin strands can be comprehensively evaluated for their number, distribution, size, and mobility and differentiated from other pathologies which may mimic them. For example, tumor bands may have a similar appearance on 2D imaging, but when cropped using 3DTTE, they appear much thicker and can be shown to infiltrate the myocardium. Cropping of pericardial effusion is also useful to look for echo reflectors within the effusion space, which signifies the presence of solid material while its absence may indicate only fluid collection. This is useful in the assessment of patients following cardiac surgery who may bleed into the pericardium. Multiple echo densities within the effusion space would suggest hematoma formation while their absence suggests only fluid or homogeneous material. Other abnormal echo densities involving the pericardium can be comprehensively studied for their exact location, extent, and size. Given the slice view of the 2D technique, it is not surprising that we found many instances in which the size of these masses was grossly underestimated by 2DTTE as compared to the 3D modality. Granulomas, which can be seen in infective diseases like tuberculosis, were easily assessed when viewed in 3D and provided a clue to the nature of the disease process. In addition, in one patient studied by us, a portion of right ventricular wall showed no inward motion during systole probably due to fibrinous adhesions, a common finding in tuberculous pericarditis. Pericardial metastases from malignant tumors such as lung carcinoma could be visualized on careful, systematic cropping of the 3D datasets. A patient with metastatic poorly differentiated lung adenocarcinoma showed an abnormal loculated appearance of a portion of the parietal pericardium. Another patient with a malignant thymoma extending into the mediastinum

Live/Real Time 3D Echocardiography, 1st edition.
By Navin C. Nanda, Ming Chon Hsiung, Andrew P. Miller, and Fadi G. Hage. Published 2010 by Blackwell Publishing Ltd.

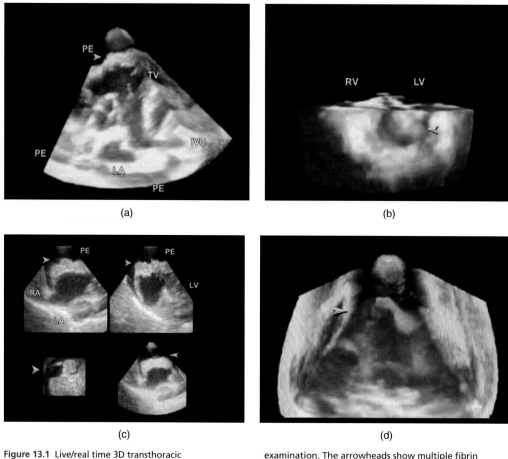

(a)

(b)

(c)

(d)

Figure 13.1 Live/real time 3D transthoracic echocardiography in pericardial effusion in a 64-year-old female with renal failure. (a) The arrowhead points to fibrin deposition over the right ventricular pericardium giving a rugged appearance. Pericardial effusion extends behind both atria (see also Movie clip 13.1 A). (b) Apical four-chamber view. Cropping from bottom displays a smooth visceral pericardium over the basal left atrial wall (arrowhead) (see also Movie clip 13.1 B). (c) Subcostal examination. The arrowheads show multiple fibrin deposits on the right atrial visceral pericardium, resulting in a rugged appearance (see also Movie clip 13.1 C). (d) The arrowhead shows a flap-like fibrin mass (see Movie clips 13.1 D Part 1 and 13.1 D Part 2). IVC, inferior vena cava; LA, left atrium; LV, left ventricle; PE, pericardial effusion; RA, right atrium; RV, right ventricle; TV, tricuspid valve. (Reproduced from Martinez Hernandez et al. [11], with permission.)

and invading the pericardium showed a huge mass involving the right ventricular pericardium, which when "cut open" by cropping showed marked inhomogenicity of tissue consistent with a malignant process.

Other benign lesions of the pericardium such as pericardial cysts may also benefit from 3DTTE. In a young man studied by us, thick band-like tissue crisscrossing the pericardial cyst was revealed on

cropping the 3D dataset. This finding was not detected by 2D imaging. This was an unusual case since the contents of pericardial cysts are usually clear without any trabeculations. The 3D technique may also be helpful in patients with constrictive pericarditis. In a female patient studied by us, 3DTTE showed extensive involvement of both the left ventricular posterior wall and the right ventricular anterior wall by calcification. The

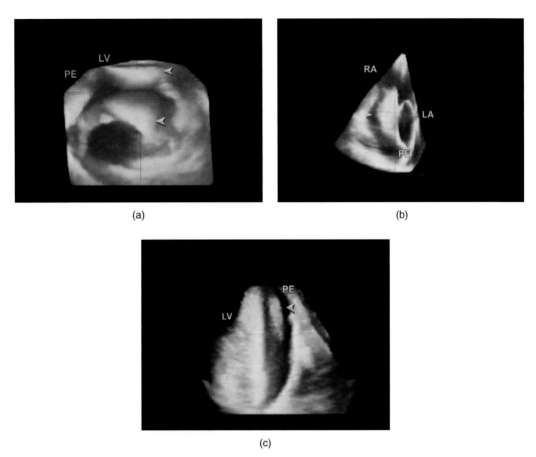

(a) (b)

(c)

Figure 13.2 Live/real time 3D transthoracic echocardiography in pericardial effusion (PE) in an 85-year-old female with congestive heart failure and ascites. (a) The upper and lower arrowheads point to visceral and parietal layers of the pericardium, respectively. Both the pericardial layers are smooth without fibrin deposition (see also Movie clip 13.2 A). (b) Right parasternal examination. The arrowhead points to a smooth visceral pericardium overlying the right (RA) and left (LA) atria (see also Movie clip 13.2 B). (c) The arrowhead shows a localized collection of fibrin over the visceral pericardium of the left ventricular free wall (see also Movie clip 13.2 C). Movie clip 13.2 D shows PE (arrowhead) extending behind the left atrium. The arrowhead in Movie clip 13.2 E points to 3D images of the falciform ligament, which is a useful landmark in distinguishing ascites from associated PE. It appears as a sheet of tissue connected to the liver rather than a linear echo mimicking a fibrin strand seen with conventional 2D imaging. The arrowhead in Movie clip 13.2 F points to the falciform ligament viewed *en face* in another patient with ascites. D, diaphragm; DA, descending thoracic aorta; IVC, inferior vena cava; L, liver; LV, left ventricle; RV, right ventricle. (Reproduced from Martinez Hernandez *et al.* [11], with permission.)

2D technique did show calcification involving these walls but its widespread extent was not delineated.

Finally, live 3DTTE imaging offers the potential advantage of better needle guidance during pericardiocentesis. Owing to its pyramidal imaging plane, finding and directing a needle can be more precise with 3D compared with 2D imaging.

We have also found 3DTTE useful in assessing other fluid collections such as ascites and pleural effusions which may be associated with pericardial effusion. Ascites is often diagnosed and differentiated from pericardial effusion by the presence of falciform ligament which connects the liver to the abdominal wall [7,8]. On 2DTTE, this often appears as a thin, mobile structure which mimics a fibrin

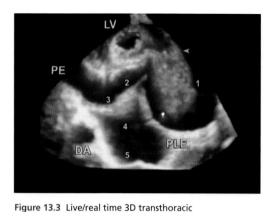

Figure 13.3 Live/real time 3D transthoracic echocardiography in an 84-year-old male with renal failure and pericardial and left pleural effusions. Cropping of the 3D dataset using QLAB software analysis package revealed a rugged visceral (#1, 2, arrowhead) and parietal (#3) pericardium as well as a rugged visceral (#4) and parietal (#5) pleura, from fibrin deposits (see also Movie clip 13.3 A). Movie clips 13.3 B and 13.3 C show similar findings using regular cropping in the same patient. Movie clips 13.3 D and 13.3 E are from a different patient with pleural effusion, shown for comparison. These show cropping to more comprehensively assess the extent of pleural effusion (PLE) and the collapsed lung (arrowhead) and their relation to the heart (H). Movie clip 13.3 F from another patient shows the attachment of collapsed lung lobes (horizontal arrowheads) to the hilum (vertical arrowheads) and its relationship to the heart (H). This patient had previously undergone pericardiectomy for constriction. Both these patients were studied from the back in the sitting position. DA, descending thoracic aorta; LV, left ventricle; PE, pericardial effusion; PP, parietal pericardium; VPL, visceral pleura; VS, visceral pericardium. (Reproduced from Martinez Hernandez et al. [11], with permission.)

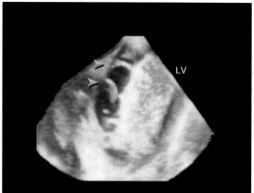

Figure 13.4 Live/real time 3D transthoracic echocardiography in a 62-year-old male with pericardial effusion developing following mitral valve replacement. The arrowheads point to fibrinous strands connecting the visceral and parietal portions of the pericardium. The accompanying Movie clips 13.4 A and 13.4 B from the same patient show both mobile and nonmobile fibrin strands. In Movie clip 13.4 A, artifacts appeared when the instrument gain was decreased and disappeared with increase in gain, emphasizing the importance of optimizing gain settings when assessing 3D images. Movie clip 13.4 B shows cropping done using the QLAB software analysis package. LV, left ventricle. (Reproduced from Martinez Hernandez et al. [11], with permission.)

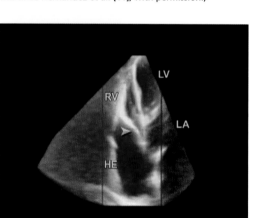

Figure 13.5 Live/real time 3D transthoracic echocardiography in a 50-year-old male with pericardial effusion compressing the right atrium. The arrowhead points to the compressed right atrium. Cropping reveals no significant echo reflectors ("solid tissue") in the effusion suggesting that it mainly comprises fluid or the hematoma (HE) is of uniform, homogeneous consistency (see also Movie clip 13.5). The patient improved after drainage of 1000 cm^3 of yellowish fluid from the pericardial cavity using a pigtail catheter. LA, left atrium; LV, left ventricle; RV, right ventricle. (Reproduced from Martinez Hernandez et al. [11], with permission.)

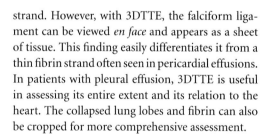

strand. However, with 3DTTE, the falciform ligament can be viewed *en face* and appears as a sheet of tissue. This finding easily differentiates it from a thin fibrin strand often seen in pericardial effusions. In patients with pleural effusion, 3DTTE is useful in assessing its entire extent and its relation to the heart. The collapsed lung lobes and fibrin can also be cropped for more comprehensive assessment.

From our experience, it is evident that 3DTTE provides additional information to that obtained by 2DTTE in patients with pericardial disorders. It has the potential to become a most useful supplement to conventional echocardiography.

Figure 13.6 Live/real time 3D transthoracic echocardiography in a 17–year-old male with a bullet injury and subsequent development of pericardial hematoma. The red dots outline a loculated component of a very large pericardial hematoma (see Movie clip 13.6 A). Movie clip 13.6 B shows a huge pericardial hematoma (arrowhead) with large multiple echolucencies consistent with fluid collections. These were not well seen on 2D imaging. LV, left ventricle; RV, right ventricle. (Reproduced from Martinez Hernandez *et al.* [11], with permission.)

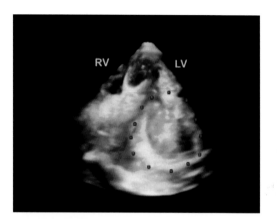

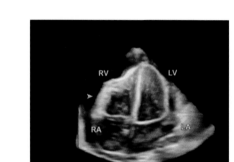

(a)

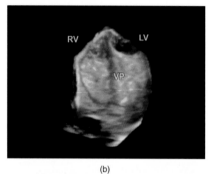

(b)

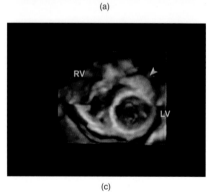

(c)

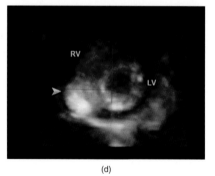

(d)

Figure 13.7 Live/real time 3D transthoracic echocardiography in a 26-year-old male with tuberculous pericardial effusion. (a) Cropping of the apical four-chamber dataset shows no inward motion of the proximal right ventricular free wall (arrowhead) during systole, probably due to fibrinous adhesions. The distal wall contracts well. (b) Examination of visceral pericardium (VP) over the ventricles demonstrates a mildly rugged appearance. Movie clips 13.7 A–B Part 1–3 show the cropping technique used to demonstrate the visceral pericardium of both ventricles. (c) A large mass (arrowhead) is seen involving the visceral pericardium of the left ventricle (LV). The etiology is not clear but it could possibly represent a tuberculous granuloma. (d) The arrowhead points to a large highly echogenic mass involving the right ventricular visceral pericardium consistent with a calcified granuloma in another patient with tuberculosis. Movie clip 13.7 C from the same patient shows a granuloma (arrowhead) involving the parietal pericardium. Movie clips 13.7 D and 13.7 E are from a different patient with purulent pericardial effusion due to methicillin-resistant *Staphylococcus aureus*. Movie clip 13.7 D shows markedly thickened and echogenic parietal (upper arrowhead) and visceral (lower arrowhead) pericardium. Movie clip 13.7 E shows an abnormal loculated appearance of the visceral pericardium (arrowhead) when viewed *en face* by cropping from the apex. LA, left atrium; RA, right atrium; RV, right ventricle. (Reproduced from Martinez Hernandez *et al.* [11], with permission.)

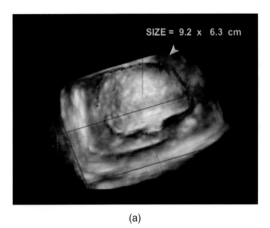

(a)

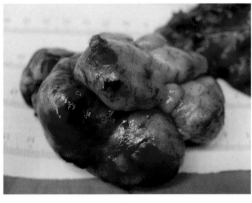

(b)

Figure 13.8 Live/real time 3D transthoracic echocardiography in a 66-year-old male with pericardial metastasis from a malignant thymoma. (a) The arrowhead shows a huge pericardial mass (bounded by red dots) measuring 9.2 cm   6.3 cm. Movie clips 13.8 A–C show the full extent of this huge mass with 3D imaging. Cutting open the tumor in its mid-portion (arrowhead in Movie clip 13.8 B) revealed solid inhomogenous tissue. The arrowheads in Movie clip 13.8 C show parietal involvement of the tumor by multiple band-like extensions. The 2D study in this patient (Movie clip 13.8 D) shows a much smaller mass (arrowhead) measuring 3.8 cm   1.5 cm attached to the right ventricular outflow tract visceral pericardium. (b) Surgical specimen. (Reproduced from Martinez Hernandez et al. [11], with permission.)

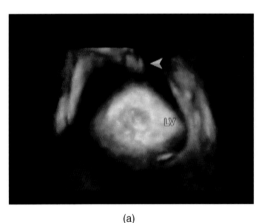

(a)

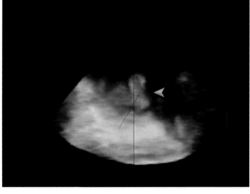

(b)

Figure 13.9 Live/real time 3D transthoracic echocardiography in a 68-year-old male with lung carcinoma. (a, b) The arrowhead points to an irregular mass in the parietal pericardium (PP) (see Movie clips 13.9 A and 13.9 B). The etiology is not clear, but it could possibly represent a pericardial metastasis. Movie clip 13.9 C shows another mass (arrowhead) located over the visceral pericardium (VP) in this patient. This type of mass (arrowhead) was also seen by 2D imaging (Movie clip 13.9 D). However, the other mass seen involving PP was not detected by this modality. Movie clip 13.9 E is from a different patient with a poorly differentiated lung adenocarcimona. The arrowhead points to a mass in the PP consistent with metastasis. This was not visualized on 2D imaging. Examination of pericardial fluid in this patient showed the presence of malignant cells. LV, left ventricle. (Reproduced from Martinez Hernandez et al. [11], with permission.)

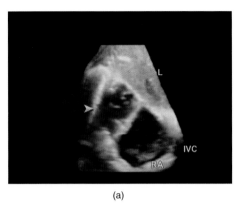

(a)

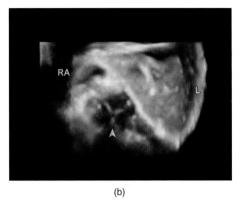

(b)

Figure 13.10 Live/real time 3D transthoracic echocardiography in a 36-year-old male with a pericardial cyst. (a) The arrowhead points to a pericardial cyst confirmed by a CT scan of the chest (see Movie clip 13.10 A). (b) Cropping of the 3D dataset demonstrates multiple band-like tissue (arrowhead) within the cyst (see Movie clip 13.10 B). Movie clips 13.10 C and 13.10 D represent 2D images which do not show multiple bands criss-crossing the cyst (arrowhead). L, liver. IVC, inferior vena cava; RA, right atrium. (Reproduced from Martinez Hernandez et al. [11], with permission.)

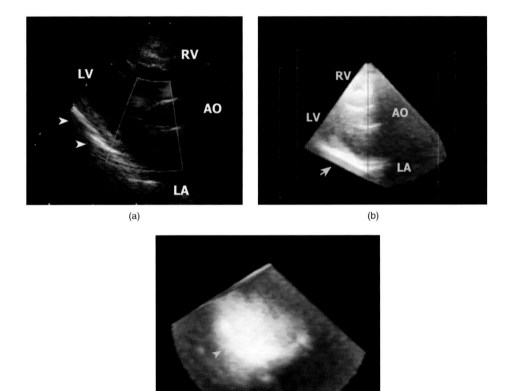

Figure 13.11 2D and live/real time 3D transthoracic echocardiography in a 53-year-old female with constrictive pericarditis. (a) 2D study. The arrowheads in the parasternal long-axis view point to an echogenic left ventricular posterior wall consistent with calcification (see Movie clip 13.11 A). (b) Represents a 3D study using QLAB software analysis package. The arrow demonstrates a highly echogenic posterior pericardium consistent with calcification. (c) When this was cropped transversely using an oblique cropping plane, widespread involvement of the left ventricular posterior wall with calcification (arrowhead) was evident. Highly echogenic calcification is visualized anteriorly also. Top and bottom arrowheads in the left upper quadrant in Movie clip 13.11 B point to anterior and posterior calcifications, respectively. The patient underwent pericardiectomy. AO, aorta; LA, left atrium; LV, left ventricle; MV, mitral valve; RV, right ventricle. (Reproduced from Martinez Hernandez et al. [11], with permission.)

References

1. Feigenbaum H, Armstrong WF, Ryan T. Pericardial diseases. In: Feigenbaum H, Armstrong WF, Ryan T, eds. *Feigenbaum's Echocardiography.* 6th ed. Philadelphia: Lippincott Williams & Wilkins; 2005:247–70.

2. Horowitz MS, Schulta CS, Stinson EB, Harrison DC, Popp RL. Sensitivity and specificity of echocardiographic diagnosis of pericardial effusion. *Circulation* 1974;50:239–47.

3. Tsang TSM, Barnes ME, Hayes SN, *et al.* Clinical and echocardiographic characteristics of significant pericardial effusions following cardiothoracic surgery and outcomes of echo-guided pericardiocentesis for management: Mayo Clinic Experience, 1979–1998. *Chest* 199:116; 322–31.

4. D'Cruz IA, Cohen HC, Prabh R, Glick G. Diagnosis of cardiac tamponade by echocardiography: changes in mitral valve motion and ventricular dimensions with special reference to paradoxical pulse. *Circulation* 1975;52:460–465.

5. D'Cruz IA. *Echocardiographic Anatomy: Understanding Normal and Abnormal Echocardiograms.* Stamford, CT: Appleton & Lange; 1996.

6. D'Cruz I, Prabhu R, Cohen HC, Glick G. Potential pitfalls in quantification of pericardial effusions by echocardiography. *Brit Heart J* 1977;39:529–35.

7. George S, Salama AL, Uthaman B, Cherian G. Echocardiography in differentiating tuberculous from chronic idiopathic pericardial effusion. *Heart* 2004;90:1338–9.

8. Hsu FI, Keefe D, Desiderio D, Downey RJ. Echocardiographic and surgical correlation of pericardial effusions in patients with malignant disease. *J Thorac Cardiovasc Surg* 1998;115:1215–16.

9. D'Cruz IA. Echocardiographic simulation of pericardial effusion by ascites. *Chest* 1984;85:93–5.

10. Cardello FP, Yoon DHA, Halligan RE, Jr, Richter H. The falciform ligament in the echocardiographic diagnosis of ascites. *J Am Soc Echocardiogr* 2005;19:1074, e3–4.

11. Martinenz Hernandez C, Singh P, Hage FG, *et al.* Live/real time three-dimensional transthoracic echocardiographic assessment of pericardial disease. *Echocardiography* 2009;26; 1250–1263.

CHAPTER 14

Live/Real Time 3D Transesophageal Echocardiography

Introduction

As of September 2007, a 3D transesophageal echocardiography (3DTEE) probe capable of live/real time 3D imaging became commercially available for clinical use in the United States [1]. This electronically steered transducer permits conventional multiplane 2DTEE image acquisition, but also offers live 3D, 3D zoom, full-volume 3D, and 3D color Doppler imaging, utilizing the matrix array technology employed in its 3D transthoracic echocardiography (3DTTE) predecessor. The clinical application of 3DTEE is similar to those described in previous chapters for 3DTTE, with the advantage of higher resolution that especially permits evaluation of valvular lesions. In this chapter, we will discuss the procedure for capturing 3DTEE images.

How to do a 3DTEE

Unlike 2D imaging where a fixed imaging plane requires the acquisition of standard views, 3D echocardiography is inherently volumetric and offers the potential for capturing a single dataset from which multiple questions can be answered through cropping. Therefore, a complete 3DTEE study involves acquisition of several full-volume datasets and then targeted acquisitions using 3D zoom and 3D color Doppler imaging. Much of the 3D datasets can be obtained hand in hand with 2D acquisition, and it is often the 2D images that guide 3D assessment. For the purposes of this chapter,

we will review a protocol for 3D image acquisition based on our 2D protocols that we established in our laboratory.

After esophageal intubation, we begin TEE imaging by finding the optimal four-chamber image in the lower esophagus. Just as in optimizing the 3DTTE image, a brief application of live 3D imaging can be useful to guide gain settings. Once the image is optimized, a full-volume 3D acquisition from the four-chamber imaging plane is acquired, permitting chamber quantification by workstation analysis later. Next, we turn our attention to the left atrial appendage (LAA) by steering the 2D plane from 0° to 90°. After evaluating the LAA with 2D and Doppler, we obtain 3D images of this structure. Here the 3D zoom feature and live 3D can be used with a small amount of online cropping to evaluate for thrombus. 3D imaging can be especially valuable in deciphering pectinate muscle from thrombus in the LAA with this technique. After acquiring 3D datasets of the LAA, we roll the probe toward the right side and into the bicaval view. Here, we evaluate for patent foramen ovale (PFO) with agitated saline injection and provocative maneuvers. While the saline injection can be acquired with live 3D, we find greater utility in using 3D color Doppler to evaluate the size and anatomy of any septal defect that is discovered. This is performed with a full acquisition with the color Doppler targeted to the defect. Later analysis will provide an *en face* view that can be cropped to visualize both sides of the defect. Imaging of the pulmonary veins completes this portion of the TEE protocol.

After accomplishing these acquisitions, we then inspect the valves. We begin with the mitral valve, which is particularly suited to 3D assessment

Live/Real Time 3D Echocardiography, 1st edition.
By Navin C. Nanda, Ming Chon Hsiung, Andrew P. Miller, and Fadi G. Hage. Published 2010 by Blackwell Publishing Ltd.

because of its saddle shape and the complex relationships between the valve, subvalvular apparatus, and myocardium. In assessing the mitral valve, we begin with a full-volume acquisition from the long-axis view again, after optimizing the 2D biplane image for the mitral valve. This will permit cropping to obtain *en face* images of the valve as well as full assessment of the subvalvular apparatus. We then obtain a 3D color Doppler dataset from the same view, targeted to any mitral regurgitation seen. To avoid stitch artifacts and to optimally perform offline analysis, live 3D zoom images are most useful. From the long-axis view, the zoom box must be adjusted to encompass the valve leaflets and hinge points in the biplane images, then live 3D zoom is engaged and a dataset is acquired. Online cropping of this image then is performed to obtain a live *en face* surgical view of the valve, which usually requires use of the steerable cropping plane. The aortic valve can serve as a guide for orientation and, by steering the *z*-plane, should be placed at the top of the imaging screen or at 12 o'clock. Once the surgical view from the left atrium is obtained, the anterior and posterior leaflets and their segments/scallops can be fully appreciated. Identification of the diseased segments/scallops from this view (as reviewed in a previous chapter) facilitates surgical decision making [2,3] (Figures 14.1 and 14.2).

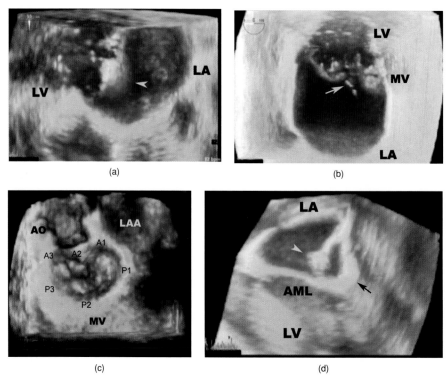

(a)

(b)

(c)

(d)

Figure 14.1 Mitral valve prolapse. The arrowhead in (a) points to prominent prolapse of A2 segment into left atrium (LA). The arrow in (b) points to a flail segment of the mitral leaflet with a torn chordae attached to it. (c) In another patient, note the extensive prolapse of P1 scallop of the posterior mitral leaflet when the mitral valve was cropped from the atrial aspect to create an *en face* view. The other two scallops of posterior mitral leaflet (P2 and P3) and the three segments of anterior mitral leaflet (A1, A2, and A3) show less extensive prolapse. (Not a surgical view where the LAA would be at 9–10 o'clock). (d, e) Mitral annular abscess. The arrowhead in (d) points to the rugged surface of the abscess cavity (arrow) located laterally. In (e), abscess cavity is viewed *en face* by cropping from bottom. (f, g) Left atrial appendage (LAA). The arrow in (f) points to echo density, possibly a thrombus, in LAA. Cropping of LAA using short-axis cuts revealed the echo density to be part of pectinate musculature (arrow in (g)). (h) Mitral valve ring viewed *en face* by cropping from the atrial aspect. The arrow points to *en face* view of Duran ring. (i) Mitral valve prosthesis (MVR). St Jude MVR viewed in open position from the atrial aspect. ((a–i) Reproduced from Pothineni *et al.* [1], with permission.) (j) Probe used for live/real time 3D transesophageal echocardiography. AO, aorta; AML, anterior mitral leaflet; LV, left ventricle; MV, mitral valve. Movie clips 14.1 C, 14.1 H, 14.1 I.

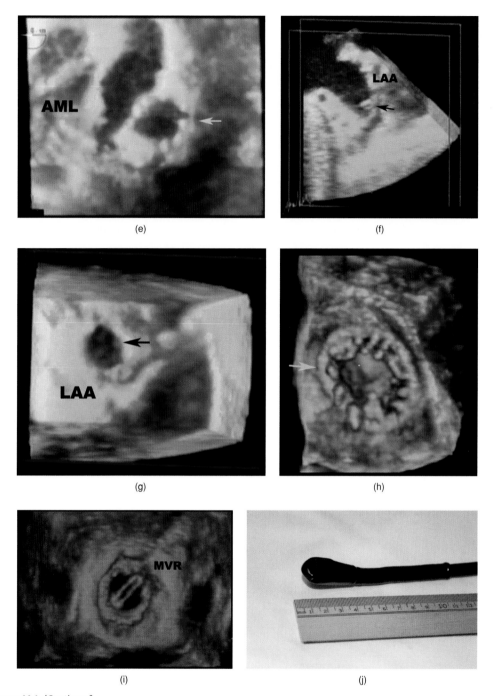

Figure 14.1 (*Continued*)

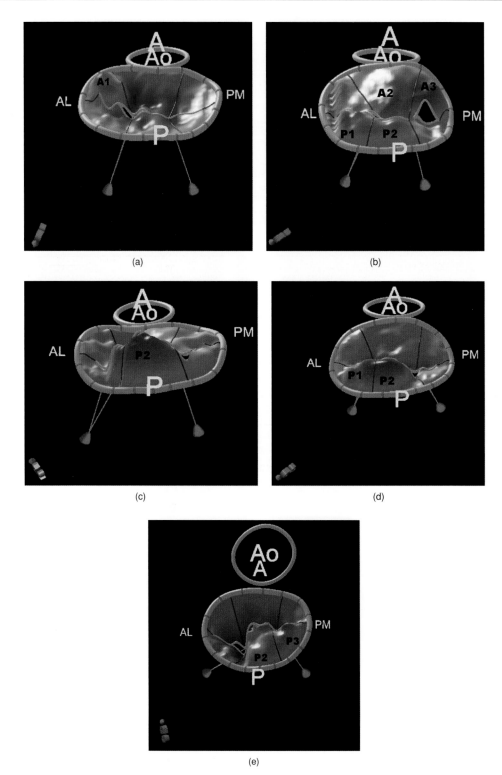

Figure 14.2 Mitral valve prolapse. The prolapsing segment/scallops can be displayed graphically using a commercially available software. (a) Isolated A1 prolapse. (b) A2, A3, P1, and P2 prolapse. (c) Isolated P2 prolapse. (d) P1 and P2 prolapse. (e) P2 and P3 prolapse. A, anterior; AL, anterolateral commissure; AO, aorta; P, posterior; PM, posteromedial commissure.

We next turn our attention to the aortic valve and follow a similar protocol as for the mitral valve. From the left ventricular outflow tract (LVOT) view at 135°, we again acquire a full volume dataset after optimization of the aortic valve image. Likewise, a 3D color Doppler dataset is acquired from this image, targeting aortic regurgitation. Again guided by the LVOT view, the aortic valve can be imaged with the live 3D zoom feature and cropped to obtain an *en face* image. The *en face* image of the aortic valve permits the best view of valve leaflet pathology and will be a useful tool for percutaneous aortic valve interventions [4]. We find that images of the aortic valve are easily acquired and are of equal or better quality than images of the mitral valve, though an early report by others suggested optimal visualization of the aortic valve in only 18% of those studied [5] (Figure 14.3).

The right-sided valves and then the aorta complete our protocol. The pulmonic valve can be seen in long-axis guided by a 2D image usually at about 90° just after acquisition of the aortic valve images. The tricuspid valve is best imaged low in the esophagus, guided by a 2D image at 0°. A similar process as for the mitral and aortic valves can be used to obtain 3D *en face* and 3D color Doppler images. Due to their distance from the probe, these valves can be challenging to image. Finally, a full-volume acquisition of the aorta can be targeted to pathology seen on 2D and can be helpful in characterizing dissection [1] (Figure 14.4).

While a complete 3D study might involve acquisitions of all of the above 3D datasets, a more focused exam is appropriate in most cases. For instance, in a patient with aortic stenosis, essential views would include a full-volume 3D dataset of the left ventricle for chamber quantification and full-volume 3D, 3D color Doppler, and 3D zoom views of the aortic valve. In this manner, a 2D and 3DTEE study can be accomplished for most clinical questions in less than 15 minutes of esophageal intubation time.

Offline analysis

A powerful asset of 3D imaging is that the dataset can be cropped to obtain any imaging plane imaginable after the patient has left the exam room. Analysis of the dataset begins at the bedside with image optimization and some cropping to ensure that the desired image is not subject to artifact. Then, more detailed analysis continues through cropping on the ultrasound system and with the use of commercial software packages such as QLAB (Philips Medical Systems, Andover, MA). Similar to 3DTTE, the 3DTEE dataset can be analyzed to quantify chamber size and function, valvular stenosis, and regurgitation, and evaluate congenital and mass lesions.

Chamber quantification

From the full-volume 3D dataset first acquired during the 3DTEE exam, analysis of left ventricular volume and regional function is accomplished, as reviewed in a previous TTE chapter. Briefly, in QLAB, four points of the mitral annulus and the apical endocardial border are selected in end-diastole and end-systole. After automated endocardial border determination, the operator proofs and edits border determination for both diastole and systole. Volume analysis is then performed, providing data on end-diastolic and end-systolic volumes, ejection fraction, and regional function in a 17-segment model.

Valvular heart disease

Similar to techniques used for 3DTTE, the 3DTEE dataset can provide planimetered valvular areas and vena contracta areas for stenotic and regurgitant valves, respectively. This is best accomplished on commercial software packages, such as QLAB. This software package provides three steerable planes to locate *en face* views of the smallest valve area at the leaflet tips from a 3D zoom or full-volume dataset and *en face* views of the vena contracta from a 3D color Doppler dataset. To obtain the best images, first orient two orthogonal planes through the long axis of the valve or regurgitant jet while the image is playing. Then align the third plane perpendicular to the first two and position it at the leaflet tips or vena contracta. Here, pausing or slowly panning through the frames can be helpful to properly place the third plane and find the most appropriate *en face* image. The short-axis or *en face* plane can then be individually viewed, zoomed, and area measured.

3DTEE especially offers incremental value in evaluating mitral valve anatomy and function. Live 3D zoom images of the mitral valve from the long-axis view can be flipped *en face*, cropped to

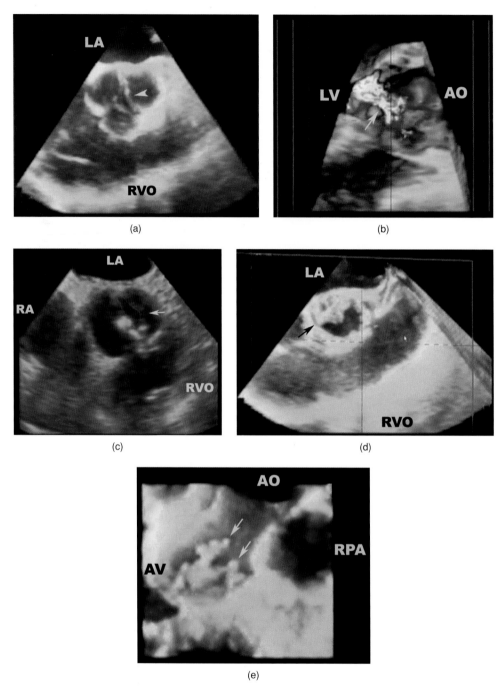

(a)

(b)

(c)

(d)

(e)

Figure 14.3 Aortic regurgitation. The arrowhead in (a) points to prominent central diastolic noncoaptation of aortic valve (AV) leaflets, which resulted in severe aortic regurgitation. This section was taken near the tip of the AV. The arrow in (b) points to vena contracta of the aortic regurgitation jet. (c) Aortic stenosis viewed by cropping from the aorta to the tips of a trileaflet AV, demonstrating fusion/calcification in the non- and right-coronary cusps with a planimetered AV area of 0.78 cm². The arrow points to the flow-limiting narrow orifice at the tip of the AV leaflets. (d, e) AV endocarditis. The arrow in (d) points to large vegetation involving the AV viewed *en face*. Note the marked destruction of leaflet tissue produced by endocarditis. The arrows in (e) show vegetations protruding into the ascending aorta. AO, aorta; LA, left atrium; LV, left ventricle; RA, right atrium; RPA, right pulmonary artery; RVO, right ventricular outflow. Movie clip 14.3 C. (Reproduced from Pothineni *et al.* [1], with permission.)

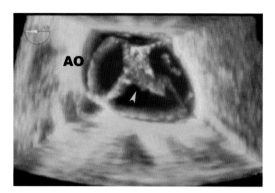

Figure 14.4 Ascending aortic dissection. The arrowhead points to the dissection flap viewed *en face*. AO, aorta. (Reproduced from Pothineni *et al.* [1], with permission.)

visualize the anterior and posterior leaflets *en face* from the left atrial perspective, and then rotated to place the aortic valve at 12 o'clock, creating the surgeon's view. Here, prolapse can be defined in the dynamic beating heart and localized to its specific segments/scallops. In comparison with 2DTEE, 3DTEE more accurately defines prolapse in this manner, with segments or scallops that prolapse appearing brighter, and can localize chordae

rupture [2,3,6,7] (Figures 14.5–14.8). It is helpful to couple this evaluation with 3D color Doppler imaging, which will also help localize the diseased segment/scallop. In offline analysis with commercial software packages, the mitral annulus can be measured and the mitral valve and subvalvular apparatus modeled to demonstrate and quantify pathologic changes. These evaluations help to empower mitral valve repair over replacement, as they provide a high-resolution, functional view of the mitral valve before it is devoid of blood as the surgeon views it in the operating suite.

In addition, we have found 3DTEE useful in evaluating other valvular lesions important to surgical planning, including endocarditis and prosthetic paravalvular regurgitation [8,9]. In correlation with surgical findings, 3DTEE provided incremental value over 2DTEE in identifying and localizing vegetations and complications of infective endocarditis such as abscesses, perforations, and ruptured chordae [8] (Figures 14.9–14.17). Likewise, 3DTEE more accurately described the location and size of paravalvular prosthetic regurgitation in another study from our laboratory [9] (Figures 14.18–14.23).

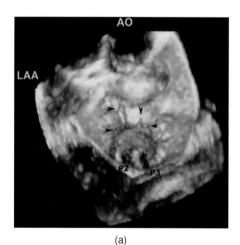

(a)

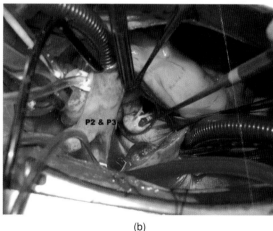

(b)

Figure 14.5 Live/real time 3D transesophageal echocardiographic assessment of ruptured chordae tendinae. (a) The arrowheads point to some of the ruptured chordae of P2 and P3 scallops of posterior mitral valve leaflet. Both P2 and P3 scallops show prominent prolapse. As viewed by the surgeon, the aorta (AO) is at 12 o'clock position and the left atrial appendage at 9 o'clock position. (b) Surgical view showing prolapse of P2 and P3 scallops with chordae rupture. LAA, left atrial appendage. Movie clip 14.5 A. (Reproduced from Manda *et al.* [7], with permission.)

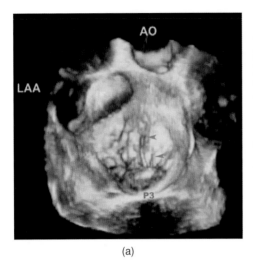

(a)

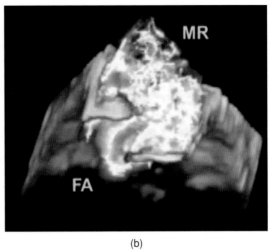

(b)

Figure 14.6 Live/real time 3D transesophageal echocardiographic assessment of ruptured chordae tendinae in another patient. (a) The arrowheads point to ruptured chordae of P3 scallop of posterior mitral valve leaflet, which shows prominent prolapse. (b) Color Doppler imaging shows severe mitral regurgitation (MR) with a large flow acceleration (FA). AO, aorta; LAA, left atrial appendage. Movie clips 14.6 A and 14.6 B. (Reproduced from Manda *et al.* [7], with permission.)

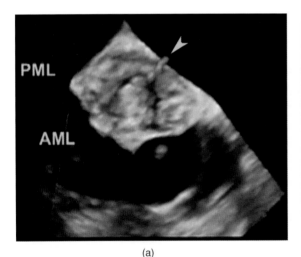

(a)

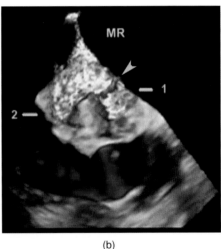

(b)

Figure 14.7 Live/real time 3D transesophageal echocardiographic assessment of ruptured chordae tendinae in a different patient. (a) The arrowhead shows a ruptured chord of severely prolapsing A2 segment of anterior mitral valve leaflet (AML). (b) Color Doppler imaging. Numbers 1 and 2 point to two jets of severe MR. The arrowhead points to the ruptured chord. MR, mitral regurgitation; PML, posterior mitral valve leaflet. Movie clips 14.7 A and 14.7 B. (Reproduced from Manda *et al.* [7], with permission.)

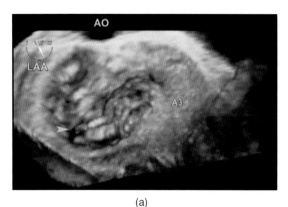

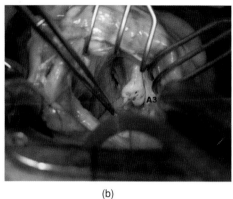

(a)

(b)

Figure 14.8 Live/real time 3D transesophageal echocardiographic assessment of ruptured chordae tendinae. (a) The arrowhead points to a ruptured chord of a markedly prolapsing A3 segment of anterior mitral valve leaflet. (b) Surgical view showing prolapse and chordae rupture of A3 segment. AO, aorta; LAA, left atrial appendage. Movie clip 14.8 A. (Reproduced from Manda *et al.* [7], with permission.)

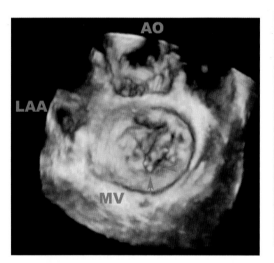

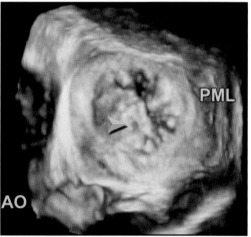

Figure 14.9 Live/real time 3D transesophageal echocardiographic assessment of valvular vegetations in a 53-year-old male. The arrows (arrowhead in the Movie clip) point to a vegetation involving the A3 segment. AO, aorta; LAA, left atrial appendage; MV, mitral valve. Movie clip 14.9. (Reproduced from Hansalia *et al.* [8], with permission.)

Figure 14.10 Live/real time 3D transesophageal echocardiographic assessment of valvular vegetations in a 76-year-old male. The arrowhead points to a perforation in the anterior mitral leaflet. The posterior mitral leaflet (PML) shows multiple vegetations and cusp destruction. AO, aorta. Movie clip 14.10. (Reproduced from Hansalia *et al.* [8], with permission.)

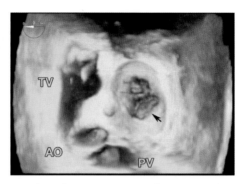

Figure 14.11 Live/real time 3D transesophageal echocardiographic assessment of valvular vegetations in a 43-year-old female. The black arrow (horizontal arrowhead in the Movie clip) points to a mitral valve vegetation involving the A1 segment and commissure. Note the presence of central perforation. Two other vegetations are also seen involving A2 and A3 segments of the anterior mitral leaflet. AO, aorta; PV, pulmonary valve; TV, tricuspid valve. Movie clip 14.11.

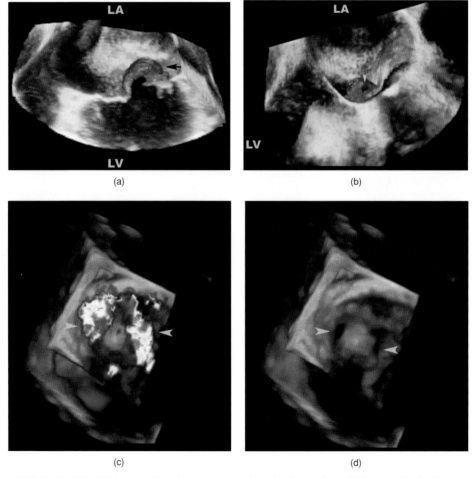

(a)

(b)

(c)

(d)

Figure 14.12 Live/real time 3D transesophageal echocardiographic assessment of valvular vegetations in a 31-year-old male. (a) The arrow points to a large irregular vegetation involving the anterior mitral leaflet. (b) The arrowhead points to a perforation in the same vegetation viewed in short axis. (c, d) The arrowheads point to two jets of mitral regurgitation (c) emanating from two large perforations (d) in the anterior leaflet in the same patient. LA, left atrium; LV, left ventricle. Movie clips 14.12 A–D. (Reproduced from Hansalia *et al.* [8], with permission.)

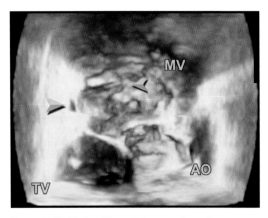

Figure 14.13 Live/real time 3D transesophageal echocardiographic assessment of valvular vegetations in a 40-year-old male. The lower arrowhead shows a mitral annular abscess. The upper arrowhead points to a ruptured chord of P3 scallop which is infected. AO, aorta; MV, mitral valve; TV, tricuspid valve. Movie clip 14.13. (Reproduced from Hansalia *et al.* [8], with permission.)

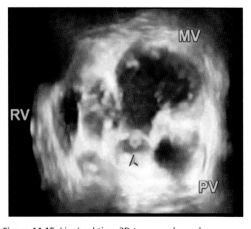

Figure 14.15 Live/real time 3D transesophageal echocardiographic assessment of valvular vegetations in a 77-year-old male. The arrowhead points to an aortic valve vegetation with a perforation in the middle. MV, mitral valve; PV, pulmonary valve; RV, right ventricle. Movie clip 14.15. (Reproduced from Hansalia *et al.* [8], with permission.)

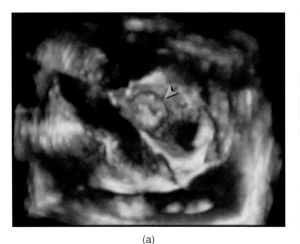
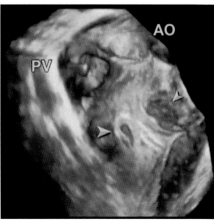
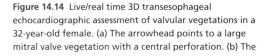

(a)   (b)

Figure 14.14 Live/real time 3D transesophageal echocardiographic assessment of valvular vegetations in a 32-year-old female. (a) The arrowhead points to a large mitral valve vegetation with a central perforation. (b) The lower arrowhead points to an annular abscess and the upper arrowhead points to the mitral valve. AO, aorta; PV, pulmonary valve. Movie clips 14.14 A and 14.14 B. (Reproduced from Hansalia *et al.* [8], with permission.)

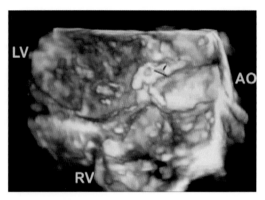

Figure 14.16 Live/real time 3D transesophageal echocardiographic assessment of valvular vegetations in a 42-year-old male. The arrowhead points to a perforation in the vegetation involving the posterior (left) cusp of bicuspid aortic valve and the other leaflet is also involved. AO, aorta; LV, left ventricle; RV, right ventricle. Movie clip 14.16. (Reproduced from Hansalia et al. [8], with permission.)

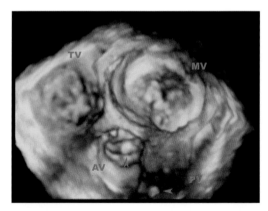

Figure 14.17 Live/real time 3D transesophageal echocardiographic assessment of valvular vegetations in a 63-year-old male. The two upper arrowheads (one arrowhead in the Movie clip) point to two vegetations involving the aortic valve (AV). A large vegetation (lower arrowhead) is also noted on the pulmonary valve (PV). MV, mitral valve; TV, tricuspid valve. Movie clip 14.17. (Reproduced from Hansalia et al. [8], with permission.)

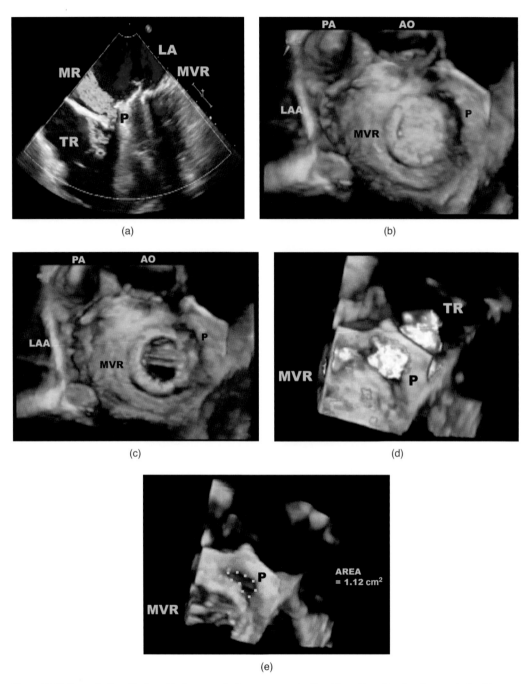

Figure 14.18 Paravalvular mitral prosthetic regurgitation in a 55-year-old male. (a) 2D transesophageal echocardiogram shows medial paravalvular (P) mitral regurgitation (MR) in this patient with St. Jude mitral valve replacement (MVR). (b–e) Live/real time 3D transesophageal echocardiogram. *En face* views. The paravalvular (P) defect is localized at 1–3 o'clock position in both systole (b) and diastole (c). Color Doppler examination (d) confirms the site of paravalvular (P) defect. The paravalvular (P) defect after color Doppler suppression is shown in (e). The defect measured 1.12 cm². AO, aorta; LA, left atrium; LAA, left atrial appendage; PA, pulmonary artery; TR, tricuspid regurgitation. Movie clips 14.18 A–E. (Reproduced from Singh *et al.* [9], with permission.)

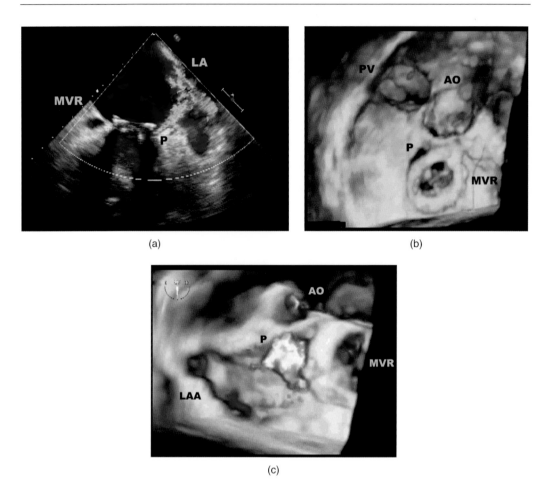

(a)

(b)

(c)

Figure 14.19 Paravalvular mitral prosthetic regurgitation in a 72-year-old female. (a) 2D transesophageal echocardiogram shows lateral paravalvular (P) mitral regurgitation in this patient with porcine mitral valve replacement (MVR). (b, c) Live/real time 3D transesophageal echocardiogram. *En face* views. The paravalvular (P) defect is localized at 10–11 o'clock position (b). Color Doppler examination (c) confirms the site of the defect. AO, aorta; LA, left atrium; LAA, left atrial appendage; PV, pulmonary valve. Movie clips 14.19 A–C. (Reproduced from Singh *et al.* [9], with permission.)

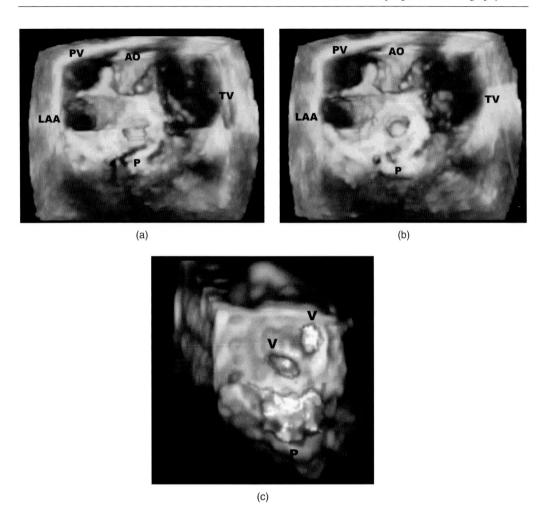

(a)   (b)

(c)

Figure 14.20 Paravalvular mitral prosthetic regurgitation in a 59-year-old female. (a–c) Live/real time 3D transesophageal echocardiogram. *En face* views. The paravalvular (P) defect is localized at 5–8 o'clock position in both systole (a) and diastole (b) in this patient with Starr Edwards MVR. Color Doppler examination (c) confirms the site of the paravalvular (P) defect. AO, aorta; LAA, left atrial appendage; PV, pulmonary valve; TV, tricuspid valve; V, valvular regurgitation. Movie clips 14.20 A–B and 14.20 C. (Reproduced from Singh *et al.* [9], with permission.)

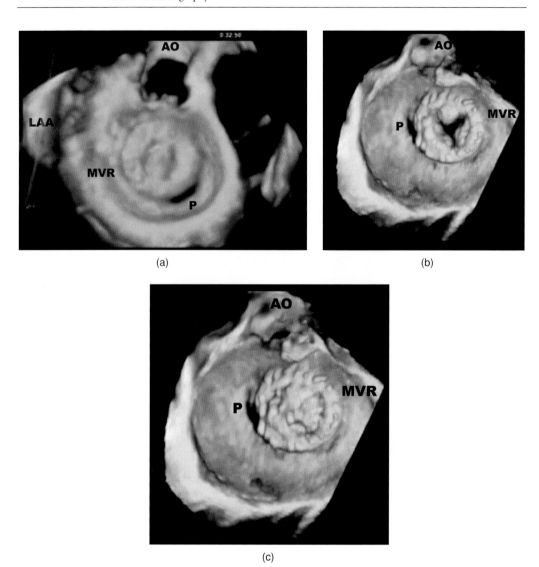

(a)

(b)

(c)

Figure 14.21 Paravalvular mitral prosthetic regurgitation in a 61-year-old male. Live/real time 3D transesophageal echocardiogram. *En face* views. (a) The paravalvular (P) defect is localized at 5 o'clock position in this patient with a metallic prosthesis. (b, c) Another elderly patient with tissue prosthesis shows the paravalvular (P) defect at 8–9 o'clock position in both systole and diastole. AO, aorta; LAA, left atrial appendage; MVR, mitral valve replacement. Movie clips 14.21 A and 14.21 B–C. (Reproduced from Singh *et al.* [9], with permission.)

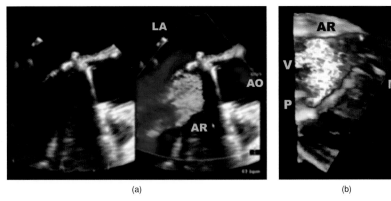

(a)

(b)

Figure 14.22 Paravalvular aortic prosthetic regurgitation in a 55-year-old male. (a) 2D transesophageal echocardiogram. In this patient with a metallic prosthesis, color Doppler signals fill the whole extent of proximal left ventricular outflow tract in diastole consistent with severe aortic regurgitation (AR). It is difficult to assess the site of AR but it appears primarily valvular, not paravalvular. (b)

Live/real time 3D transesophageal echocardiogram. Paravalvular (P) regurgitation is located at 7 o'clock position. Two jets of valvular (V) regurgitation are also visualized within the confines of the prosthesis. In Movie clip 14.22 B, IAS is interatrial septum. LA, left atrium; MV, mitral valve. Movie clips 14.22 A and 14.22 B. (Reproduced from Singh et al. [9], with permission.)

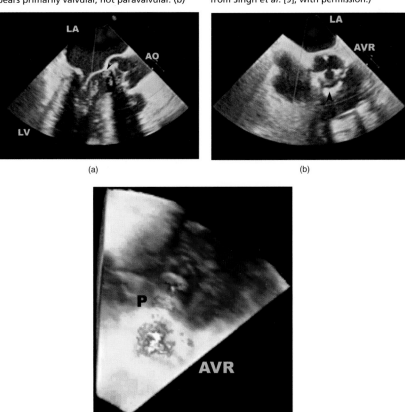

(a)

(b)

(c)

Figure 14.23 Paravalvular aortic prosthetic regurgitation in another patient. (a, b) 2D transesophageal echocardiogram. Both posterior (a) and anterior (b) paravalvular (P) regurgitation jets (arrowhead) are seen in five-chamber and short-axis views, respectively, in this patient with a tissue aortic valve replacement (AVR)

(c) Live/real time 3D transesophageal echocardiogram. A large paravalvular (P) defect is seen anteriorly at 1 o'clock position. AO, aorta; LA, left atrium; LV, left ventricle. Movie clips 14.23 A–C. (Reproduced from Singh et al. [9], with permission.)

Congenital heart disease and mass lesions

Since 3DTEE permits high-resolution images of cardiac structures from any perspective and retains complex spatial relationships with the surrounding anatomy, it is ideally suited to evaluate congenital lesions. 3D echocardiography accurately evaluates the size and shape of atrial and ventricular septal defects and the surrounding rim of tissue to empower and guide decisions for intervention [4,10,11]. 3D color Doppler datasets can be cropped and analyzed on QLAB to provide *en face* views of the defect. We found that circumference of the defect was an important measurement to provide a retrofitted "stretched diameter" (circumference/pi) for septal occluder sizing [10]. With 3DTEE, the defects can be seen at high resolution with live 3D or 3D zoom as well, and these modes can provide direct guidance during intervention.

Offline analysis is also very helpful in evaluating the size and anatomic relationships of mass lesions. From 3DTEE datasets, the size and attachment points for vegetations, tumors, and thrombi can be precisely obtained. Using the steerable three planes in QLAB, measurements of the largest dimension and a minor cord of a mass lesion permits accurate follow-up that is not subject to the limitations of 2D imaging. Volumes of vegetations or masses may also be assessed using an offline software and this may be a more useful and accurate parameter of their size than measurement of dimensions. Echocardiographic "dissection" of a mass lesion by serial cropping is also helpful to define areas of hemorrhage as in myxoma or lysis as in resolving thrombus (Figure 14.24).

Taken together, the offline analysis of 3D datasets offers tremendous potential for insight into complex valvular and myocardial diseases that will increase our confidence in describing these lesions.

Intraoperative applications

The potential for 3DTEE was first realized in the operating suite with the surgeon's view of the mitral valve [2]. As mentioned above, high-resolution 3D images of the mitral valve from the left atrial perspective accurately define segment/scallop prolapse and mitral annulus size, which empowers surgical decision-making. This is an image that was not

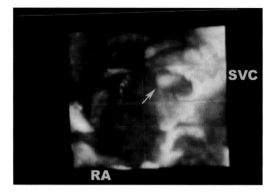

Figure 14.24 Superior vena cava (SVC) thrombus. Cut section of the SVC reveals a thrombus protruding into the right atrium (RA). Movie clip 14.24. (Reproduced from Pothineni *et al.* [1], with permission.)

possible until recently, with surgical decisions previously being made upon the flaccid appearance of the valve under direct inspection. By localizing prolapse and facilitating repair of the valve preoperatively, 3DTEE will become an indispensable tool in the surgical treatment of mitral valve disorders.

For the aortic valve, the 3DTEE exam not only assists in the quantification of stenosis/regurgitation, but also can be very valuable in the assessment of subvalvular stenosis (Figure 14.25). Further, postoperative evaluation of prosthetic function and evaluation for paravalvular insufficiency can be fully appreciated with 3DTEE.

Guidance of percutaneous cardiac interventions and future directions

3DTEE has the potential to empower percutaneous approaches to congenital and valvular lesions that are just developing. Live/real time 3D imaging is capable of providing a "virtual operating suite" for implantation of septal occluders, percutaneous valve repair or replacement, and electrophysiological procedures under direct 3D visualization. Whereas 2D imaging with TEE or intracardiac echocardiography requires scanning through several imaging planes to mentally reconstruct catheter placement and anatomy, live/real time 3D imaging enables exact visualization of the pathologic lesion *en face*, as a surgeon might view it, along with percutaneous devices.

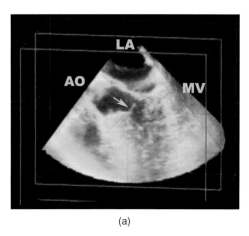

(a)

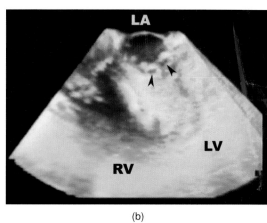

(b)

Figure 14.25 Discrete subaortic membranous stenosis viewed in long axis (a) and short axis (b) by cropping from the ventricular aspect. The arrow points to the subaortic ridge. The arrowheads in (b) point to two areas of discrete subaortic stenosis viewed *en face*. AO, aorta; LA, left atrium; LV, left ventricle; MV, mitral valve; RV, right ventricle. Movie clip 14.25 A–B. Reproduced from Pothineni *et al.* [1], with permission.)

The most promising application in this regard is percutaneous aortic valve replacement, which is commonly being performed with 3DTEE guidance [4]. In this procedure, aortic balloon valvuloplasty is first performed and then a stent-based valve prosthesis is implanted. By obtaining a live 3D view of the aortic valve *en face*, immediate valvuloplasty success can be measured. Then, using short- and long-axis images, live 3DTEE guides proper placement of the prosthesis with careful attention to the anterior mitral leaflet on the ventricular aspect and the coronary arteries on the aortic aspect. Finally, *en face* images and 3D color Doppler images gauge procedural success. 3DTEE also provides incremental value over 2DTTE in percutaneous mitral valve repair using the Alfieri technique.

Since 3DTEE is a safe, portable, minimally invasive imaging modality that provides spatial understanding of complex cardiac pathology and guidance of interventional devices, it has great potential to bridge the imaging, operating, and catheterization suites. As more interventions move toward less invasive techniques, a live 3D high-resolution imaging technique should play a central role.

Summary

With the advent of live/real time imaging, 3DTEE has finally moved from a research tool to a power-ful imaging modality that will become instrumental in evaluating valvular lesions, congenital defects, and percutaneous or surgical interventions in clinical practice. Historically, our laboratory first described 3DTEE imaging in 1992 [12], and we were the first to report our experience with live/real time 3DTEE in 2007 [1]. Our early experience already demonstrates tremendous value for answering difficult clinical questions with images that complement the 2D exam, but sometimes provide perspectives that were previously impossible to obtain. Further experience in live 3D imaging and in cropping 3DTEE datasets will empower investigations and interventions at the forefront of cardiovascular medicine.

References

1. Pothineni KR, Inamdar V, Miller AP, *et al.* Initial experience with live/real time three-dimensional transesophageal echocardiography. *Echocardiography* 2007;24:1099–1104.
2. Ahmed S, Nanda NC, Miller AP, *et al.* Usefulness of transesophageal three-dimensional echocardiography in the identification of individual segment/scallop prolapse of the mitral valve. *Echocardiography* 2003;20:203–9.
3. Grewal J, Mankad S, Freeman WK, *et al.* Real-time three-dimensional transesophageal echocardiography in the intraoperative assessment of mitral valve disease. *J Am Soc Echocardiogr* 2009;22:34–41.

4. Balzer J, Kuhl H, Rassaf T, *et al.* Real-time trans-esophageal three-dimensional echocardiography for guidance of percutaneous cardiac interventions: first experience. *Clin Res Cardiol* 2008;97:565–74.

5. Sugeng L, Sherman SK, Salgo IS, *et al.* Live 3-dimensional transesophageal echocardiography: initial experience using the fully sampled matrix array probe. *J Am Coll Cardiol* 2008;52:446–9.

6. Patel V, Hsiung MC, Nanda NC, *et al.* Usefulness of live/real time three-dimensional transthoracic echocardiography in the identification of individual segment/scallop prolapse of the mitral valve. *Echocardiography* 2006;23:513–18.

7. Manda J, Kesanolla SK, Hsuing MC, *et al.* Comparison of real time two-dimensional with live/real time three-dimensional transesophageal echocardiography in the evaluation of mitral valve prolapse and chordae rupture. *Echocardiography* 2008;25:1131–7.

8. Hansalia S, Biswas M, Dutta R, *et al.* The value of live/real time three-dimensional transesophageal echocardiogra-phy in the assessment of valvular vegetations. *Echocardiography* 2009;26:1264–73.

9. Singh P, Manda J, Hsiung MC, *et al.* Live/real time three-dimensional transesophageal echocardiographic evaluation of mitral and aortic valve prosthetic paravalvular regurgitation. *Echocardiography* 2009;26:980–987.

10. Mehmood F, Vengala S, Nanda NC, *et al.* Usefulness of live three-dimensional transthoracic echocardiography in the characterization of atrial septal defects in adults. *Echocardiography* 2004;21:707–13.

11. Zekry SB, Guthikonda S, Little SH, *et al.* Imaging vignette: percutaneous closure of atrial septal defect. *J Am Coll Cardiol Cardiovasc Imaging* 2008;1:515–17.

12. Nanda NC, Pinheiro L, Sanyal R, Rosenthal S, Kirklin J. Multiplane transesophageal echocardiographic imaging and three-dimensional reconstruction. *Echocardiography* 1992;9:667–76.

CHAPTER 15

The Challenges of Volume Ultrasound: Real Time Full-Volume Imaging

Kutay Ustuner and Matthew Paul Esham
Siemens Healthcare Sector, Ultrasound Business Unit, Mountain View, CA, USA

Introduction

One of the fundamental attributes that makes ultrasound unique among medical imaging modalities is its being real time. This is a tremendous advantage over other imaging modalities such as computed tomography or magnetic resonance imaging, and is particularly important in clinical applications where temporal information, accuracy, or resolution is as critical as spatial information, accuracy, or resolution. Examples of echo applications where temporal information is critical include imaging cardiac wall motion and blood flow and in monitoring cardiac procedures such as valve replacement and ablation. The real time nature of ultrasound also enables clinicians to have direct interactive contact with the patient during scanning.

The key performance measure of real time imaging systems is the information rate. This simple measure unifies many well-known image quality determinants such as temporal resolution, field of view, penetration, detail resolution, and contrast resolution.

In fact, the information rate of an imaging system defines the upper boundary for achievable image quality and exam efficiency, and therefore drives the diagnostic confidence and speed of workflow. Given this high information rate volumetric ultrasound imaging upper boundary, performance in any of

Live/Real Time 3D Echocardiography, 1st edition.
By Navin C. Nanda, Ming Chon Hsiung, Andrew P. Miller, and Fadi G. Hage. Published 2010 by Blackwell Publishing Ltd.

the image quality parameters can be improved by trading off performance in others through various controls and presets provided to the user. Operators of ultrasound imaging systems frequently use these means such as frequency, image width, line density, etc., to select the trade-offs that are correct for the particular clinical application or patient. For example, imaging frequency is increased to improve detail resolution, trading off penetration and temporal resolution. The image width or display depth can be reduced to improve temporal resolution, trading off field of view, and so on.

As new clinical applications and imaging techniques emerge, the information rate of existing platforms has become the bottleneck. Today, real time volumetric imaging is the most challenging application of all as expanding the field of view from a 2D slice to a full 3D volume is not possible without significant trade-offs in temporal detail, and contrast resolution and penetration, unless the system information rate is increased dramatically. In addition, the performance of many specialized imaging techniques such as spatial and frequency compounding, elasticity imaging, and contrast agent imaging are also limited by the system information rate. These techniques require multiple pulse/echo events per line of sight to gather information on parameters such as angle or frequency dependence of the tissue response, nonlinearity or stiffness of tissue, and contrast.

Therefore, the limited information rate imposes trade-offs in field of view, temporal resolution, or image quality.

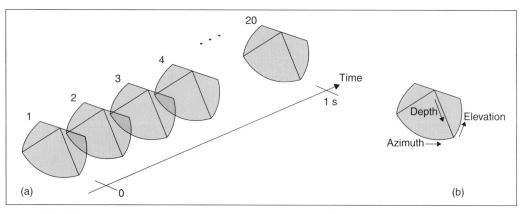

Figure 15.1 (a) Volume rate is given by the number of volume images formed per second. (b) Volume size is given by the image width in lateral dimensions—azimuth and elevation—and the penetration depth.

Reducing speckle or clutter increases contrast resolution, and therefore information. *Speckle* is the acoustic noise generated by unresolvable microstructures. Due to the coherent or phase-sensitive nature of ultrasound beam formation, echoes from multiple scatterers within each resolution cell volume interfere constructively, i.e., in-phase, and destructively, i.e., out-of-phase, and create a random pattern called speckle. Speckle is an additive noise for B-mode. When an object has nine or more unresolvable scatterers within a resolution cell volume, it generates a fully developed speckle. Speckle is a formidable challenge to detectability of otherwise resolvable structures. Techniques such as compounding that reduce speckle variance are critical to the detectability of resolvable structures. *Clutter* is the acoustic noise resulting from scattering from off-axis resolvable and unresolvable structures. It prevents the detectability of on-axis resolvable structures. Second harmonic imaging is the most effective technique used today to reduce clutter.

Information rate

To extend the discussion, information rate needs to be defined and the contributing properties well understood. For real time volume imaging engines, the information rate or information per second, is given by the information per volume times the temporal resolution:

$$\text{Information rate} = \text{information/volume} \\ \text{temporal resolution}$$

Temporal resolution is the ability to detect motion and is given by the volume rate, or the number of volumes formed per second (frame rate or frames/second for 2D imaging). See Figure 15.1a for a graphical depiction of information rate. The information per volume in turn is given by the volume size times the information density, or the information per unit volume (e.g., per cubic centimeter).

$$\text{Information/volume} = \text{volume size} \\ \text{information density}$$

Volume size is given by the image width in the two lateral axes, azimuth and elevation, and the penetration, the deepest depth with information:

$$\text{Volume size} = \text{width in azimuth} \\ \text{width in elevation} \quad \text{penetration}$$

Information density is a measure of detectability of tissue echogenicity variations. It is directly proportional to the detail resolution and contrast resolution and is given by:

$$\text{Information density} = \text{detail resolution} \\ \text{contrast resolution} = \frac{\text{CNR}^2}{\text{resolution size}}$$

where CNR is the contrast-to-noise ratio.

Detail resolution determines the detectability of closely spaced acoustic inhomogeneities. It is inversely proportional to the resolution cell size or the volume of the point spread function.

Contrast resolution, which should not be confused with image contrast, determines the detectability of resolvable structures and is a measure of how low the acoustic noise levels are. The contrast resolution measure is the CNR:

$$\mathrm{CNR} = \frac{\bar{I}}{\sigma}$$

where $\bar{I}$ is object's average brightness representing the average echogenicity, or the information. We assume unity $\bar{I}$ to keep the measure object independent. σ is the point-wise standard deviation of acoustic noise. For simplicity we here assume that the dynamic range of the platform is sufficient to prevent saturation or clipping, and the quantization is not a dominant source of noise.

To summarize, the information rate is directly proportional to detail, contrast and temporal resolution (volume or frame rate), and field of view (volume or frame size). The information rate unifies these well-known information parameters into one extremely valuable measure for real time imaging systems. To improve any one of the information parameters without a trade-off in others requires a platform with higher information rate.

Furthermore, in addition to the potential information rate limitation of the system, the body may impose limitations on one or more of the parameters as well. For example, in echocardiography, detail resolution is limited by the acoustic window size between the ribs which determines the maximum aperture size, and by the penetration requirements of the application which determine the imaging frequency. For echocardiography, an increase in information rate directly translates into improvements in volume rate, volume size, and/or contrast resolution.

Real time 3D imaging versus stitched image acquisition

The imaging engines of today's 2D ultrasound systems do not have sufficient information rate to achieve real time full-volume 3D imaging and are forced to perform partial volume sampling of the target organ. In systems not built to support the information rate required to do full-volume image acquisition, cardiac structures are acquired over a series of two to four heart cycles and an offline application builds the final volume from four sub-volumes. In this workflow, any variance from beat

to beat will cause the images to misalign during the reconstruction phase. This rules out the use of stitched image acquisition in patients with arrhythmias as well as any respiratory movement, greatly reducing potential patient population as well as tying the system to the electrocardiogram (ECG).

Real time full-volume image acquisition is freed from these limitations, however, and does not require the use of an ECG for acquisition. This has multiple benefits, including reducing the temporal window required for acquisition as well as enabling volume color flow evaluation.

Data size and density

As full-volume imaging continues to mature and the workflow shifts from 2D to 3D, we face several issues and multiple opportunities. With the increased data density provided by real time full-volume acquisition comes a much larger file size. In order to resolve the data size issue, a volume image must rely on its ability to reference specific cut planes and reference them for future use. This bookmarking allows a single volume to appear on the viewing station as multiple views, while the

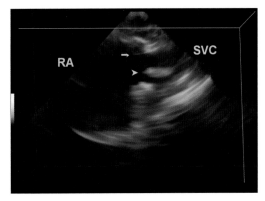

Figure 15.2 Real time full-volume scanning. The arrowhead points to a thrombus located in the superior vena cava (SVC) imaged using the right parasternal approach. The vertical arrow shows a vestige of the right-sided sinus venous valve which is located at the junction of the SVC and right atrium (RA). Movie clip 15.2 A shows the thrombus protruding into the RA. The vertical arrow points to a line in the SVC. Other notations are similar to the figure. Movie clip 15.2 B shows the thrombus (arrowhead) viewed *en face*. These studies were done at the University of Alabama at Birmingham Echocardiography Laboratory.

system is storing only the primary volume and pointers. The ability to reference the generated planes from bookmarks becomes a critical feature to ensure study size remains within the limits of existing network capacity. With the advent of bookmarks, a single full-volume image can be referenced for multiple slice views while the system need only store the volume dataset and the corresponding pointers.

Automated tools to segment and present the data from within the volume become the key to utilizing the data in an organized fashion. The ability for the system to intelligently create multiple subviews from a single volume unlocks the increased data density of the volume capture.

Conclusion

The greatest practical differentiator of ultrasound is its real time imaging capability. The infor-

mation rate of existing platforms, originally designed for real time 2D imaging, have become insufficient for emerging new applications such as real time volumetric imaging. On these platforms, a full-volume cardiac image is formed in a repeated progression stitching multiple subvolumes acquired over multiple heart cycles and then reanimating the composite volume. This leads to loss of information on arrhythmic cardiac motion. In addition, discontinuities at the stitch boundaries limit the diagnostic utility of the images. To prevent stitch boundary artifacts, the patient has to hold his/her breath, adversely affecting the workflow, or rendering it impossible as in the case of stress echo. Recently introduced platforms such as the Siemens Acuson SC2000 (Siemens Healthcare, Mountain View, CA) resolve these information rate limiting steps by providing a system architecture built for real time full-volume imaging (Figure 15.2).

CHAPTER 16

3D Wall Motion Tracking as the Ultimate Technology for Wall Motion Analysis

Tetsuya Kawagishi MS[1], William Kenny RDCS[2], Berkley Cameron RDCS[2] and Willem Gorissen RDCS[1]

[1] Ultrasound Systems Division, Toshiba Medical Systems Corp., Tochigi, Japan
[2] Toshiba America Medical Systems, Inc., Tustin, CA, USA

Introduction

Wall motion analysis by echocardiography is increasingly used to assess coronary artery disease [1,2] and to qualify candidates for cardiac resynchronization therapy [3,4]. Tissue Doppler imaging (TDI) was developed to quantify the motion of the myocardium, but TDI has the limitation of Doppler angle dependency. To overcome this limitation, 2D speckle tracking was adopted. 2D speckle tracking is more robust and widely used in clinical situations but there is still the problem of out-of-plane motion of the heart. Cardiac motion orthogonal to the B-mode plane causes the replacement of tissue imaged on the 2D image. Replacement of tissue decreases the accuracy of 2D speckle tracking. This is not a limitation of speckle tracking but of 2D echocardiography. Echocardiography has been expanded to 3D, and recently 3D speckle tracking has been developed and released for clinical use (Toshiba Artida™, Wall Motion Tracking [5,6], Toshiba Medical Systems Co., Tochigi, Japan).

Speckle tracking

Speckle tracking is an application of a pattern-matching technique to an echo image. In 2D speckle tracking, template images are set around the myocardium in the starting frame. Generally, about 1 cm^2 is used for the template size. In the next frame, the template is moved where the speckle pattern of the template matches the speckle pattern of the image. Movement vectors are defined according to the movement of the templates between subsequent frames. New templates are created for tracking each subsequent frame. Matching processes are repeated frame by frame, and all local movements during the cardiac cycle are assessed (Figure 16.1).

In 3D speckle tracking, cubic templates are used to track the regional myocardial motion in three dimensions. Matching of 3D speckle patterns between the subsequent volumes is repeated during the cardiac cycle (Figure 16.2). 3D speckle tracking overcomes the issue of out-of-plane motion like in 2D imaging because all data remain within the voxel. Good image quality and high volume rates are important to the accuracy of 3D tracking. Artifacts should be removed as much as possible and frame rates should be kept high enough to minimize the change of the speckle pattern.

Wall motion analysis

Strain value shows the shortening and expansion of the myocardium and is independent from

Live/Real Time 3D Echocardiography, 1st edition.
By Navin C. Nanda, Ming Chon Hsiung, Andrew P. Miller, and Fadi G. Hage. Published 2010 by Blackwell Publishing Ltd.

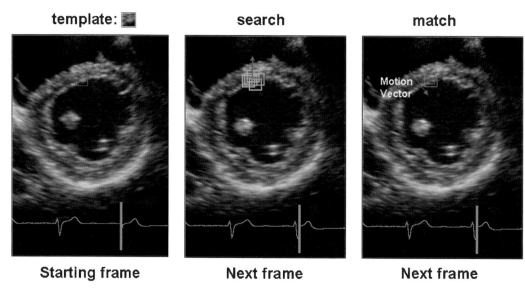

Figure 16.1 Schema of 2D speckle tracking.

heart motion like tethering. Strain is preferred for diagnosis of regional myocardial function. Radial, transversal, longitudinal, and circumferential strains are defined for the assessment of cardiac motion.

In the calculation of strain, pairs of points are defined in the initial volume and movements of the points are tracked. Regional strain values are derived from the ratio of the differences in displacement of points between the initial volume and the ending volume. Usually, the end-diastolic frame is selected as the initial frame. By extracting different components of the displacement from the tracking result, every kind of strain can be calculated simultaneously with one 3D echo dataset by one 3D speckle tracking analysis. This results in

3D speckle tracking being more efficient than 2D speckle tracking.

In 3D speckle tracking, not only can strain be calculated but also twist, torsion, and rotation are available simultaneously (Figure 16.3). Moreover, the volume estimation and ejection fraction of the left ventricle and the myocardium are possible with the 3D tracking result. For segmental analysis, values of wall motion parameters are averaged in segments and drawn on the time graph. For intuitive understanding of disease areas, the parameter value is color coded and displayed in various parametric imaging, multiplanar reconstruction, motion vector, wire frame, endocardium projection, and polar map (Figure 16.4).

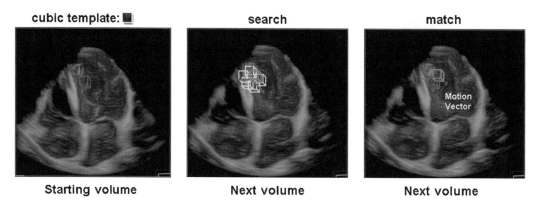

Figure 16.2 Schema of 3D speckle tracking.

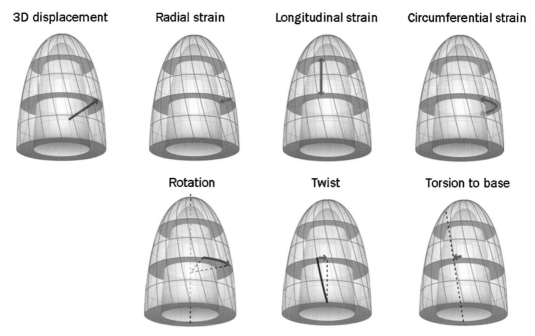

Figure 16.3 Wall motion parameters calculated by 3D speckle tracking.

Validation studies about wall motion parameters calculated from 3D speckle tracking are undergoing and some of them are published [7–9].

Clinical application

Examples of the clinical applications in regards to infarction are shown in Figure 16.5. These images are snapshots of radial strain parametric imaging at end-systole. Positive values of radial strain are represented as warm colors and negative values are represented as cold colors. Normal regions are displayed as warm colors and infarcted areas are shown as cold colors. The extent of infarction in 3D space is easily estimated with the parametric imaging.

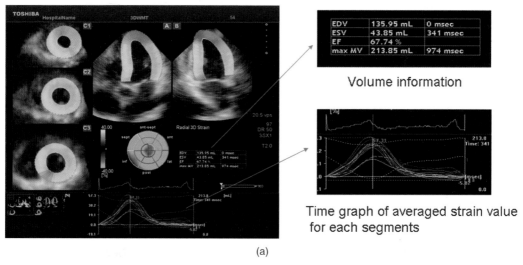

(a)

Figure 16.4 (a) Multiplanar reconstruction and polar map (*Continued next page*).

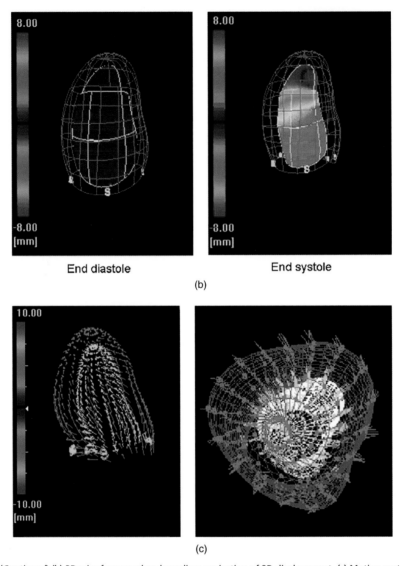

(b)

(c)

Figure 16.4 (*Continued*) (b) 3D wire frame and endocardium projection of 3D displacement. (c) Motion vectors with/without wire frames.

Figure 16.6a shows longitudinal strain analysis in the case of left bundle branch block. In a healthy case, longitudinal strain of each segment is synchronous at end-systole. In this case, the dyssynchrony of systolic motion is clearly represented on the graph. Parametric imaging of time-to-peak strain is also available. The time-to-peak strain value in the cardiac cycle is color coded and displayed on the myocardium (Figure 16.6b). Abnormal synchronous motion is captured on multiplanar reconstructed images.

Segmentation technology

In 3D speckle tracking, the endocardial and epicardial borders must be identified to start the tracking. Manual setting of these is cumbersome from a clinical workflow point of view. With the latest automatic tracking technologies, operators only have to set three points. Two points are set at the mitral valve annulus and one point at the apex, and then the ultrasound machine automatically traces the endocardial and epicardial borders in 3D

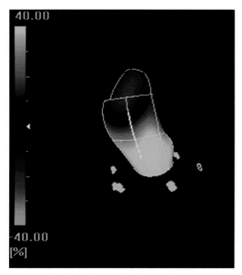 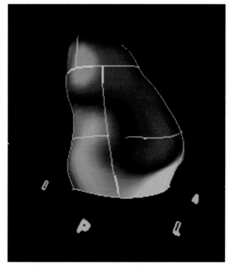

Anterior infarction   Inferolateral infarction

Figure 16.5 Clinical application to infarction. (Courtesy of Prof. H.J. Nesser in Linz.)

space. This automated technique saves the operator time and improves workflow. The automated segmentation is based on 3D edge detection technology.

Summary and perspective

3D speckle tracking is angle-independent and gives all parameters of strain, volume, and ejection fraction simultaneously. This new technology will en-hance echocardiography by quantifying cardiac wall motion.

3D speckle tracking has the potential to bring echo to a new era, by providing information about 3D wall motion that has not been able to be looked at before by echocardiography. For example, fractional area change of the regional endocardium during the cardiac cycle is one of the new parameters from 3D speckle tracking (Figure 16.7) and may give insight to the recent discussion about sheet structure of the myocardium.

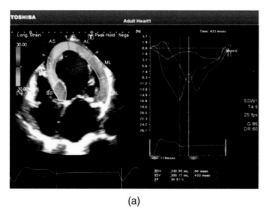

(a)

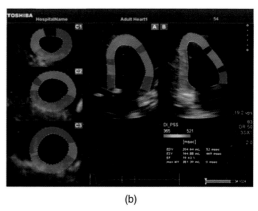

(b)

Figure 16.6 Dyssynchrony assessment with time graph and parametric imaging of time to peak: (a) Time curve measurement; (b) dyssynchrony imaging. (Courtesy of Dr. Pérez de Isla L in Madrid.)

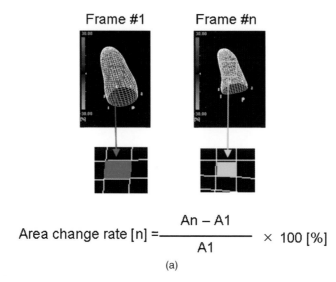

$$\text{Area change rate } [n] = \frac{An - A1}{A1} \times 100 \, [\%]$$

(a)

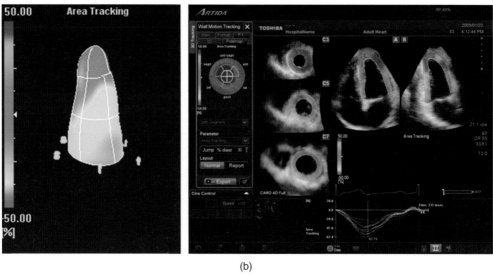

(b)

Figure 16.7 (a) Fractional area change of endocardium. (b) Example of analysis with fractional area change in a healthy case.

References

1. Katsuhisa I, Makoto I, Tamaki S, *et al*. Exercise-induced post-ischemic left ventricular delayed relaxation or diastolic stunning. *J Am Coll Cardiol* 2009;53(8):698–705.

2. Katsuhisa I, Tamaki S, Makoto I, *et al*. Abnormal regional left ventricular systolic and diastolic function in patients with coronary artery disease undergoing percutaneous coronary intervention clinical significance of post-ischemic diastolic stunning. *J Am Coll Cardiol* 2009;54(17):1589–1597.

3. Masaki T, Bouchra L, Hidekazu T, *et al*. Echocardiographic speckle tracking radial strain imaging to assess ventricular dyssynchrony in a pacing model of resynchronization therapy. *J Am Soc Echocardiogr* 2008;21(12): 1382–1388.

4. Hidekazu T, Hideyuki H, Samir S, John Gorcsan III. Usefulness of three-dimensional speckle tracking strain to quantify dyssynchrony and the site of latest mechanical activation. *Am J Cardiol* 2010;105(2): 235–242.

5. Yasuhiko A, Tetsuya K, Hiroyuki O, Tomoyuki T, Masahide N. Accurate detection of regional contraction using novel 3-dimensional speckle tracking

technique. *J Am Coll Cardiol* 2008;51(10, Supp A): 903–253, A116.

6. Tetsuya K. Speckle tracking for assessment of cardiac motion and dyssynchrony. *Echocardiography* 2008;25(10): 1167–1171.

7. Yoshihiro S, Tomoko I, Yoshiharu E, *et al.* Validation of 3-dimensional speckle tracking imaging to quantify regional myocardial deformation. *Circ Cardiovasc Imaging* 2009;2:451–459.

8. Hans-Joachim N, Victor M, Willem G, *et al.* Quantification of left ventricular volumes using three-dimensional echocardiographic speckel tracking: comparison with MRI. *Eur Heart J* 2009;30:1565–1573.

9. Leopoldo Pérez de I, David Vivas B, Covadonga Fernández-Golfín, *et al.* Three-dimensional-wall motion tracking: a new and faster tool for myocardial strain assessment: comparison with two-dimensional wall motion tracking. *J Am Soc Echocardiogr* 2009;22:325–330.

Index

Note: Page numbers with italicized *f* and *t* refer to figures and tables.